FS	focal spot		QC	quality control
Gd	gadolinium		QDE	quantum detection efficiency
Gy	Gray		R	resistance: Ohm
H & D	Hurter and Driffield		R	roentgen
HEW	Health, Education, and Welfare, Department of		Ra	radium
			Rad	radiation-absorbed dose
HVL	half-value layer		RAO	right anterior oblique
I	iodine		RBE	radiation biologic effect
I	electrical current; amperage		Re	rhenium
ID	identification		Rem	dose equivalent
keV	effective kilovoltage		RPM	revolutions per minute
kV	kilovoltage		RPO	right posterior oblique
kVp	kilovoltage peak		Se	selenium
La	lanthanum		Sec	seconds
LAT	lateral		SI	International System
LAO	left anterior oblique		Si	silicon
LET	linear energy transfer		SID	source image detector distance
LPO	left posterior oblique		Sv	Sievert
LSF	line spread function		T	time
mA	milliampere		Th	terbium
mAs	milliampere second		TFD	target film distance
Mo	molybdenum		TOD	target object distance
MPD	maximal permissible dose		TLD	thermoluminescent dosimeter
MRI	magnetic resonance imaging		US	ultrasound
MTF	modulation transfer function		V	volt
NEMA	National Electrical Manufacturers Association		V	electromotive force; voltage
			W	tungsten
Ni	nickel		W	watt
OFD	object film distance		WHO	World Health Organization
PA	posterior anterior		Y	yttrium
Pb	lead		Z	atomic number
pV	peak voltage			
QA	quality assurance			

Producing Quality Radiographs

Producing Quality Radiographs

Angeline M. Cullinan
R.T.(R.), F.A.S.R.T

Director of Education
School of Radiologic Technology
The Genesee Hospital, Rochester, New York

ILLUSTRATIONS
ARNOLD L. GÓMEZ

Rochester, New York

 J.B. LIPPINCOTT COMPANY   Philadelphia

London · Mexico City · New York
St. Louis · São Paulo · Sydney

Acquisitions Editor: Lisa A. Biello
Sponsoring Editor: Delois Patterson
Manuscript Editor: Virginia M. Barishek
Indexer: Angela Holt
Design Director: Tracy Baldwin

Designer: Adrianne Onderdonk Dudden
Production Manager: Kathleen Dunn
Production Coordinator: Caren Erlichman
Compositor: Ruttle, Shaw & Wetherill, Inc.
Printer/Binder: The Maple Press Company

6 5 4 3 2 1

Library of Congress Cataloging-in-Publications Data

Cullinan, Angeline M.
  Producing quality radiographs

  Includes index.
  1. Radiography, Medical.   2. Radiography, Medical—
Quality control.   I. Title.   [DNLM: 1. Quality Control.
2. Technology, Radiologic.   WN 160 C9669p]
RC78.C84   1987   616.07'572   86-21141
ISBN 0-397-50778-X

The author and publisher have exerted every effort to ensure that drug selection and dosage set forth in this text are in accord with current recommendations and practice at the time of publication. However, in view of ongoing research, changes in government regulations, and the constant flow of information relating to drug therapy and drug reactions, the reader is urged to check the package insert for each drug for any change in indications and dosage and for added warnings and precautions. This is particularly important when the recommended agent is a new or infrequently employed drug.

In memory of my father, Patrick A. Baratta,
who helped me to recognize the value
of an educational goal at an early age

and

to my mother, Venus D. Zuercher,
whose personal sacrifices later helped
me to more than achieve that goal.

Preface

A consistently high-quality radiograph with minimum exposure of patient and personnel depends on proper exposure factors and processing conditions. The skill of the radiographer can have the greatest influence on the final image. Any adjustment in technique can significantly affect image quality. The evaluation material in Chapter 14 should help radiographers judge their work and make appropriate corrections when needed.

Radiation physics, radiation protection, and quality assurance are interlaced with the principles of radiographic exposure. Radiographic technique is not a simple topic, but I hope that I have made this book easy to read and understand. Some of the material in this book has been condensed, to serve as a reminder of lessons previously learned.

Considerable space is devoted to the description of radiographic equipment. A full operator control panel as well as schematic functions of the x-ray circuit are illustrated in Chapter 2, "The X-Ray Generation System" (see Fig. 2-7).

Chapter 15, "Related Terminology," is more than a glossary. The terms found in this chapter are defined only as they relate to radiography. Elaborate explanations of physics are replaced by simple definitions whenever possible.

Topics such as modulation transfer function are introduced in one page or less. Since entire books have been devoted to sensitometry, only sensitometric illustrations of practical value are used. (See Chapter 11, Fig. 11-4.) It is hoped that this approach will stimulate additional interest in these topics.

Almost 200 new illustrations and tables are contained in this textbook. Related technical concepts are presented as composite illustrations. Some of the legends are lessons in themselves when considered with the illustration.

Elaborate cross referencing is used with some subjects because of the interdependent nature of the material. For example, it is difficult to discuss contrast without understanding the effect of kilovoltage, scatter radiation and control, differential absorption, contrast media, sensitometry, and so forth. If another illustration will support the material, it is also cross referenced.

A short parenthetic definition often follows a technical term. For example, when the term *increased kilovoltage* is used, *(penetration)* might follow. The most appropriate definition in the context of the topic is used, for example, some of the terms often associated with increased kilovoltage are *(decreased contrast)*, *(increased scatter)*, *(shorter wavelength)*, and *(hard radiation)*.

The format of this book should enable instructors to organize their material easily to fit their needs and the needs of their students. Instructors often have to put aside planned lessons to respond to students' questions. The interrelated subjects in this textbook should give the instructor this flexibility, as well as easy access to related topics. The cross reference feature helps to integrate the material.

As far as possible, and within the constraints of the topics, I have tried to follow the content recommendations in the Curriculum Guide of the American Society of Radiologic Technologists and the Guidelines for the certification examination set by the American Registry of Radiologic Technologists.

Diagnostic medical imaging has changed dramatically in recent years; newer imaging modalities are now common. Therefore, a portion of Chapter 6 highlights some of the more widely accepted imaging techniques that are not essentially radiographic in nature. New diagnostic medical imaging procedures will probably not replace conventional radiography. Technologies using optical disks, high-density magnetic storage devices, and so forth will coexist with conventional radiography.

Professional skills must continually be refined to take advantage of new improvements in x-ray film, techniques, positions, and the like to produce quality radiographs.

Angeline M. Cullinan, R.T.(R.), F.A.S.R.T.

Acknowledgments

I find the writing of these acknowledgments a most pleasant task for it gives me the opportunity to recognize those who contributed to my learning: in my formal training, Sister Mary Francis, R.S.M., R.T. and Dr. R.J. Killhullen, at the Mercy Hospital, Wilkes-Barre, Pennsylvania; in one-to-one sessions with physicians and fellow radiographers; in refresher courses, continuing education lectures, and related publications. A special acknowledgment is due to two radiologists who greatly influenced my professional growth: Dr. Joseph Bruno, Wilkes-Barre, Pennsylvania and Dr. Harold J. Isard, Philadelphia, Pennsylvania.

After many years of learning, it is often difficult to identify exactly where one has learned specific information, but there is one source that I can readily identify. Anyone who has had even a brief technical discussion with Jack Cullinan knows that it is always a learning experience. I have had a unique advantage. Our conversations for more than 30 years have often included some aspect of radiologic technology. Thank you, Jack, for being a source of reference as well as my sounding board. Your time and suggestions in the writing of this textbook are greatly appreciated.

I gratefully acknowledge the following for their advice and suggestions: Arthur Haus and Kal Vizy of the Eastman Kodak Company; and Drs. Derrace Schaffer, Herman Wallinga, and David Millet, Department of Radiology, The Genesee Hospital, Rochester, New York. Thanks to Josh Porte, R.T.(R.); Janice Elliott, R.T.(R.); Dawn Estay, R.T.(N.); and Shelly Degan, R.T.(R.) for helping me to select some of the specialty images.

I would be remiss if I did not acknowledge my students, past and present. I am proud to say that they are not willing to accept an answer without an explanation. Since no instructor can have all of the answers, the technical questions raised by my students often stimulated me to new research. Chapter 15, "Related Terminology," is an outgrowth of their requests for a list of terms.

A special thank you to the illustrator, Arnold L. Gómez, whose quick grasp of the material presented to him helped to express my thoughts visually.

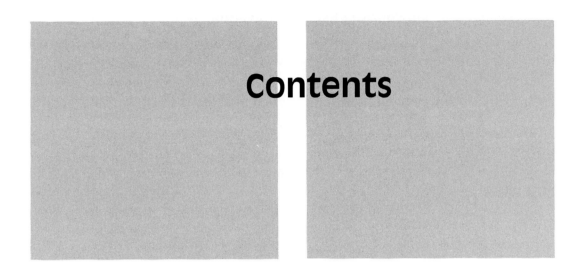

Contents

1 Production and Characteristics of X-Radiation

X-RAYS, discovered by Wilhelm Conrad Roentgen on November 8, 1895, are a part of the electromagnetic spectrum. Professor Roentgen, a physicist, working with a vacuum tube in his darkened laboratory at Wurzburg University, Germany, noted that a plate on his workbench coated with a fluorescent material (barium platinocyanide) fluoresced even though it was some distance from the completely covered Crookes tube. Investigating this phenomenon, Professor Roentgen discovered and recorded several properties of this new ray, which he called "X" because it was previously unknown. The phenomenon recorded by Roentgen had been previously observed by others but had not been investigated further or documented.

One cannot address the problems encountered in the production of quality radiographic images without a working knowledge of how x-radiation is produced; therefore, the purpose of this chapter is to review basic physics information and to summarize previously acquired physics knowledge. In-depth coverage of physics is not possible in a single chapter and is not the intent of this textbook.

Characteristics of X-Rays

The following characteristics of x-rays can be demonstrated by experimentation. X-ray photons:

1 Possess no mass.
2 Are electrically neutral.
3 Are invisible.
4 Travel at the speed of light in a vacuum.
5 Cannot be focused by a lens.
6 Are highly penetrating. (See Chapters 11 and 12.)
7 Travel in straight lines in a divergent beam when emanating from a focal point. (See Chapters 4 and 11.)
8 Produce secondary and scatter radiation. (See Chapter 5.)
9 Can cause certain substances to fluoresce. (See Chapters 3, 6, and 8.)
10 Can expose photographic or radiographic film. (See Chapter 8.)
11 Have an extended medically useful range of wavelengths and energies. (30 kVp—long wavelength, low energy for soft tissue studies such as

mammography [see Chapters 7 and 11] to 150 kVp—short wavelengths, high energy for latitude imaging techniques such as chest radiography). (See Chapters 11, 12, and 14.)

12 Can convert themselves to heat when passing through matter.

13 Can ionize gases and remove orbital electrons from atoms. This is known as *ionization*.

14 Can produce biological changes by means of induced molecular alterations.

Energy And Work

Energy (the ability to perform work) exists in nature in many forms, such as kinetic energy, potential energy, thermal energy, chemical energy, electromagnetic energy, and molecular energy.

Energy is involved when one moves objects, heats them, and causes them to emit light and to take part in chemical reactions. Work occurs when a force is exerted on the mass of an object over a given distance. The force on a body (work) must overcome the inertia (tendency of a body at rest to remain at rest) that is inherent in all matter.

IMPORTANT: Energy can be changed from one form to another. For example,

Electrical energy can be converted to light, radio waves, heat, and motion and can cause chemical changes. It can be converted into electromagnetic energy such as light, radiowaves, or x-radiation.

Mechanical energy can be converted to heat and electrical energy or to motion of objects.

Chemical energy can be converted to light, heat, mechanical energy, and electrical energy.

Radiant energy can be converted to heat and electrical energy, can cause chemical changes, and can be used to transmit messages.

Nuclear energy can be converted to light, heat, motion, and electrical energy.

Matter

Matter is any substance that is composed of atoms and that occupies space. The amount of matter contained in an object is assessable by means of its mass. Depending upon its surroundings, mass can change in size, shape, and form. For example, water, ice, and vapor have the same atomic number but are represented in different forms.

IMPORTANT: Matter and energy are interchangable in form. This was demonstrated by Albert Einstein in his famous derivation that yielded $E = MC^2$

Elements

Matter is made up of only relatively few kinds of elementary particles. All known substances are made up of a combination of these elementary particles. The number and arrangement of the elementary particles determines the atomic structure of an elemental atom. Three of the elementary particles of the atom—the proton, neutron, and electron—are the basis of simple atomic structure (Fig. 1-1). Elements are classified according to their atomic numbers, which is the number of protons in their central nucleus.

Each element has characteristics that distinguish it from other elements. These characteristics determine whether the element can participate in certain chemical reactions,

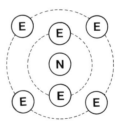

Figure 1-1 Atomic Structure
A typical atom consists of a nucleus (N), which contains protons (positively charged), neutrons (no charge), and electrons (E; negatively charged). The electrons orbit around the nucleus. In a stable atom (not ionized), the number of electrons must be equal to the number of protons in the atom.

This representation of the atom carbon does not depict the true sizes of the nucleus and electrons. In actuality, neutrons and protons each constitute 1838 times more mass than does the electron.

whether it is a good or bad conductor, whether it is a nonconductor or insulator or a superconductor, and so on.

Atomic Number and Mass Number

The nucleus contains almost all the mass of the atom; both neutrons and protons are comprised of 1838 times more mass than the electron. The number of protons in the nucleus is called the *atomic number, (Z)*. The total number of protons and neutrons in the nucleus is called the *atomic mass number, (A)*.

The diameter of an atom is about 100,000 times greater than the diameter of its nucleus. A high-speed electron interacting with matter can go through the mostly empty space of many atoms before interacting with any part of an atom.

Electrical Charges

The atom has been described as a minature solar system, with the sun as its nucleus and electrons orbiting around it (Fig. 1-2). However, there is an important difference: Planets are held in orbit around the sun by gravitational forces. Electrons, which are negatively charged, revolve around the nucleus at high speeds and are held in orbit by balancing the attraction of the positive charges of the pro-

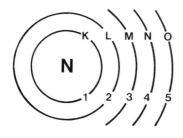

Figure 1-2 *Electron Shell Arrangement and Binding Power* *The binding force on the electron shells holding the electrons in orbit around the nucleus weakens as the number of shells increase. Numbers 1 to 5 are used to illustrate shell numbers. Five electron shells labeled K, L, M, N, and O (spectroscopic designations) are shown. The K shell possesses the strongest binding power. The electrons in the K shell require the most energy to dislodge from orbit, whereas the electrons in the peripheral shells are easier to displace.*

tons and the repulsion forces (centripetal and centrifugal) created by the velocity of the rapidly spinning and revolving electrons.

The charges of the nucleus come from its protons, which possess a positive electrical charge, and these are balanced by an equal number of the negative electron charges in the outer portion of the atom. The charges of the protons (+) and the charges of the electrons (−) are equal in quantity but differ in charge. Neutrons, which do not have net charge, also reside in the nucleus in quantities sufficient to stabilize the nuclear forces.

In radiologic physics, you learned about electron interactions with the target of the x-ray tube. (See Chapter 4.) The x-rays, in turn, interact with matter and are absorbed or scattered by its atoms. (See Chapter 5.) In your studies, you have also encountered moving charged particles, which involve the phenomenon of electrodynamics as in a flowing electrical current. (See Chapter 2.)

Energy Levels

The electrons in atoms are arranged in energy levels (shells) in a complex system derived from quantum theory. The shells are labeled K, L, M, N, and so on, with the K shell being closest to the nucleus and possessing the greatest binding force (Fig. 1-2).

The number of shells present in each atom is dependent upon the atomic structure of the atom. There is a maximum number of electrons permissible in each shell. Up to two electrons are permitted in the K shell, 8 in the L shell, 18 in the M shell, 32 in the N shell, and 50 in the O shell. (See Chapter 13.)

IMPORTANT: Electrons may move or be made to move from one energy shell to another. Whenever a vacancy occurs in an energy shell, movement of an electron to a lower energy shell is almost always accompanied by the emission of energy. Movement to a higher energy shell occurs only with the absorption of energy and is called *excitation*. These energies are typically photons of electromagnetic energy or light.

Ionization

An atom in its normal non-ionized state contains an equal number of protons and elec-

trons. The number and arrangements of the electrons in a neutral atom establishes the chemical and electrical properties of the atom.

The number of protons in the nucleus establishes how many electrons an atom must have to remain electrically neutral and stable. If an electrical change occurs in an atom as the result of a gain or loss of an electron, the atom will become ionized.

There are several interactions of significant importance to radiography that can cause an atom to gain or lose an electron. For example, atoms can be ionized:

1 By electron bombardment of matter.

2 By x-ray bombardment of matter.

3 By reaction with the emissions from radioactive substances.

4 By release of electrons by thermionic emission. (See Chapter 4.)

5 By bombardment of specific elements by light.

6 By nuclear capture of a K electron.

7 Chemically.

Electromagnetic Radiation: Wave and Particle Theories

Electromagnetic energies that are present in space as bundles of electrical and magnetic fields are arranged in nature in an orderly fashion according to the wavelength of their energies.

When we speak of long and short wavelength in the portion of the x-ray spectrum in which medical x-rays are found, we are limiting our discussion to a range from approximately 0.1A to 0.5 A (0.01 nm–0.05 nm) (Fig. 1-3).

When this energy is transported through space, it is referred to as electromagnetic radiation and travels in the form of waves (generally illustrated by a sinewave-like oscillation) at the speed of light, about 186,000 miles per second (Fig. 1-4).

Electromagnetic radiation includes cosmic rays, gamma rays, x-rays, ultraviolet rays, visible light, infrared rays, radio waves, and electrical field waves.

The sinewave oscillation can be characterized by:

1 Amplitude (the height of the wave from crest to average or from valley bottom to average).

2 Wavelength (the distance from one crest to another; the distance between two corresponding points on the wave).

3 Frequency (the number of crests or valleys passing by a specific point in a given unit of time).

The smallest particle of any type of electromagnetic radiation is called a *photon* or a *quantum* and is thought of as a small bundle of energy having no mass and no charge.

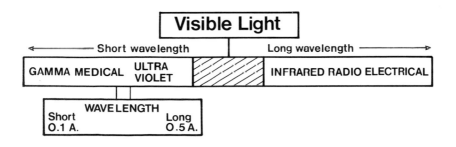

Figure 1-3 **The Relationship of Medical X-ray to the Electromagnetic Spectrum** *The electromagnetic spectrum in this abbreviated illustration runs from gamma radiation (short wavelength) to electrical waves (long wavelength). Within the medical x-ray portion of the spectrum, we speak of short wavelengths (0.1 Angstroms) to long wavelengths (0.5 Angstroms).*

In the medical x-ray range, a short wavelength will be produced with high kilovoltage values (increased penetration), whereas a long wavelength will be generated by low kilovoltage values (decreased penetration).

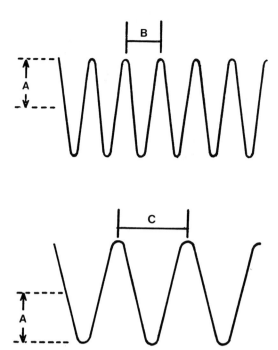

Figure 1-4   Sinewave
Electromagnetic energy is transported through space in the form of sinewave-like oscillations. This energy travels at the speed of light (about 186,000 miles per second) and can be schematically illustrated.

Components of the sinewave include amplitude, wavelength, and frequency. Amplitude refers to the height of the wave from crest to mean value (A). Wavelength describes the distance from one crest of the wave to another and represents the distance between two corresponding points on the wave (B and C). Frequency is determined by the number of crests or valleys passing through a specific point in a given time. In comparing B to C, one will note the increase in the number of wavelengths in B (increased frequency) compared with that of C. Shorter wavelengths (B) will result in increased frequency of the wave.

The energy of the photon emitted from a radiation source is directly proportional to the frequency or inversely proportional to the wavelength of the radiation.

Production of X-Radiation

X-rays are produced when rapidly moving electrons interact with the nucleus of the at-oms of a target (anode) of the x-ray tube. (See Fig. 4-3).

The source of the electrons is the filament (cathode) of the x-ray tube, which when heated to incandescence causes electrons to "boil off" in a process known as *thermionic emission*. The potential difference (voltage) between the terminals of the cathode (−) and the anode (+) pulls the "released electrons" from the vicinity of the filament across the tube to strike the anode. The electrons' energy is converted into heat and x-ray energy when the electrons strike the anode. X-ray beam intensity is influenced by both tube current (mA) and the applied voltage (kVp). The milliampere setting determines the heat of the filament, therefore, the number of "released electrons" available for interaction with the target. The range of the applied voltage (kVp) determines the wavelength and thus energy of the x-ray photons. (See Chapters 2, 11, and 12.)

Interactions

Electron Interactions With the Target of the X-Ray Tube

When electrons interact with the atoms of the target (anode) of the x-ray tube, the following occur (Table 1-1):

1 *More than 99% of the energy is converted to thermal energy (heat).* The remaining energy is divided among bremsstrahlung and characteristic radiation. Heat is produced by the energy derived from the movement of the atoms and their quick return to a normal state. The greater the kinetic energy (energy of motion or vibration) the greater the temperature.

2 *Production of bremsstrahlung radiation* (a braking action as the electrons interact with the target). This process involves electrons that grazingly pass by the heavy nuclei of the metallic atoms in the target material. The attraction between the electrons (negatively charged) and the nuclei (positively charged) cause the electrons to be deflected and decelerated from their original path and lose some of their energies. Since energy cannot be destroyed, the energies lost by the electrons are transformed and emitted as x-ray photons (Fig. 1-5).

This radiation is known as general radia-

TABLE 1-1. Electron Interaction With the X-ray Target

Action	Effect	Amount
Incident electrons collide with atoms in target	Heat	99% or greater
Electrons approach strong positively charged nucleus	Bremsstrahlung (braking radiation); electron deviated from its path; loses some kinetic energy into equivalent x-ray energy of varying intensities	90% of remaining 1%
Interaction of inner orbital electrons	Charateristic radiation; produces radiation characteristic of the energy level differences of the target atoms	10% of remaining 1%

tion, the continuous spectrum, white radiation, or bremsstrahlung radiation. The most commonly used term is *bremsstrahlung*.

The considerable rate of deceleration causes the emission of short wavelength radiation (x-rays). As deceleration (braking action) varies, so does the intensity of the resultant x-ray energy. In the 80 kVp to 100 kVp range, using a tungsten target, these bremsstrahlung rays constitute about 90% of the radiation emitted as x-rays.

Increasing the voltage generates an increased number of x-rays with shorter wavelengths and therefore a more energetic or penetrating beam.

3 *Characteristic radiation.* Characteristic radiation occurs as electrons emitted from the hot filament collide with the atoms of the target and displace structural electrons from any inner shell of the target atom. Approximately 10% of the x-radiation emitted at 80 kVp to 100 kVp is characteristic radiation. The incoming electron must be of sufficient strength to dislodge any inner shell electron by overcoming its binding force. Electrons from other shells move in to fill this lower level vacancy. The x-ray photons emitted by this action have wavlengths equal to the differences in energy between the various shells involved in the interaction. The excess energy resulting from the electron transition to a K shell is usually emitted as an x-ray photon (Fig. 1-6).

If this interaction occurs in the innermost shell (K), the wavelength of the characteristic radiation is determined by the composition of the target material and the binding power of the K shell of the atoms in the target. To produce characteristic radiation with a tungsten target, at least 70 kVp is required for K shell interaction because the K shell electron of tungsten is held with 69.53 keV.

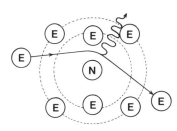

Figure 1-5 Bremsstrahlung Radiation
When an electron moves into the proximity of the nucleus of an atom, the attraction between the electron (negatively charged) and the nucleus (positively charged) causes the electron to be deflected from its original path. A "braking" action occurs when the electron collides with the atom of the target of the x-ray tube. The electron will lose some of its energy. The fact that energy cannot be destroyed results in the lost energy of the electron being transformed to and emitted as an x-ray photon. This radiation is commonly called bremsstrahlung radiation. *In German, bremsstrahlung means "braking radiation."*

IMPORTANT: Characteristic radiation can be produced in the production of x-rays when the electrons interact with the target material and can also be produced as a secondary effect when x-rays interact with matter (subject being radiographed). Characteristic radiation produced in the interaction of x-rays with matter is usually referred to as secondary radiation and is a form of scatter. (See Chapter 5.)

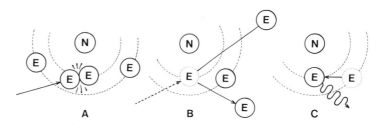

Figure 1-6 Characteristic Radiation

When an electron is emitted from the cathode of the x-ray tube and it collides with any inner shell electron of the target atom (A) and overcomes its binding force (B), an electron from another shell will fill this vacancy (C). The x-ray photon generated by this action has wavelength proportional to the difference in energies of the various shells involved in this interaction (C).

TABLE 1-2. X-ray Photon Interactions With Matter

Energy Range	Where	X-Ray Photon (wavelength, direction)	Effect
Low	Interacts with target atom	No change	Classical scattering (Thompson, coherent)
Moderate	Interacts with inner shell electron, which is quickly absorbed	X-ray absorbed; generally not scattered	Photoelectric effect (Figure 1-7)—absorption of x-ray; production of photoelectron The photoelectric effect is responsible for differential absorption. Secondary effect (Figs. 1-6 and 1-7)—characteristic radiation also produced.
Moderate	Interacts with outer shell electron	Change in direction with reduced energy	Compton effect (Fig. 1-8)—ionizes atom, produces scatter radiation.
High (E > 1.1 MeV)	Incoming photon in the vicinity of the nucleus	Photon disappears	Pair production positive and negative electrons are created from the energy transformation.
High	Photon escapes electron interaction	Absorbed by nucleus	Photodisintegration; nuclear fragments emitted; great variety available

<u>**IMPORTANT:**</u> Only photoelectric effect and Compton effect are significant in the production of diagnostic radiographic images.

X-Ray Interaction With Matter

The interaction of x-rays with matter is significant in radiology. Every effort must be made to reduce the amount of non-useful ionization of patient tissue by x-ray bombardment. This can be accomplished by the careful use of highly specialized equipment, radiographic accessories, superior techniques, and optimal radiation protection methods.

The following types of x-ray energies are important to diagnostic radiology:

1 Primary x-rays or photons emitted by the x-ray tube.

2 Scattered x-rays or photons produced when primary photons collide with electrons in matter.

3 Remnant radiation or the rays that pass through the patient striking the image detector.

Theoretically, there are many possible x-ray interactions with matter, five of which are usually described in x-ray physics textbooks (Table 1-2).

When x-rays pass through matter, the interactions continue until the primary energy and the energies of the secondary and characteristic radiations are spent.

Two x-ray interactions with matter of significant importance in the production of a radiographic image are:

1 Photoelectric effect (absorption) (Fig. 1-7).

2 Compton effect (scatter) (Fig. 1-8).

Any interaction depends on the x-ray photon energy and the atomic number (Z) of the absorber.

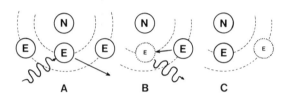

Figure 1-7 Photoelectric Effect

When an inner shell electron of an atom is struck by an x-ray photon (A), the photon may give off all of its energy. This photon collision causes photoelectric effect (absorption).

The electron struck by the x-ray photon is emitted as a photoelectron and is quickly absorbed. The electron ejected as a photoelectron is quickly replaced by another electron from any outer shell

(B) or any "free" electron. The x-ray energy (characteristic radiation, a secondary effect) emitted is determined by the binding energies of the shells participating in this event.

The vacancy created in the outer shell by the movement of an electron to fill the inner shell results in an atom with a deficiency of one electron (ionized) (C).

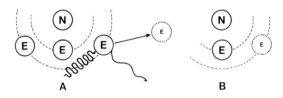

Figure 1-8 Compton Effect

When the kilovoltage value is increased, the incoming x-ray photon has increased energy. This photon can strike an electron in an outer shell and be deviated from its original path with a reduction in energy (A). The photon (x-ray) will then travel in a different direction, but with less energy (Compton) (A). The process can be multiplied if the incident photon retains part of its energy and the

remaining energy becomes a recoil electron. This interaction is called Compton effect of scattering, and many secondary collisions may occur with additional Compton and recoil electrons being generated. If the incoming photon is of sufficient energy to dislodge the electron, in addition to giving up some of the photon energy, the recoil electron (ejected electron) causes a vacancy in the outer shell and the atom becomes unstable (ionized) (B).

ABSORPTION OF RADIATION

X-ray photons possess no mass. When the x-ray photon collides with the inner shell electron of an atom, the photon may give off all its energy, and the collision causes the photoelectric effect (absorption) along with ionization.

The photoelectric effect occurs mainly when low to moderate x-ray energies interact with high atomic absorbers (such as bone or barium) and is a contributing factor to the differential absorption and contrast on the recorded image. (See Chapter 11). The x-ray image results from the radiation being absorbed totally, partially, or not at all. This effect is known as differential absorption (Fig. 1-9).

SCATTER

If the incoming x-ray photon has increased energy (resulting from increased kilovoltage applied to the x-ray tube), the x-ray photon, when striking an electron, gives up part of its energy and is deviated from its original path with reduction in energy. Part of the incident x-ray energy is retained, and the remaining energy goes to a recoil electron as kinetic energy. This interaction is called *Compton effect,* or *scattering.* The scattered photons may have other secondary collisions and eject more Compton or recoil electrons until their energy is finally spent (Fig. 1-8).

Photons are scattered in all directions (spatial) at low energies, with most scattering occurring in a forward direction at high energies.

With an increase in potential (higher kVp), the production of scatter radiation rapidly increases. (See Chapters 11 and 12.)

In the diagnostic range, the scattered photons retain most of their energy and frequently reach the film screen system, producing mostly undesirable supplemental radiographic densities. (See Chapter 5.)

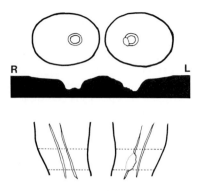

Figure 1-9 Differential Absorption
There are five basic medical radiographic densities: air, fat, water (soft tissue), bone, and metal. Air is the most radiolucent and will result in the blackest image. Bone, metal, or positive contrast agents absorb all or most of the x-radiation and are seen as lighter radiographic shadows. A cross section is shown through bilateral central portions of the femurs. Note the absorption differences between soft tissue and the osseous structures. The right femur is normal, and a density difference can be traced between the soft tissues and the femur. The left femur exhibits a destructive lesion of the bone with some soft tissue involvement. Note the irregularity of the density tracing. The medial aspect of the left femur is destroyed by disease; therefore, significantly less x-ray is absorbed. The lateral aspect of the left femur is still a mirror image of the lateral aspect of the right femur.

In the diagnostic energy range, Compton scattering is the most common type of x-ray interaction with matter.

IMPORTANT: For a quality radiograph, it is imperative that scatter radiation be controlled by the radiographer.

Production and control of scatter radiation is discussed in Chapter 5.

2 The X-Ray Generation System

ELECTRICAL energy conversion into electromagnetic (x-ray) energy occurs in the x-ray generator and tube system. The function of the x-ray circuitry and the application of technical factors (kilovoltage, milliamperage, and time) are closely interrelated. The radiographer should be aware of the basic components and functions of this x-ray system. In this chapter, electrical and magnetic principles are reviewed in a simplified manner. Schematics of a typical x-ray circuit are presented as an aid to understanding what happens when technical factor selections are made.

A Review of Some Basic Electrical Terms

Electrical Circuit

An electrical circuit is used to gather, carry, or use flowing electron energy. A circuit must have a source of electrical power capable of doing work, must be able to use the electrical energy to perform work, and requires a path to carry the electron flow from the source to where it will be used (load).

A simple electrical circuit carries current in a closed path and must possess the following:

1 Potential difference (V) from start to end of path.
2 Current or electron flow (I).
3 Electrical resistance (R).

Electrical charges may be static (at rest) or dynamic (in motion). The presence of an electromotive force (EMF) (voltage) will cause electrons to move along the surface of a conductor, a material whose outer valence shell and an adjacent excited shell or conduction band overlap. This situation makes electrons available for flow whenever a voltage drop is put across the material.

When a conductor is made into a closed path (uninterrupted), a circuit is formed and electrical current will flow. A break in the circuit can be achieved with switches that are used to control the length of time that the current may flow. Fuses or circuit breakers are protective devices that open at preset levels of current and thus prevent circuit overloading and or damage.

Electrical energy is carried through the circuit by electrical current (electrons in motion). The measurement of the amount of electrons flowing from the source is called *amperage,* or the number of electrons per unit, per unit cross-sectional area.

An EMF causes the electrons to flow in a particular direction. The electromotive force is defined and measured between two points or terminals by a unit known as the *volt*. Often the terms potential difference or voltage are substituted for the term *electromotive force*. Potential difference exists because there is an excess of electrons maintained at one end of the conductor and a deficiency of electrons at the opposite end. Voltage is measured with an instrument called a *voltmeter*. In radiography, high voltages—measured in terms of kilovoltage, where 1 kV = 1000 volts—are needed. Kilo always means *one thousand* when used as a prefix with units of measurement.

Current measured in amperes must overcome the opposing force of resistance. Resistance comes about from the impeding effects of conductor atoms to the flow of the electrons. An ammeter is used to measure current. Small amounts of electrical current are measured in milliamperage (1/1000 of an ampere).

There is resistance (opposition) to the electron flow in all circuits, with some absorption and thus loss of energy.

The resistance of a conductor is directly proportional to the resistivity of the material of which the conductor is formed. It is also directly proportional to the length of the conductor, but inversely proportional to the width (cross-sectional area) of the conductor.

Resistance is also affected by changes in temperature of the conductor. Resistance measured in ohms is inherent in all conductors at normal temperatures. Some materials are good conductors, whereas others are not as good. Some materials do not conduct and are thus referred to as *insulators*. Some materials are almost able to conduct and do so with little help; these are known as *semiconductors*. *Superconductors* lose all their resistance at very low temperatures, close to absolute zero. Resistance is the cause of a conductor heating up when in use.

Rheostats are controls used to add resistance to the circuit to adjust incoming voltage and amperage values.

The relationships of voltage and amperage to resistance can be expressed by Ohm's law. These formulas can be found in Chapter 13.

TYPES OF CIRCUITS

Current flows from one terminal to another in a simple circuit.

When current flows through several components or terminals, these components can be arranged in a series or in a parallel fashion. In a series circuit, the current will pass consecutively through each individual component. With a parallel circuit, current flow is divided among the branches of the circuit.

When using Ohm's law and related formulas, voltage, amperage, and resistance in parallel or series circuits can easily be computed. (See Chapter 13.)

Electrical energy in the form of voltage and amperage is usually supplied by commercial power companies and delivered as oscillating or alternating current. A single source of power is known as a *single-phase supply*. Three separate, but interconnected, power sources produce a three-phase supply (Fig. 2-1).

Electrical energy can be stored for future use in condenser plates or capacitor discharge devices. Batteries can also be a source of electrical current, converting chemical energy to electrical energy. (See Chapter 3.)

Electromagnetics

Electromagnetics deals with the physical relationships between electricity and magnetism.

Electrical current is always surrounded by a magnetic field. The magnetic field exists only while the current is flowing. By the process of electromagnetic induction, current can be induced in a second wire if the wires cut through the magnetic field lines produced by an electrical current. The force in a second wire loop is directly proportional to the number of turns in the first wire loop. Since both coils are not electrically connected, placing a second coil of wire adjacent to the first coil induces an electrical current in the second coil by mutual induction.

When the wire of a conductor is coiled, a helix is formed. A helix with alternating current flowing through it is called a *solenoid*. The solenoid (an electromagnet) has a strong magnetic field in its center when current is flowing through the coil's wire.

TYPES OF ELECTRICAL CURRENT

There are two types of current: alternating and direct current.

Alternating current of sinusoidal waveshape results from the application of an alternating voltage, with its polarity and values

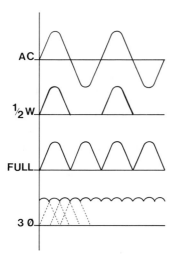

Figure 2-1 Waveforms
Alternating (oscillating) current is the electrical energy form supplied by commercial power companies. Alternating current (AC) is depicted as a sinusoidal wave shape. Alternating current reverses its polarity at regularly occurring intervals— typically, 60 times per second (60 Hz) in the United States.

Since only the positive impulses of an alternating current can be stepped up to kilovoltage for use in a radiographic tube, the negative impulses must be suppressed or rectified in some manner. Self rectification (1/2W) uses the x-ray tube as a rectifying source to suppress the negative impulse of the alternating current. Full wave, four rectifiers (Full) converts negative impulses to positive impulses to produce 120 positive impulses per second. The alternating current is changed to direct current. When three separate but interconnected power sources are used instead of a single source of electrical current, three-phase (3 Ø) current is supplied. Multiphase generators use either 6 or 12 rectifiers to convert three-phase current into almost ripple-free direct current.

reversing direction at regularly occurring intervals, typically 60 times /second (60 Hz) in the United States (Fig. 2-1).

The direction of flow does not change with direct current. Direct current may be steady, or it may fluctuate or be said to be intermittent (Fig. 2-1).

Constant potential is a voltage that shows no fluctuation from its maximal amplitude and is said to be ripple free.

X-Ray Generators

An x-ray generator using electrical current from a commercial power source, a battery, or a mechanically driven generator transforms this energy into milliamperage and kilovoltage values. Circuits using complex electrical and magnetic principles produce x-radiation suitable for diagnostic purposes.

The x-ray generator must be capable of producing very short exposure times. Variation in power delivered by way of the x-ray tube permits the radiographer to control several technical factors. Note that x-ray tube ratings must be matched to the power output of the generator. (See Figs. 4-7 and 4-8.)

The X-Ray Circuit

The x-ray circuit is divided into subsections called *primary* (low voltage) and *secondary* (high voltage) *circuits* (Figs. 2-2 and 2-3).

The primary circuit consists of:

1 *Main switch.* Power is turned off and on from an electrical source. A variation in power supply can occur, particularly in mobile units; therefore, it is important to monitor incoming line voltage. Line voltage compensation is automatic in some units.

2 *Fuses or circuit breakers.* These are used to prevent equipment overload or tube damage.

3 *Autotransformers.* They are used to control voltage supplied to the primary of the step-up transformer, providing for minimal variations in kilovoltage.

4 *A pre-reading voltmeter.* Kilovoltage is determined by the amount of voltage supplied to the step-up transformer and is present only when the exposure is being made. A pre-reading voltmeter indicates the amount of voltage being sent to the primary of the step-up transformer (Table 2-1). The kilovoltage value selected is indicated on the control panel.

5 *Timer and exposure switches.*

6 *Filament circuit.* This provides thermal energy for the heating of the filament of the x-ray tube.

7 *Filament ampmeter.* This is used to measure filament current.

8 *The primary coil of the step-up transformer.*

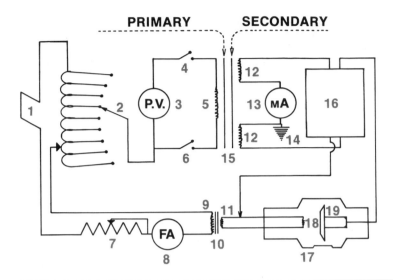

Figure 2-2 X-Ray Generating Systems
The x-ray generating circuit is divided into a primary (low voltage) and secondary (high voltage) circuit. The primary circuit consists of (1) a main switch, (2) an autotransformer, (3) a prereading voltmeter, (4) fuses or circuit breakers, (5) a primary coil of the step-up transformer, (6) a timer, including exposure switches, (7) a filament circuit rheostat (used to vary current to primary of step-down transformer for use in illuminating filament of x-ray tube), (8) a filament ampmeter, (9) a primary coil of the step-down transformer, (10) a step-down transformer, and (11) a secondary coil of the step-down transformer.

The secondary or high-voltage circuit consists of (12) the secondary of the step-up transformer, (13) a milliampmeter, (14) a ground, (15) step-up transformer, (16) a rectification system, (17) the x-ray tube ([18] cathode, [19] anode), including shockproof grounded cables to conduct high voltage from the secondary of the step-up transformer to the tube. The rectification schematic of this x-ray circuit can be found in Figure 2-5. Solid state rectifiers are used to illustrate the rectification segment since valve tubes (vacuum tubes with illuminated filaments) are no longer in common use. When and if valve tubes are used, step-down transformers are required in the rectification system

---

TABLE 2-1. Voltage To Kilovoltage*

Pre-reading Voltmeter	1:700 Step-up Transformer	1:1000 Step-up Transformer
50 V	35 kVp	50 kVp
80 V	56 kVp	80 kVp
100 V	70 kVp	100 kVp
120 V	84 kVp	120 kVp

*A pre-reading voltmeter displays the voltage selected by means of the autotransformer to be sent to the primary of the step-up transformer during the x-ray exposure. The voltage is stepped up to a kilovoltage value as determined by the ratio of the transformer.

The secondary or high-voltage circuit consists of:

1 *The secondary coil of the step-up transformer.*

2 *The milliampmeter,* used to measure tube current.

3 *An mAs meter,* to measure mAs values at short time intervals.

4 *Shockproof (grounded) cables,* which conduct high-voltage current from the secondary of the step-up transformer to the x-ray tube.

5 *The x-ray tube.* (See Figs. 4-1 and 4-2.)

Transformers Used in X-ray Circuits

Transformers require alternating current for their operation. A transformer does not produce energy; it transforms voltage and current by way of the ratios of their respective windings.

By placing a coil of wire with current flow-

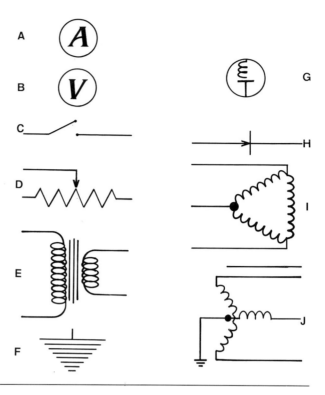

Figure 2-3 Schematic Representation of Some of the Components of an X-Ray Circuit
The filament ampmeter is usually designated in the circuit by a circular meter containing the symbol A (A).

A voltmeter is similarly indicated by the symbol V used for its identification (B).

A circuit breaker or a timer is often represented as an open-ended switch (C).

A rheostat (D), used to vary electrical current to the primary of the step-down transformer, is shown.

A step down transformer with a greater number of turns in the coils of the primary as opposed to the secondary windings is represented by E.

The universal symbol for ground is shown in F.

Vacuum tubes contain a filament and flat an-ode and can be used for rectification of alternating current to direct current (G).

A solid state rectifier is represented by H.

Three-phase transformers used for three-phase equipment generate a more homogenous x-ray beam. Three separate circuits are required in an x-ray machine using three-phase power, one for each phase. Each circuit requires its own transformer, rectifiers, line voltage compensator, and so on. In the high-tension transformer, the primary coils are wound around separate arms of a core common to all three transformers. A "Delta" configuration (I) depicts this arrangement of the coils. The secondary high-tension coils have a common center, each coil radiating outward in a "star" pattern (J). (See Figure 2-4.)

ing through it (solenoid) adjacent to a second coil of wire, an air core transformer is formed. This is the simplest type of transformer.

To form an open core transformer, soft iron bars are placed in both the primary and secondary coils. The cores are not electrically connected; they just conduct field lines.

A continuous laminated iron bar forming a rectanglar annulus is used to support the primary and secondary windings in a closed core transformer. Again, there are no electrical connections between the coils.

A continuous laminated iron bar forming a rectangular figure eight with the primary and secondary wires wound around the center support is called a *shell core transformer*.

When alternating current is applied to one coil of a transformer, it induces a changing

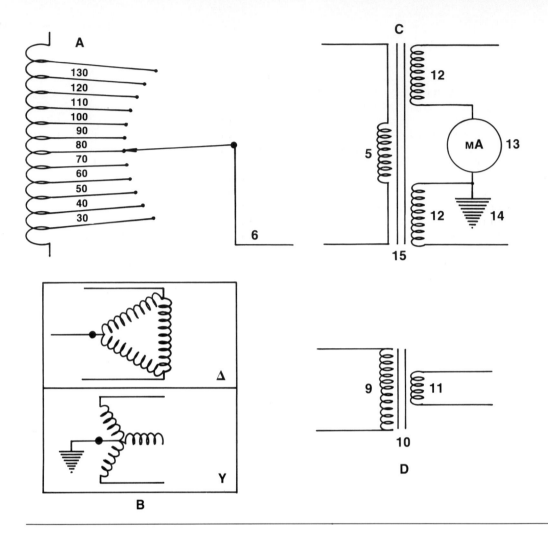

Figure 2-4 Schematic Representation of Transformers Used in an X-Ray Circuit *The numerical designations listed on Figure 2-2, X-Ray Generating Systems, are also used in this illustration.*

A single coil with primary and secondary windings is required for an autotransformer (A). When kilovoltage is selected for a specific technique, differing amounts of primary voltage (30–130 volts in this illustration) are tapped from the contacts of the autotransformer. Each tap can provide a specific primary voltage to be sent to the primary of the step-up transformer (5) via the timer (6), where the voltage will be stepped up to a preselected kilovoltage level. (See Table 2-1.) Although kilovoltage selection is made on the primary side of the high-voltage transformer (5), kilovoltage is only produced during the actual x-ray exposure. "Delta" and "star" transformer windings (used with three-phase circuits) are shown in insert B. (Also see Figure 2-3.)

A step-down transformer (D,10) is used to supply the voltage to the filament of the x-ray tube. This independent transformer steps down the pre-

selected amount of current needed to illuminate the filament of the x-ray tube. A rheostat is used to vary the current to the primary of the step-down transformer (9) so that milliampere values can be adjusted for various radiographic techniques. In practice, multiple rheostats are included in the filament circuit to accommodate various mA settings.

The high-voltage, step-up, transformer (C, 15) steps up the voltage selected from the autotransformer (A) to the required kilovoltage needed to generate x-radiation. (See Table 2-1.) The secondary of the high voltage transformer (12) is center tapped. One half of the voltage is generated by the upper portion of the high-voltage transformer, and the remaining half is generated by the lower portion. Because of this arrangement, an mA meter (13) can be maintained at near ground potential (14), making it possible to measure the actual current flowing through the x-ray tube.

The relationship of the transformers to the x-ray circuit can be better appreciated in Figure 2-2.

magnetic field within the iron core. This, in turn, induces an alternating current in the second coil. A ratio exists between the primary and secondary currents and is related to the number of turns in the wires in the individual coils. A transformer can be used to increase or decrease the voltage of alternating current.

Voltage is changed to kilovoltage by a step-up transformer, which operates on the principle of mutual induction to change the voltage ratio (Fig. 2-4).

If more turns exist in the wire of the primary coil than in that of the secondary coil, voltage will be reduced (stepped down) (Fig. 2-4).

An autotransformer is easy to recognize in a circuit schematic. The primary and secondary windings of the autotransformer are connected in series with no electrical insulation between the primary and secondary sides. A large number of contacts (taps) are attached to the different turns of the transformer. Voltage values are taken from these taps to be supplied to the primary of the step-up transformer (Fig. 2-4 and Table 2-1).

A concise description of this material can be found in "Practitioner Educational Package, Transformers, and Autotransformers" published by the American Society of Radiologic Technologists, Albequerque, New Mexico.

There is some power loss in a transformer. Some types of power losses include:

1 *Copper losses.* Losses arising from inherent resistance in the wire.

2 *Eddy current losses.* Heat losses resulting from swirling currents in the transformer core (solid iron bar). A laminated silicon steel sheet core will reduce eddy current loss.

3 *Hysteresis losses.* As the magnetic field constantly changes direction, it is physically impossible for the core's magnetic domain to continually align itself with the magnetic field, since remanent inductions persist.

Three-phase equipment requires special transformer windings to accomodate the three separate sources of alternating current. The primary circuit is triplicated (three autotransformers, three primary circuits to the autotransformers, and so on) (Fig. 2-3*I* and *J*).

The Filament Circuit

A step-down transformer is used in the filament circuit (Figs. 2-2 and 2-3C). The filament circuit carries the relatively high amperage needed to heat the filament to produce thermionic emission. (See Chapter 4.) Resistance in the filament circuitry is varied by choke coils or rheostats. These resistors can be used to vary the amount of current (milliamperage, 1/1000 ampere) so that filament heating (thermionic emission) can be controlled.

The High-Voltage Circuit

The step-up transformer is a part of both the low-voltage circuit and the high-voltage circuit. The primary of the step-up transformer is in the low-voltage circuit, whereas the secondary of the step-up transformer is located in the high-voltage circuit. The high-voltage transformer steps up the voltage from the autotransformer. The secondary of the high-voltage transformer is "center tapped" to allow an mA meter to be installed at near-ground potential. In this "center-tapped" position, the mA meter can measure the actual current flowing through the x-ray tube (Fig. 2-2).

Rectification

Transformers require alternating current to produce the mutual induction needed for their function. The x-ray tube, however, is most efficient when a unidirectional high-voltage (DC) current is used. Current is made unidirectional for use by the x-ray tube by means of rectification systems (Fig. 2-3G and H).

Rectification changes alternating current from the secondary of a step-up transformer into direct current (Fig. 2-5).

In a single-phase cycle (60 Hz current), the voltage varies from zero to the maximal kVp selected. A single-phase, single-pulse x-ray generator uses the x-ray tube to suppress the inverse half cycle (negative impulse) of current. The x-ray tube functions as a rectifier; it controls when electrons can flow from cathode to anode. Using single-phase current, every other impulse (positive) produces x-radiation. When the tube current is in the negative phase, electrons cannot flow from cath-

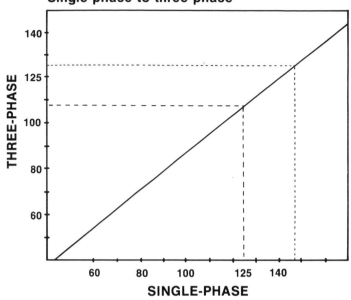

KILOVOLTAGE CONVERSION-
Single-phase to three-phase

Figure 2-6 Kilovoltage Conversion, Single-Phase to Three-Phase *When making technique conversions from single-phase to three-phase equipment, changes in kVp settings are usually desirable to obtain similar radiographic results. (See Chapter 12.) Since three-phase x-ray is virtually ripple-free as opposed to single-phase x-ray (100% ripple), technique adjustments are often required, particularly if similar radiographic density and contrast are to be maintained. (See Chapter 11.) To match radiographic densities, kilovoltage values must be adjusted. Note three-phase 125 kVp (fine-dotted line) must be **raised** to 147 kVp, single-phase. Single-phase 125 kVp (dashed line) must be **lowered** to 108 kVp three-phase for comparable densities. If the kilovoltage values are adjusted as shown, comparable contrast is also maintained. (The values in this chart are extrapolated from the data of G.J. Barone and E.D. Trout reported in Radiology 100:663, Sept. 1971. Courtesy of The Eastman Kodak Company, Rochester, NY)*

an automatic exposure device (AED). The reduction in mA continues until the AED terminates the exposure.

The X-ray Tube

Within the x-ray circuit, the incoming electricity is passed through switches, timer, meters, transformers, rectifiers, and the x-ray tube.

The x-ray tube is a major component of the x-ray circuit, converting electrical energy into electromagnetic energy. (See Chapter 1 and Figs. 4-1 and 4-2.) Conditions necessary for the production of x-radiation include:

1 There must be a source of electrons (a heated filament).

2 The electrons must be made to move rapidly across the x-ray tube from cathode to anode (owing to applied kilovoltage).

3 The rapidly moving electrons must be stopped suddenly (target bombardment).

Selection of appropriate technical factors determines the quality (type) and quantity (amount) of radiation needed to produce a quality image. (See Chapter 12.)

Controlling Exposure Factors

The selection of factors required to produce a quality radiograph is made at the control panel (Fig. 2-7) after consulting a technique

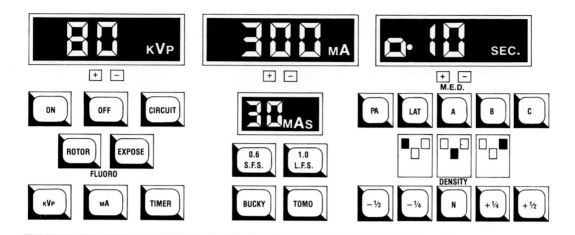

Figure 2-7 Operator Controls of an X-Ray Machine *This representation of a control panel is divided into three segments. Kilovoltage and related circuits (left); milliamperage, focal spot–size selection (center); and timer control (right).*

Depending on the equipment design, these controls can be presented in many configurations. Additional meters such as tube load limits, heat displays, and a direct readout of the fluoroscopic examination time are often found on control panels.

Kilovoltage can be raised or lowered (left) as required to adequately penetrate the part being examined. A power "On" and "Off" button and a circuit breaker are shown. The rotor control as well as the expose button is situated beneath the kilovoltage readout in this illustration. At bottom, left side, fluoroscopic kilovoltage and milliamperage stations are presented. A fluoroscopic timer that can be set to limit the length of the fluoroscopic procedure is also shown.

In the center of the illustration, the milliampere meter (readout) is shown. Milliamperage can be raised or lowered depending upon technical needs. A high milliamperage value combined with a short exposure time is sometimes needed to overcome motion. The selection of a moderate milliampere value often permits the use of a small focal spot. The focal spots represented in this panel are 0.6 mm and 1.0 mm in size. Directly above focal spot selection indicators, an mAs meter is shown. This device is required when extremely short exposures are used so that an ac-

curate reading of the milliampere seconds used can be obtained. In the center of the panel, below the focal spot size selection, are the Bucky "On" and "Off" buttons and a tomographic selector control.

To the right is the timing section of the control panel. The time values can be raised or lowered by the radiographer, or an automatic exposure device can be selected for specific studies. Specific indicators for the chest (PA or lateral) or other Bucky stations are shown. Table Bucky is represented by A; the upright Bucky by B; and the radiographic component of the fluoroscope by C. These selectors are used to activate the appropriate AED. The darkened sensors (left, right, or center) indicate the specific sensor to be selected for the part under study. (See Figs. 2-9 and 2-12.)

In the lower portion of the timer section on the control panel, density adjustment controls (−, N, +) are shown. The center button, labeled N, is intended for use when a normal or preselected density is desired. The (−) panel can be adjusted for a 1/4 or 1/2 decrease in density. The (+) settings can be adjusted in a similar fashion for an increase in density. This density variation control is to be used when an increase or decrease in density is required on a specific AED study. When an examination must be repeated, image density should be able to be adjusted by the use of the (−) or (+) settings. In practice, this is not always so. (See Fig. 2-11.) Review minimal response time information in the timer section of this chapter.

chart. Three major exposure controls are used by the radiographer.

The first, milliamperage (current), determines the number of electrons available to flow across the x-ray tube. This setting is

needed to produce "released electrons" in a process known as *thermionic emission* (see Chapter 4) and controls the intensity of the beam. (See Chapter 11.)

The second, kilovoltage, determines the

high voltage applied across the x-ray tube and, as a result, the speed of the incoming electrons and thus the energy of the x-ray photons, usually described by kVp. (See Chapter 11.)

The third, time, determines the total time during which x-radiation is produced, usually given in seconds. (See Chapter 11.) The timer is situated between the autotransformer and the primary of the step-up transformer.

Timers

A timer is used to initiate and terminate an x-ray exposure. Exposure timers include the spring-driven mechanical timer (limited to 1/10th second or longer), the synchronous or motor-driven timer, usually not reliable for exposures shorter than 1/20th second and thus not in common use, and electronic or impulse timers. Most electronic timers operate at 1/120th second or less.

EVALUATION OF THE TIMER OF A SINGLE-PHASE, FULL-WAVE RECTIFICATION SYSTEM

A radiographer can check the accuracy of the timer of a single-phase, full-wave rectified

unit by using a spinning top. A circular lead disc approximately 3 in. in diameter with a small hole (1/16th in.) in the outer portion of the disc is mounted on an axis so that it can spin freely. The flat surface of the disc is placed parallel to an x-ray cassette. An x-ray exposure is made while the disc is rotating. Since most of the x-ray waveform produces little or no density, only the peak of each individual pulsation is recorded on the radiographic film as a black dot. Each 1/120 second exposure will produce a single black dot on the radiograph. For an exposure of 1/10th second (single-phase, full-wave rectification) with a properly calibrated timer, 12 individual black dots (exposures) will result. A timer that is not functioning properly may produce more or less than 12 dots at 1/10th second. A failure in the rectification system, resulting in single-phase, nonrectified current, will produce half the number of dots per exposure, since the unit is operating at 60 positive impulses per second (half wave) instead of 120 positive impulses per second (full wave) (Fig. 2-8).

Three-phase radiographic timers require sophisticated tools for evaluation. If a spinning top were used with a three-phase generator, a continuous line (arc) of density

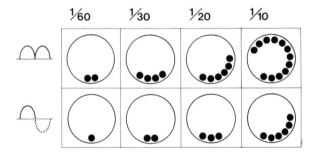

Figure 2-8 Timer Accuracy Test
Timer accuracy can be checked on a single-phase full-wave or half-wave rectified unit by the use of a spinning top. The spinning top test is a reliable method for checking timer accuracy. The spinning top is a circular lead disc, approximately 3 in. in diameter, with a small hole, 1/16 in., in the outer portion of the disc. The disc is mounted on an axis and made to spin freely with the flat surface of the disc parallel to the cassette. When the x-ray exposure is made with the disc rotating, the peak of each individual pulsation of a waveform is recorded on the radiographic film as a black dot. Each 1/120th second exposure will produce a single black dot on the radiograph if the timer is operating accurately. Typical short radiographic exposures (1/60th, 1/30th, 1/20th, and 1/10th second) are shown for single-phase, full-wave and single-phase half-wave exposures. Note that since the current is not rectified in half-wave rectification, only half the number of dots appear on the processed radiograph.

would result on the test radiograph. This is due to almost ripple-free waveform throughout the length of the exposure.

Timer tests tools include a template that can be used to measure the arc of the continuous line of density produced with three-phase equipment. The length of the arc gives an indication of the exposure time used to perform the test. An oscilloscope is suggested to accurately check the timer of a three-phase unit.

Automatic Exposure Device

An automatic exposure device (AED) should help to assure the radiographer of exposures of consistent density. The exposure is initiated by the radiographer, but the AED determines the length of exposure. Positioning skills are essential to properly position the part being examined to the phototimer or ionization sensor (Fig. 2-9).

PHOTOTIMER STRUCTURE AND ACTION

The phototimer consists of a highly light-sensitive phototube, optically and electrically connected to a fluorescent pick-up screen. A signal to the photomultiplier tube is amplified by an associated electrical circuit and terminates the radiographic exposure when a predetermined quantity of fluorescent light has reached the photocell. Another type of automatic timer uses an ionization chamber and a complex electronic circuit to terminate the exposure. Ionization chambers operate similarly to phototimers. They are affected by kilovoltage, milliamperage, focal film distance, size of patient, and exposure length. Ionization chambers sense remnant radiation to determine the exposure length.

An AED (phototimer or ionization chamber) can be installed in front (entrance) or behind the grid (exit) in either the table or upright Bucky (Fig. 2-10).

Newer automatic exposure devices, whether light-sensitive (phototimers) or radiation-sensitive (ionization chambers) are capable of exposures as low as 0.002 second (2 msec).

As with the phototimer, the correct sensor must be selected for specific body parts (Fig. 2-9).

Conventional radiographic cassettes have a sheet of lead foil behind the posterior intensifying screen to absorb backscatter. (See Fig.

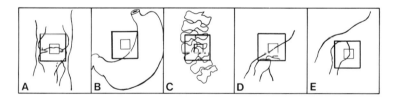

Figure 2-9 Automatic Exposure Device: Sensor Positioning Relationships The sensor of an automatic exposure device must be properly centered to the part under study to achieve a predetermined film density. Over or underexposed images can result if a patient is not properly centered to the pick-up screen (fluorescent screen or ionization sensor). Some older phototimers use large (usually 4 in. square) or small (usually 1.5 in.–2 in. square) apertures for specific body parts. Improper centering to either scanner negates the effectiveness of the phototimer.

This illustration shows the relationship of small and large sensors to body parts. Similar difficulties occur when using an ionization chamber. Both small and large apertures are properly centered to the knee (A). Both apertures are centered to the soft tissue structures of the abdomen (B), rather than the dense barium-filled stomach; a slightly underexposed radiograph may occur. The lumbar spine does not completely cover either scanner in the lateral position (C). The patient should be positioned slightly posterior. Both scanning devices are outside the osseous structures of the shoulder (D). An underexposed radiograph should result. A primary beam leak should also occur in this image. (See Fig. 2-12.) Since both scanning devices are situated within the dense muscular-osseous structures of the shoulders (E), a properly exposed radiograph should be obtained.

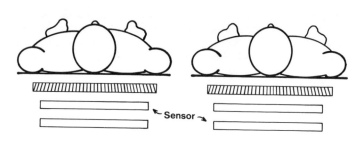

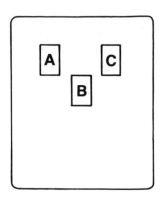

Figure 2-10 Automatic Exposure Device: Sensor Placement *Two different types of AED sensor placement are shown. (left, center.) On the left, the sensor is positioned beneath the grid but above the cassette (entrance-type sensor). In the center, the sensor is positioned beneath the grid and the cassette (exit-type sensor). The x-ray beam must pass through both the grid and the back of the cassette to strike this sensor. The use of strap-type cassettes with an exit sensor can result in overexposed radiographs. If the straps are inadvertently positioned over the AED, remnant radia-*

tion may be absorbed by the straps, resulting in a longer exposure time than is desired.

A typical illustration of the sensor configurations used for automatically exposed chest studies is shown on the right. Sensors must be selected so that either the PA or lateral images will be properly exposed. (See Fig. 2-7 for control panel sensor selection options.) One or more sensors are used for the PA chest AED. The middle sensor is usually preadjusted to produce a proper lateral chest density.

8-12.) Phototimer cassettes were originally designed without lead foil to avoid detection problems with exit-type sensors. In practice, most cassettes contain posterior lead foil sheeting, and phototimers are appropriately adjusted.

If older style cassettes having dense metallic closure straps are used with the exit-type detectors and the straps are inadvertently positioned over the phototimer pick-up cell, remnant radiation may be absorbed by the straps, resulting in longer exposure times than desired (Fig. 2-10).

Two important principles associated with automatic exposure controls are (1) minimal response time, and (2) back up time.

MINIMAL RESPONSE TIME

The minimal response time (minimal reaction time) of an AED represents the time required for the shortest possibe automatic exposure. The use of faster screen film combinations that produce greater film blackening per unit of exposure can accentuate minimal response time difficulties. (See Table 8-1.)

IMPORTANT: The minimal response time is independent of the quality or quantity of the x-ray beam.

When a patient requires less x-radiation than the minimal response time is capable of delivering at a predetermined kilovoltage and milliamperage setting, some type of technical factor adjustment must be made. Since the timer cannot terminate an exposure quicker than the minimal response time of the unit, milliamperage or kilovoltage must be lowered. A common error, particularly in chest radiography, is the lowering of kilovoltage. When kilovoltage is lowered, shorter scale contrast is produced. (See Chapters 11 and 12.) The lungs become blacker, while osseous structures and the mediastinum may appear chalk-like. Instead of a chest quality image, a rib or thoracic spine radiograph is produced. Lowering of the milliampere value to overcome this problem is recommended (Fig. 2-11).

A density adjustment control is present on the console for use with most automatic ex-

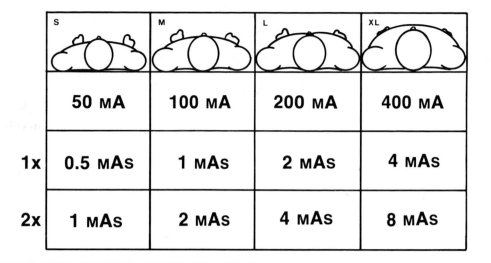

	S	M	L	XL
	50 mA	100 mA	200 mA	400 mA
1x	0.5 mAs	1 mAs	2 mAs	4 mAs
2x	1 mAs	2 mAs	4 mAs	8 mAs

Figure 2-11 Lowest mAs Possible With a Minimal Response Time of 1/100 sec at Two Different Screen Film Speeds When a high mA station is used for a radiograph, the minimal response time of an automatic exposure device may result in too high an mAs value for a proper density. This is often a problem when examining the chest of a small patient in the PA or AP position. The AED is not able to terminate an exposure faster than the minimal response time of the unit. A **minus** density selection on the AED control cannot overcome minimal response time difficulties in this situation. (See Fig. 2-7.)

Four representative patient sizes are shown. The radiographic density required for the larger patient would exceed 1/100th second exposure for proper density. The smaller patients require less mAs for proper exposure. Since the AED cannot terminate faster than 1/100th second in this example, higher milliampere values will result in higher mAs values than may be needed for the smaller patients. The use of a faster speed screen film combination compounds this problem. By lowering the mA value, the proper mAs can be achieved by the AED since it can remain activated for longer than the minimal response time. The AED can make the correct decision regarding density. Lowering kilovoltage will also help overcome the effect of minimal response time limitations but will result in shorter scale contrast. Although this might be desirable in some examinations (iodinated contrast studies or osseous examinations), it can result in blackened lung fields and chalk white ribs in a chest study. High mAs values will blacken the lung fields of a small patient. Low mAs values used with a large patient will increase the length of exposure and can result in patient motion or organ motion on the image. The mAs values must be raised or lowered according to patient size when attempting to overcome minimal response time limitations.

posure timers (see Fig. 2-7). The control is generally set on NORMAL density to produce the accepted departmental standard. Changes in density should occur when the MINUS or PLUS density stations are used.

IMPORTANT: If a radiograph is overexposed because a shorter exposure time is not possible (owing to minimal response time limitations), the use of the MINUS density station is not effective. No change in image density can occur.

BACK-UP TIME

The back-up time represents the maximal exposure that an AED will permit for a given mA and kVp value. The back-up time is generally set by the manufacturer within the instantaneous load capacity of the x-ray tube. On some units, the back-up time can be manually selected on the control panel by the radiographer. The settings (manual or automatic) must fall within the tube manufacturer's recommendations for instantaneous loading (See Fig. 4-7).

The back-up timer settings help avoid additional x-ray exposure to the patient as well as damage to the x-ray tube.

If a patient is positioned for a table Bucky radiograph and the chest x-ray sensor is energized in error, the x-ray beam will exit from the radiographic tube through the patient to the table AED. Since the table Bucky sensor is not energized, the x-ray tube would give off x-radiation until the radiographer realized the error or until the x-ray tube was destroyed. The reverse situation could also occur. The patient could be positioned for chest radiography and the table Bucky sensor could be activated in error. In either situation, the patient would receive detrimental unnecessary radiation.

Another misuse of the AED is the use of a cross-table (horizontal beam) technique, with the inadvertent selection of an AED station. In this situation, an AED sensor is not available to terminate the exposure.

If a patient is protected with a lead shield or if sandbags are used to support an injured limb and if the sensor were covered, the exposure might not terminate properly.

A primary beam leak can undercut the image, causing the premature termination of the exposure (Fig. 2-12). (See Figs. 9-4 and 9-5.)

In theory, an AED eliminates the need to measure part thickness or to calculate milliampere second values. Many automatic exposure technique charts use optimal or fixed kilovoltage values. (See Chapter 12.) The AED does not minimize the skills needed by radiographers. Knowledge of surface anatomy and the relationship of one organ to another help to avoid body part/sensor misalignment (Fig. 2-9).

SPECIAL USES FOR AUTOMATIC EXPOSURE DEVICES

Some unusual uses for AEDs include:

1 *Mobile exposure control.* Components of a typical AED used with a mobile unit include a control display module and an ion chamber

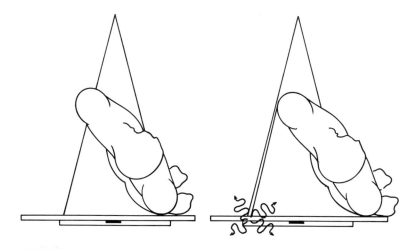

Figure 2-12 *The Effect of a Primary Beam Leak on an Automatic Exposure-Controlled Image* *When a patient is properly positioned to an AED sensor, remnant radiation as well as scatter radiation determines the amount of exposure to the radiographic film (left). If a patient is mispositioned so that a primary beam leak occurs (primary radiation striking the tabletop or chest Bucky), the AED may not produce a proper density. As the primary beam strikes the tabletop or upright holder, scatter radiation is generated in all directions (spatial). Some of this scatter strikes the sensor. Since an AED can only sense preselected densities, the scatter can cause the phototimer or ionization chamber to terminate prematurely. An underexposed radiograph would result. A primary beam leak, with image undercutting, could lead one to believe that the AED is not functioning properly. The AED is not able to distinguish between primary, remnant, or scatter radiation. In actuality, the AED is working as designed, since it is sensing a preselected density value.*

detector paddle. This paddle is used on the exit side of the cassette and must be centered properly to the area of interest. An AED will help to maintain consistent image quality over a broad range of kilovoltages and patient sizes. Density variations that could require retakes can be reduced by the use of an AED at the bedside.

2 *Mammography.* An AED on a dedicated mammographic unit will compensate for the density difference in atrophic, more radiolucent breasts (decreased exposure) vs. dense, fibrocystic breasts (increased exposure). (See Chapter 7.)

3 *Image intensifiers.* The image intensifier uses a type of automatic control for fluoroscopy as well as cineradiography. (See Chapters 6 and 9.) This device, known as an *automatic brightness control* (ABC) adjusts technical factors as areas of the body with large density differences are scanned. For example, when the right lower segment of the lung (radiolucent) is being examined and the fluoroscope is moved below the diaphragm into the right upper quadrant of the abdomen (radiodense) for evaluation of the liver, the brightness control will automatically adjust either milliamperage or kilovoltage, or both, to produce a proper fluoroscopic density.

3 Radiographic and Fluoroscopic Imaging Equipment

INHERENT limitations in imaging equipment can affect the selection of technical factors and patient positioning and can influence the making of a quality radiograph. In this chapter, emphasis will be placed on the image-producing characteristics of permanently installed and mobile x-ray equipment rather than the design of specific units.

Equipment calibration prior to the use of any radiographic unit is essential.

Before attempting to operate any type of radiographic equipment a data sheet should be made available to the radiographer. Information necessary for optimal operation of x-ray equipment includes:

1 The manufacturer's recommendations for tube "warm-up" procedures. (See Chapter 4.)

2 The maximal permissible mA and kVp values permitted for a single exposure (instantaneous load). (See Fig. 4-7.)

3 An understanding of heat unit concepts (see Fig. 4-8), particularly when more than one radiographer performs a procedure. Gastrointestinal or tomographic studies can generate large amounts of heat, taxing the anode thermal capacity of an x-ray tube.

4 Focal spot size. (See Fig. 4-2.) One should know whether focal spot size is automatically determined for specific mA stations or whether the radiographer must make the selection.

5 Timer consideration. (See Chapter 2.) When an automatic exposure device (AED) is used, both minimal response time and back-up time limitations should be known. (See Fig. 2-11.)

6 Filtration. (See Fig. 4-9.) If added filtration is removed (for a study such as mammography), it must be replaced for conventional radiography.

7 Grid characteristics. (See Fig. 5-11.) Grid ratio, radius, and lines per inch for each grid in use should be known.

8 Collimation. (See Fig. 5-6). One should be aware of all beam-limiting accessories that can be used with the collimator.

9 List of radiographic accessories. The radiographer, with the aid of a checklist, can quickly identify deficiencies in room supplies. Adequate supplies and tools can help to expedite patient flow.

10 Availability of oxygen and suction. Emergency aids are often wall mounted, requiring only replacement of the disposable portions of the emergency equipment.

11 Listing of telephone and emergency code numbers.

Equipment Maintenance

A minor variation in one component of the imaging chain can have a major effect on the radiographic image. Several minor variations in equipment standards, each within acceptable tolerances, can collectively produce a degraded radiographic image. Everything may seem to have been done correctly or at least within specifications, and yet radiographic quality may not meet departmental standards. Attention to each component of the imaging chain will improve radiographic quality.

Quality assurance (QA) techniques help to "fine tune" imaging equipment and accessories. Records must be maintained when modifications are made to the equipment. These records can be used to evaluate room downtime as well as repair costs per room.

QA techniques are mandatory in many states. At a conference of The World Health Organization in 1980, in Germany, the following definition for QA was developed: "Quality assurance is the organized efforts by staff to insure the consistent production of adequate diagnostic information at the lowest possible cost with minimum exposure to both patients and personnel to radiation." It is imperative that QA tests be documented, updated, and continually available for reference. Carefully maintained records become valuable for future evaluations of the equipment.

Attention should be given to:

1 *The maintenance and monitoring of x-ray film processors.* Quality control tests include developer and fixer solutions temperature readings, careful attention to replenishment rates, sensitometric evaluation of the developer activity, appropriate safelights, and cleanliness of equipment and work areas. (See Chapter 10.)

2 *X-ray equipment calibration.* Tests for focal spot size, timer accuracy, and linearity of milliampere settings and kilovoltage calibration are important. The quality (kVp) and quantity (mAs) of the x-ray beam greatly influence the making of a quality radiograph.

3 *Scatter control.* Grid ratio, focus, and alignment must be evaluated. Periodic x-ray evaluation of the grid for damage (see Fig. 5-15) as well as collimator shutter pattern alignment (light source to x-ray source; see Fig. 5-7) should be checked.

4 *Recording media control.* Testing for film screen contact as well as fall off in screen speed should be an ongoing procedure. Screen cleaning should be scheduled at regular intervals. (See Chapter 8.) When images are made from the output phosphor of an image intensifier, its resolution should also be evaluated.

5 *Care of protective devices.* Apron racks should be installed in every room and on mobile units so that these garments can be hung correctly to minimize damage.

6 *Protection.* Patient and personnel exposure information should be carefully recorded.

Occasionally, radiographs of marginal quality must be accepted for interpretation. Because of the nature of the examination or the condition of a patient, it may not be advisable to repeat a study. When accepting marginal quality radiographs, care must be taken to avoid the lowering of departmental standards. A small carcinoma that is undetected as the result of poor technique will continue to grow and may metastasize. A false-negative report could delay treatment.

Quality Assurance Testing

A regular schedule should be adopted for QA testing on all radiographic equipment (Table 3-1). Test tools should be reliable to guarantee accurate, reproducible results. Each component of the radiographic system should be subjected to the following QA guidelines:

1 There should be specific materials and equipment available for each test.

2 A QA specialist should be familiar with the test equipment and understand how to evaluate and interpret the results of the tests.

3 Test procedures should be standardized to ensure reproducible results.

4 Preventive maintenance schedules should be set up to detect minor variations in equipment.

5 Corrective procedures should be initiated and carried out whenever test results indicate a deviation from normal.

6 Records should be maintained for each piece of equipment for which a problem is indicated and should include the date, corrective action, date of action, and so on. This record will help to document recurrent problems and to check variations in equipment that may occur between scheduled tests. A retake analysis program should be used to evaluate all repeat radiographs to help identify the reasons for additional exposures. The repeat analysis program will help to identify topics that could be addressed in in-service programs.

QA test tools are available from several manufacturers. Instructions for the use of the tools, descriptions of the tests and test results, and suggestions for monitoring test evaluations are included with each test tool.

Although noninvasive tests can be performed by a radiographer, invasive tests (requiring electrical attachment of the test tools to the imaging equipment) should be performed by qualified service personnel.

Some Radiation Protection Considerations

Most radiation received during one's lifetime will be due to manmade radiation. Health care workers are issued radiation safety monitoring badges or dosimeters if they are employed in areas where studies using radiation for diagnosis or treatment are performed.

Personnel can be protected from radiation by the use of lead barriers in walls, windows,

TABLE 3-1. Basic Quality Assurance Tests

Test	Tools	Comments
Processor function and replenishment; Documentation of sensitometric properties or radiographic film	Sensitometer Densitometer Stepwedge Graduated beakers	Changes may affect density, contrast, and fog level on processed radiographs.
Screen film contact (sharpness)	Wiremesh	Poor screen film contact affects radiographic detail.
Beam alignment	Alignment test tool or 4 small objects (coins)	Misalignment can cause "cut-off" on one or more sides of the radiograph. (See Fig. 5-16.)
Timer accuracy	Spinning Top (single phase) Motor-driven Spinning top (three phase) Oscilloscope (three phase)	Timer accuracy can be determined by number of dots recorded in a given time (See Figure 2-8). If spinning top used for three-phase equipment, an arc (continuous line) results. Requires a template for evaluation Requires qualified service personnel for performance of test
kV accuracy mA accuracy	Test cassettes	Performed to check calibration of equipment; kilovoltage; milliampere stability; timer accuracy
mA accuracy	Stepwedge Direct reading dosimeter	Performed to check mA linearity
mA accuracy	Oscilloscope	Requires qualified service personnel for performance of test
Beam quality	Dosimeter Filters	Performed to check for half-value layer

(continued on next page)

TABLE 3-1. Basic Quality Assurance Tests (continued)

Test	Tools	Comments
Automatic exposure reproducibility	Stepwedge Ruller Containers Water Densitometer	Performed to determine whether phototimer or ionization chamber exposures are consistent
Grid uniformity		Grid radiographed to check for damage. (See Fig. 5-15.)
Grid alignment	Phantom	Performed to check for tube alignment to the grid (Bucky) in the table (Can also be a visual check) (Figure 3-3).
Focal spot size	Pinhole camera	Performed to determine effective focal spot size of focal spots greater than 0.3 mm
Focal spot size	Star test pattern Direct exposure prepacked film Stand to mount test tool	NEMA requires star test pattern to evaluate focal spots 0.3 mm or smaller (fractional focal spots). Central ray alignment is critical for accurate measurements.
Optical system (fluoro, image intensifier)	Wiremesh segments Phantom	Performed to evaluate resolution or loss of resolving power from the output phosphor; also exposure rates and brightness levels
TV (mirror optics), fluoro, image intensifier	Aluminum blocks Penetrometer (with holes)	Performed to evaluate low-contrast structures
Automatic brightness control	Dosimeter Aluminum blocks	Performed to evaluate ability of brightness control to adjust to patient size or thickness of part
Safelight	Stopwatch Film mask	Improper safelight filter or wattage can add supplemental density to film (fog)
Viewbox	Lightmeter Mask	Performed to check for percentage and uniformity of transmitted light through the glass panels

doors, movable lead shields, and lead sheeting. Radiation dosage to personnel can also be reduced by increasing the distance between the operator and the x-ray source. Exposure control cords should be long (up to 12 feet) on mobile equipment to permit the operator to stand at a greater distance from the x-ray source and should be very short on permanently installed units to ensure that an exposure cannot be made from outside the control booth. X-ray personnel should wear lead aprons and gloves whenever they may be exposed to primary or scatter radiation. Fluoroscopists should consider protective eyeglasses and thyroid shields in addition to a lead apron and gloves.

Other methods of monitoring radiation include:

1 *Direct reading pocket ionization chambers.*

2 *Thermolucent dosimeters (TLD),* which can be placed in the path of the primary beam, and can be used to monitor entrance skin exposure (ESE) from medical and dental x-rays.

Patients can be protected from excess radiation in several ways:

1 *Filtration.* Filters remove soft (long wavelength) radiation that would be absorbed by the patient but does not produce any useful information on the radiograph. (See Chapter 4.)

2 *Beam limiting devices.* Restriction of the x-ray beam to the area of interest. (See Chapter 5.)

3 *Shielding.* Like collimation, shielding restricts the field size and can selectively protect radiosensitive areas. All patients with reproductive potential are entitled to gonadal shielding. Many accessories can be used for protective purposes, including pelvic lead sheeting or a lead shield attached to the colimator. (See Fig. 5-7.) Occasionally, special coverage of the thyroid gland or lenses of the eyes is indicated. (See Chapter 7.) At the bedside, the patient adjacent to any patient being radiographed should be considered. People accompanying a patient are also at risk. Hospital personnel as well as visitors are entitled to radiation protection.

Leakage radiation from the x-ray tube is a concern and should not exceed 100 mR/hr/meter from the source when the machine is operating at maximal output.

4 *Selective positioning.* Some patient positioning techniques reduce dosage to radiosensitive areas. For example, in the anteroposterior (AP) position for skull tomography, the primary beam (unattenuated) enters through the lens of the eyes. With the patient in the posteroanterior (PA) position, remnant radiation (attenuated) exits through the lens of the eyes. The use of the PA position for scoliosis studies minimizes dosage to the breasts of female patients. (See Fig. 4-11.)

5 *The ten-day rule.* Attention to the menstrual cycle of women in the childbearing years can reduce the possibility of radiation exposure to a fetus.

6 *Exposure factors.* The use of proper technical factors such as an optimal kilovoltage technique ensures adequate penetration of the part under study with decreased absorbed dosage. (See Chapter 12.)

7 *Use of high-speed screen film combinations whenever possible.* Rare-earth technology significantly lowers radiation dosage without compromising the image. (See Chapter 8.)

8 *Avoid repeat radiographs.* Careful attention to technical details and positioning prior to the making of an exposure can often eliminate the need for repeat examinations.

A personal monitoring program has been developed by Personal Monitoring Technol-ogies, Rochester, New York, in which members who are enrolled in the program carry a credit card-size card that contains several TLDs. One TLD is reserved to monitor background radiation. Prior to the x-ray examination, the member presents the card to the radiographer, who tapes a TLD in the x-ray field. Following the study, the TLDs are returned to the monitoring service for evaluation. A report of the radiation received from the x-ray examination and the control TLD (background) are sent to members enrolled in the program.

Types of Radiographic Equipment

Radiographic equipment can be either permanently installed or mobile. Permanent installations include conventional radiographic rooms (Fig. 3-1) as well as radiographic/fluoroscopic rooms (Fig. 3-2) equipped with either a conventional fluoroscope (see Chapter 8) or an image intensifier. (See Figs. 6-1 and 6-2.) Image intensified fluoroscopic units usually house a spot film device or a spot film photographic camera in tandem with the intensifier. (See Fig. 6-2.)

Permanently installed dedicated units include chest imaging equipment and conventional neuro (head) units.

Mobile or bedside machines can be operated from a conventional power source, can be condenser discharge energized, or can operate from a self-contained battery system. Mobile image intensifiers are useful in the operating room or for special fluoroscopic-controlled procedures such as catheter placement. The "C-Arm" intensifier is described in Chapter 6. (See Fig. 6-4.)

Mechanical/Electrical Considerations

When assigned to a radiographic room, a visual check of the following should be made:

1 *Mechanical stability of the x-ray tube.* Vibration in the tube crane can produce image unsharpness.

2 *Bucky stability.* If the Bucky tray vibrates during exposure, image sharpness will deteriorate.

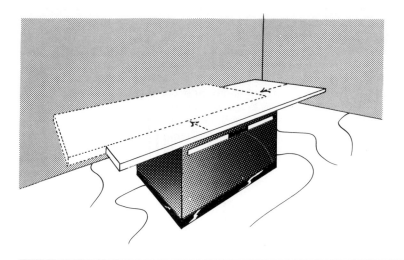

Figure 3-1 Permanently Installed Radiographic Equipment   *A horizontal radiographic table is shown with a floating or moving tabletop. Patient positioning is easier for both the patient and the radiographer with a floating tabletop. Some tables can be elevated or lowered so that patient litters can be abutted to them for patient* transfer.

In this illustration, the tabletop is shown moved from its normal position, illustrated by dotted segments and arrows. When the patient is placed on the table, the floating tabletop can be moved to center specific body parts to the table Bucky.

3 *Equipment locks.* Bucky tray locks and tube crane locks should be checked, since a malfunctioning lock may result in vibration in either the crane or Bucky tray.

4 *Condition of the electrical cables.* Through rotation for horizontal beam studies, the tube cables may become entwined, putting stress on tube connections. A hanging cable, rubbing against the equipment or a wall, may fray.

5 *Control panel function.* Meters, dials, and so on must be observed for fluctuations, since minor changes in output may affect radiographic density. Radiation output changes may reflect tube aging or a need for calibration of the equipment.

6 *Tube crane/Bucky alignment.* Indicators for alignment of the x-ray tube to the grid (see Chapter 5) and focal film distance must be accurate. When a tube is rotated from its normal position for a horizontal beam radiograph and then returned to its conventional position, misalignment can occur. A minor tilt against the grid (one or two degrees) may cause grid cutoff. (See Chapter 5.) A simple tube realignment adjustment is shown in Fig. 3-3.

Permanent Radiographic Installations: Routine Radiographic Equipment

Tables

A permanently installed radiographic room includes a table that can be fixed in the horizontal position, can vary in position (motor-driven; Fig. 3-2) to a full upright position, or can be adjusted to the Trendelenburg position (head lower than feet). Tables with dual 90-degree capability are associated with fluoroscopic/radiographic procedures.

Floating tabletops make the positioning of the patient easier for both patient and radiographer (Fig. 3-1). Some tables can be elevated or lowered to permit litter alignment to the tabletop for ease in patient transfer to the table.

Of particular interest is the geometric relationship of the table top to the Bucky tray (TT/BT). This distance can be as great as 13 cm, significantly increasing object film distance. There is also a difference in object film distance if a grid cassette is used instead of a

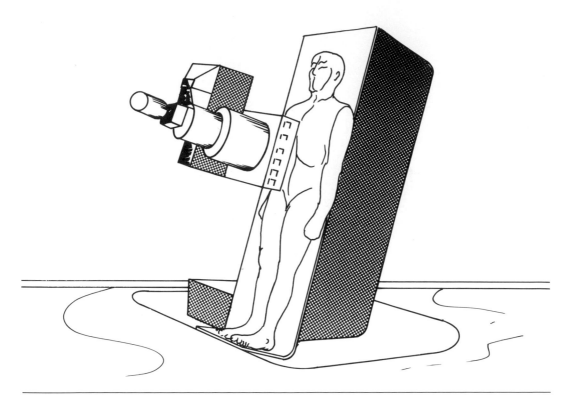

Figure 3-2 Fluoroscopic Radiographic Unit *Some permanently installed radiographic/fluoro- scopic units can either be used in the horizontal position or be motor driven to a full upright po- sition. Most units can be adjusted to the Trende-* *lenburg position (head lower than feet). Some ta- bles have a dual 90-degree capability. In this illus- tration, the table is almost 90 degrees upright as the patient is elevated for horizontal beam fluo- roscopic spot film evaluation.*

table Bucky technique. (See Figs. 11-11 and 11-12.)

Tube Cranes or Tube Stands

A birail tube stand often limits the making of an exposure to the x-ray table (Fig. 3-4). A ceiling-mounted tube crane can be moved over greater distances and can accommodate non-grid exposures or grid cassette exposures on a litter if the patient cannot be transferred to the x-ray table (Fig. 3-4).

Upright Cassette Holders

Most upright cassette holders can be used with several size cassettes. A typical upright cassette holder holds cassettes 14 in. × 17 in. in size for chest or abdominal radiography. These units can be equipped with either a fine-line stationary grid or a Bucky (Fig. 3-5). Some wall-mounted holders can accept a 14 in. × 36 in. cassette for upright radiography of the vertebral column (scoliosis study) or full-length lower extremity evaluation. (See Figs. 4-11 and 4-12).

Timers

Radiographic timers, including AEDs were described in Chapter 2.

Generators

X-ray equipment varies in output. Some units can generate up to 1500 mA or greater as well as high kilovoltage levels (150 kVp or greater).

IMPORTANT: When a unit is rated at a high kilovoltage value as well as a high mA

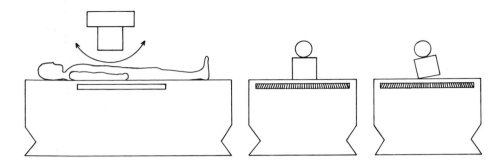

Figure 3-3 X-Ray Tube/Bucky (Grid) Relation-ships *Birail tubestands or ceiling-mounted tube cranes can be used in many positions, for example, for horizontal cross table radiography.*

When the tube is rotated in its housing and then returned to its normal position, misalignment can occur. A minor tilt (1 or 2 degrees) against the grid can result in grid cutoff. (See Fig. 5-16.) It is good practice to check grid/tube alignment prior to the making of a radiograph. A simple tube re-alignment adjustment may be required prior to the making of a radiograph. This problem or any technical problem can be compounded when the radiographic equipment is used by more than one radiographer. When the radiographer stands on the side of the table (adjacent to the Bucky tray opening), tube angulations to the head or foot of the table are easy to visualize (left). Unfortunately, tube rotation to or away from the radiographer is hard to detect visually (right). By standing at the end of the table and lowering the radiographic tube and collimator so that the flat surface of the exit portion of the collimator is flush with the x-ray table, one can guarantee tube/grid alignment (center).*

value, it is usually not possible to use both maximal values at the same time.

The selection of a specific type of generator (single-phase or three-phase) is determined by imaging needs and is directly related to the cost of the equipment. Specific information on x-ray generators can be found in Chapter 2.

Mobile Radiographic Equipment

Portable Equipment

Even though portable x-ray equipment is mobile by nature, all mobile x-ray equipment should not be considered portable. If an x-ray machine can be packed into a small carrying case and transported to an area of need, it can be called portable. Most portable (trans-portable) x-ray units are lightweight and can be quickly assembled. Mobile imaging services use this type of equipment to examine patients at home, in a nursing home, or in other remote locations.

Portable equipment requires some type of power source (AC current). Milliamperage and kilovoltage outputs are always limited (10 mA or greater, 85 kVp maximum) on portable equipment. The oil-filled lead-lined head contains an x-ray tube, a step-up transformer, and a step-down transformer. A small control unit contains the main switch and a rheostat to vary current (mA). A handheld mechanical timer is usually used to make an exposure. This type of inexpensive timer (often found on older dental units) will rarely operate accurately below 1/10th second. Because of low mA output, long exposure times are usually required. The 1/10th second timer limitation is a problem when performing a chest examination because of cardiac motion. A timer of this nature can rarely be used for pediatric studies.

The use of rare-earth screen film combinations (600 speed or greater) brings exposure times to acceptable levels. AEDs may be used with mobile equipment. (See Chapter 2.)

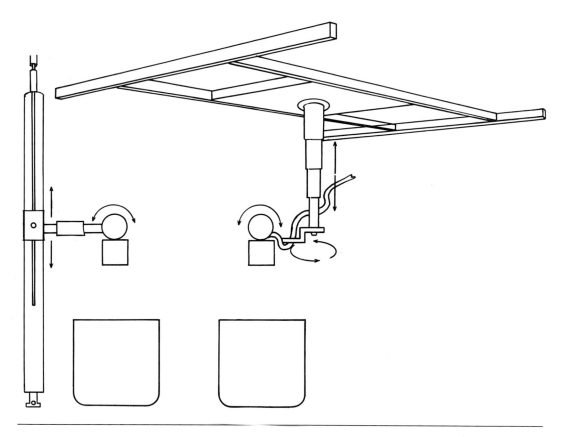

Figure 3-4 Radiographic Tube Holders
Birail, fixed tubestands (left) limit the mobility of the x-ray tube. The tube usually can be moved back and forth in a single direction on its rails from one end of the table to the other. The tube may be moved off center to the Bucky (left or right) for non-Bucky radiographs. It is often difficult to examine a patient on a litter with a birail tubestand unless clearance for the litter is available at one end of the table.

A ceiling-mounted tube crane (right) can be moved over a greater distance to accommodate non-Bucky exposures on a litter if the patient cannot be transferred to the x-ray table. The mobility of the tube crane is limited only by the dimensions of the ceiling-mounted crane rails. Some of these cranes can be moved the full length and width of the radiographic room. This mobility can be particularly helpful when lateral horizontal beam radiographs such as skull, hip, or trauma examinations are requested. Decubitus examinations are also easier to perform with a ceiling-mounted tube crane.

Mobile Equipment

An electrical supply is required for both mobile and portable equipment.

Lengthy heavy cables are needed if low output mobile units are linked to an electrical outlet. A voltage drop or change in an incoming line voltage may cause variations in exposure. In areas such as the emergency ward or intensive care unit, special electrical lines can be installed to minimize this problem.

IMPORTANT: Line voltage regulator adjustments are critical with mobile radiographic units because of possible variations in current.

Many mobile units use batteries for the generation of x-radiation as well as transport

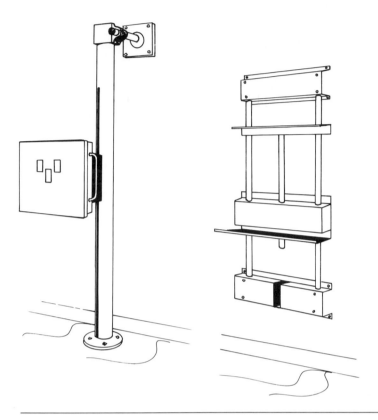

Figure 3-5 Wall-Mounted Cassette Holders
The basic types of wall-mounted cassette holders include (left) *a counterbalanced Bucky. This device houses either a moving grid (Bucky) or a fine line stationary grid for upright radiography of the chest, skull, and abdomen. An AED sensor pattern is shown in this illustration as part of an automatic exposure device. (See Fig. 2-10.)*

A standard cassette holder is shown at the right. Tracks are used to hold the cassette in place.

A grid track is also available on most cassette holders to hold a stationary grid for upright chest or abdominal radiography. It is important that grid focus be considered when using a grid with this holder. Most abdominal or osseous structure studies are exposed at a 40-in. FFD. Chest radiographs are made using a 72-in. FFD. If the focal range of the grid is not correct for the study, image cutoff can occur. (See Fig. 5-16.)

(motor drive). Battery-operated mobile units eliminate the need for special power lines at the bedside. These units use nickel–cadmium storage batteries. A conventional power supply is used to charge the batteries when the unit is not in use.

The principles of x-ray generation as outlined in Chapters 1, 2, and 4, apply to portable and mobile radiographic units (Fig. 3-6).

It is difficult to produce an ideal radiograph in a mobile situation. Trauma patients with multiple injuries are particularly difficult to examine. A patient's condition will often dic-

tate positioning limitations. The critically ill patient in the intensive care unit may not be able to be elevated to the preferred upright position for a chest study or may not be able to inspire fully for maximal ventilation of the lungs. (See Figs. 12-8, 14-15.) Occasionally, an angled projection, with less than optimal inspiration, must be taken (Fig. 3-7).

Unless the patient can be put into the true upright position and a horizontal beam can be used, an optimal chest radiograph is not produced. It might be advisable to make a supine radiograph for better control of posi-

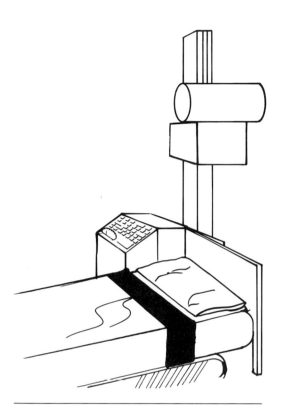

Figure 3-6 Mobile Radiographic Unit
A typical high-output mobile radiographic unit is shown. Newer mobile units can be either capacitor discharge units or battery operated. With the battery-operated unit, a rotating anode tube is used with a conventional light beam collimator. The radiographic tube is positioned parallel to the flat surface of the bed. Central ray is therefore perpendicular to the bed and any cassette that would rest upon the surface. Shortened focal film distances are often the norm. Even when the proper FFD is possible, it is difficult to center to a grid cassette. The weight of the patient or the flexible nature of the mattress often produces cassette rotation and grid cutoff. (See Fig. 5-16.)

Many patients cannot be positioned flat or supine for mobile chest radiography, so the bed is raised toward the upright position. Rarely is the patient positioned 90 degrees erect as in conventional chest radiography. Positioning difficulties can occur. See Figure 3-7 for positioning during mobile chest radiography. See Figure 3-8 for air–fluid interface evaluation. Improper grid placement can result in grid cutoff. (See Fig. 5-16.)

tioning and inspiration. This modification in positioning may produce an image with less motion, since the patient is not in an unstable (uncomfortable) position.

IMPORTANT: A horizontal beam technique is required to demonstrate an air–fluid level in the chest, abdomen, or sinus cavities (Fig. 3-8).

Capacitor Discharge Unit

A capacitor (condenser) is a device for accumulating and holding a charge of electricity. Capacitor or condenser discharge mobile units use a conventional electrical source to charge a high tension capacitor. A quantity of electricity is stored in the capacitor (condenser) prior to exposure. When the timer is activated, electricity is discharged through the x-ray tube, producing x-radiation.

IMPORTANT: Capacitor units do not maintain a constant kilovoltage value throughout the length of the exposure. For every one mAs used during an exposure, these units will gradually drop, in effect, one kVp. When a specific mAs value is used, for example 20 mAs at 80 kVp at the end of the exposure, there has been a gradual drop of kilovoltage from 80 kVp to 60 kVp. A portion of the exposure is made at lower kilovoltage levels. According to Thompson (Practical Approach to Modern X-Ray Equipment, Little, Brown and Company, Boston, 1978) voltage drops off approximately one kVp per one mAs during exposures that are longer than 10 msec (1/100th second). The capacitor discharge unit is very efficient when low milliampere second values are used, since only a minor drop in the kilovoltage occurs.

The unit should be charged immediately prior to use. Because the charge can leak rapidly from the capacitor, it is not recommended that a unit be charged in one area and used in another area. A power source should be available in the vicinity of the examining area.

Battery-operated units have significantly more output than capacitor discharge units and do not drop in kilovoltage during the exposure as milliampere seconds are increased. Radiation output approximates a

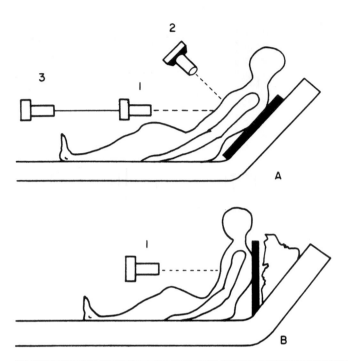

Figure 3-7 Focus Film Distance Variations
An erect bedside examination of the chest is difficult to perform. If the patient is unable to sit completely erect (A), the x-ray tube can be positioned at an appropriate FFD (2) to ensure proper film blackening. Unfortunately, with this position (2), an air–fluid interface cannot be demonstrated. (See Fig. 3-8.)

Often it is easier to move the x-ray tube to the foot of the bed (3), producing almost a 2× increase in the FFD. When the patient remains in the semi-erect position (A) with the tube in its normal position (1), a distorted apical lordotic radiograph results.

Once the tube is positioned with the patient partially erect, the cassette should be used as a lever to elevate the patient to the full upright position. A pillow can be wedged behind the cassette to maintain the erect position (B).

With the exception of 2,A, any of the aforementioned horizontal tube positions can be used to demonstrate an air–fluid level within the chest. If air–fluid levels are to be demonstrated, every effort must be made to place the patient in a fully erect position at the appropriate FFD. Central ray must remain parallel to the floor.

three-phase generator (12-pulse rectification). (See Chapter 2.) Nickel–cadmium batteries are used for exposure as well as for mobility (motor-drive assist). The battery source can be recharged from an electrical outlet. A capacity of 10,000 mAs per charge is possible.

IMPORTANT: If the battery charge falls off, an inconsistency in generator output may be noticed between exposures. Newer units monitor the condition of their batteries, automatically compensating for power changes. More consistent exposures are possible.

Field Emission Units

Conventional radiographic tubes use a heated filament to emit electrons. (See Chapter 4.) A field emission tube emits electrons from a metal plate. The metal plate is electronegative, with a high voltage potential between it and its anode. When a sufficiently strong electrical field is applied to this plate, there is an emission of electrons.

Field emission mobile units using a microprocessor control can operate at up to 240 kVp. Short exposure times are also possible, reducing radiographic blurring owing to patient or organ motion.

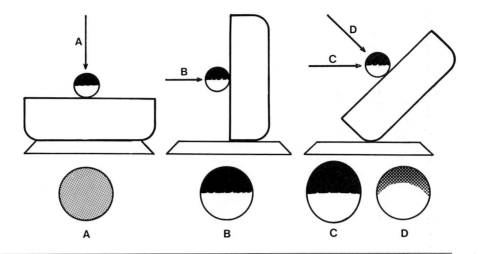

Figure 3-8 Air–Fluid Level Demonstration

For an air–fluid level to be seen on a radiographic image, central ray must be parallel to the floor (horizontal beam technique). In this illustration, a conventional supine radiograph is made (A). *Note the air–fluid level in the circular object on the radiographic table. Air is represented by the blackened superior portion of the circle, fluid by the whitened inferior portion of the circle. Below this illustration, a diffuse gray object representing the radiographic image is shown. The air–fluid interface has not been demonstrated. In the full upright position, there is no change in the air–fluid position within the circular object, but the horizontal beam central ray* (B) *is able to demonstrate the air–fluid interface without distortion. When the table is in the semi-erect position* (right), *the air–fluid level will still remain parallel to the floor. When the central ray* (C) *is used, a distorted elliptical, almost egg-shaped pattern results. Because a horizontal beam technique is used, an air–fluid level is demonstrated. When an attempt is made to avoid this distortion* (D), *the x-ray beam does not enter parallel to the air–fluid interface, failing to demonstrate this important diagnostic sign.*

When it is impossible to place a patient in the fully erect position for a study of this nature, a lateral decubitus radiograph can be taken to demonstrate an air–fluid interface. This positioning approach is helpful in demonstrating free fluid in the chest or sinus cavities, obstruction of the bowels, and for air–barium contrast studies. Grid placement must be an ongoing concern. (See Figs. 5-18 and 5-19.)

Technical Considerations for Mobile Examinations

Patients are often radiographed many times during their hospitalization. Sequential examinations (sometimes several times per day) are common practice. Sequential labeling of the radiographs is important, because if the examinations are of high quality, subtle findings between examinations can be appreciated.

The principles of scatter control outlined in Chapters 5 and 11 also apply at the bedside.

The use of a grid at the bedside can result in focusing difficulties. Variations in focal film distance are an ongoing concern. Central ray can be difficult to align to the center of a grid. Because the mattress and cassette are not always flat, lateral decentering of the grid can occur. Low-ratio grids are often used at the bedside to minimize these problems. (See Table 5-1.)

IMPORTANT: When a non-grid study is made at the bedside, tight beam collimation is mandatory for scatter control.

Radiation Dosage Considerations

Some factors that must be considered regarding reduction of radiation dosage when performing a mobile examination are:

1 The exposure control switch should be connected to a long cord (up to 12 feet) to help avoid radiation exposure to the radiographer.

2 A lead apron should be worn by anyone attending these procedures.

3 Additional radiographs should not be made to avoid a return trip for a possible repeat examination.

4 Gonadal shielding should be used on all patients with reproductive potential. Concern regarding the possibility of pregnancy of the patient, other patients in the area, or hospital personnel reflects a professional attitude.

5 Mobile units should not be overlooked when QA tests are being made. Many of the tests used for permanent installations can be used for mobile equipment. The electrical source cables as well as the tube cables of the mobile unit should be evaluated regularly for signs of wear or damage.

IMPORTANT: Extension cords or adaptor plugs should not be used unless approved by hospital safety officials.

Mobile Radiographic Fluoroscopic Units

Operating room, critical care, or emergency procedures often require the use of a mobile radiographic/fluoroscopic unit. These units have a C arm configuration and can be linked with videotape, videodisk, or other image storage systems. (See Fig. 6-4.) An image intensifier enables the physician to see a fluoroscopic image in "real" time. Confirmation radiographs are often made following the fluoroscopic evaluation.

Other Mobile Units

Mobile imaging systems are no longer limited to conventional radiography. Mobile ultrasonographic equipment, as well as gamma cameras (nuclear medicine), are used for medical imaging.

Permanent Installation: Radiographic/Fluoroscopic Units

For some examinations, static imaging (radiography) must be supplemented by organ motion evaluation (fluoroscopy). A fluoroscope is used for this purpose.

The use of a conventional fluoroscopic screen requires dark adaptation of the eyes and total room darkness because of the low light level of the fluoroscope. (See Chapter 8.) Modern fluoroscopic units use image intensifiers rather than a conventional fluoroscopic screen (Fig. 3-9). Image intensifiers are operated in almost normal room light in tandem with a television viewing system. (See Figs. 6-1 and 6-2.)

Conventional fluoroscopic screens are made of zinc cadmium sulfide crystals that phosphoresce yellow-green when excited by x-radiation. Zinc cadmium sulfide phosphors exhibit lag (afterglow), which persists for a short period of time after the activating source has ceased. The emissivity range of the phosphor matches the color sensitivity of the human eye. Similar in nature to the phosphors used in intensifying screens (see Chapter 8), fluoroscopic screen phosphors also absorb x-ray energy and convert it to visible light.

The fluoroscopic tube is usually mounted beneath the radiographic table. X-radiation passes through the table top, through the patient, striking the fluoroscopic screen. A fluoroscopic spot film mechanism that holds a cassette is a major component of a fluoroscopic installation. The cassettes can vary in size. Some spot film devices can use cassettes as large as 14 in. × 14 in. The film can be exposed as single frame or divided into several segments by a built-in lead masking system, making multiple sequential imaging possible. (See Fig. 5-2.) When an area of interest is seen, the fluoroscopist can bring the cassette, from the park position, into the x-ray field, make an exposure, and then return the cassette to its parked position (Fig. 3-9).

Low milliampere values (1 mA to 5 mA) are used for fluoroscopy; conventional milliampere values (200 mA or greater) are used for spot film radiography.

Foot switches are sometimes used to activate the fluoroscope or to make radiographic images (screen film radiographs, cut or roll film images). (See Chapters 6 and 9.) Foot switches should be protected from contaminants that might cause the switch to stick in the closed position and produce prolonged fluoroscopy.

Most fluoroscopic/radiographic rooms use an image intensifier in place of a conventional fluoroscopic screen. Photographic cameras (70

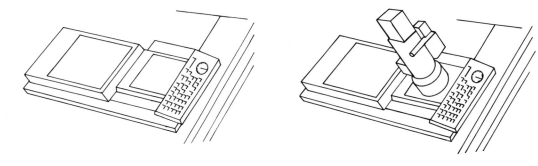

Figure 3-9 *Conventional Fluoroscopic Tunnel vs. Image Intensifier Attachment* *Fluoroscopic screens requiring dark adaptation of the eyes were used for years, prior to the advent of the image intensifier. The low light level of the fluoroscope (left) produced a dimly illuminated image for the fluoroscopist. The patient was examined in a darkened room, and radiographs were made using a spot film tunnel. Single or multiple frame studies per cassette were possible. When an area of interest was seen on the fluoroscopic screen, the radiologist brought the cassette into position, and a spot film radiograph was made. The modern fluoroscopic spot film tunnel (right) is similar in design for spot film purposes but uses an image intensifier for fluoroscopic guidance. Under almost normal room light conditions, the radiologist can view the fluoroscopic procedure on mirror optical viewers or on a television screen. Fluoroscopic spot films are made in a similar manner. The cassette is brought into the x-ray field, an exposure is made, and the cassette is returned to its parked position. Because of the high light output of the image intensifier, photographic-type fluoroscopic spot films can be made using a strip or cut film camera. (See Figs. 6-1 and 6-2.) The size of the image intensifier input phosphor (6 in.–15 in.) determines the area of the patient that can be imaged with a photographic spot film device. Using the conventional spot film tunnel with screen film cassettes, the field size can be varied to the size of the cassette. Most spot film devices use either 8 in. × 10 in. or 9 1/2 in. × 9 1/2 in. cassettes. Some newer models use 14 in. × 14 in. cassettes, producing almost full-size radiographic images from a fluoroscopic spot film tunnel.*

mm to 105 mm) can be used with an image intensifier as a substitute for screen film cassettes. These photographic images are restricted to the field size of the output phosphor of the intensifier. (See Figs. 6-2, 9-11, and 9-12.)

Permanent Installation: Dedicated Radiographic Units

Specialized units dedicated to specific examinations where high patient volume is present, expedite workflow.

The Dedicated Chest Unit

Dedicated chest radiographic units are designed with a film transporting mechanism, a pair of intensifying screens, a magazine housing unexposed film (usually 100 sheets or more), and a receiving cassette for the exposed radiographic film. They can be linked directly to an automatic processor so that a conventional chest radiograph can be made and viewed in less than 2 minutes. The x-ray tube moves in synchrony with the film changer. As the changer is adjusted in height, the tube tracks correspondingly. (See Chapter 14.)

A bar can be mounted above the changer to help stabilize the patient in the lateral position. Patients are instructed to lift their arms above their heads and to use the bar as a steadying aid.

The Head Unit

The dedicated head unit (neuro) is used for routine radiography of the skull, sinuses, mastoids, facial bones, and some other small body parts.

Major advantages of the head unit include patient comfort, ease in positioning, and the ability to demonstrate air–fluid levels (Fig. 3-8). For critically ill patients, the head unit can be used in a recumbent position.

Stereoradiography

When viewing three-dimensional structures in two dimensions (a radiograph), an image lacks the third dimension (depth).

To produce radiographs that give the effect of depth, two slightly different projections must be made. The patient must remain in exactly the same position for both exposures. The tube is moved off-center (a predetermined distance) prior to the first exposure. After the first exposure, but prior to the second, the tube is moved an equal distance (past center) in the opposite direction. Tube shift can be either manual or automatic. See Chapter 13 for stereo shift distance formula.

IMPORTANT: The stereo shift of the tube must always be in the direction of the grid lines to avoid grid cutoff. (See Fig. 5-16.)

Both images are evaluated on a stereoscopic viewer and are reflected by a combination of mirrors that are arranged so that each eye simultaneously sees only one image. The brain converts both images to a single image, giving the illlusion of depth.

Stereo radiographs are used to separate superimposed structures. Tomography with its "separating capacity" is another method for separating superimposed structures.

Tomography

Tomographic equipment and techniques are presented in Chapter 7.

IMPORTANT: Tomographic attachments can be installed on routine radiographic equipment. A centimeter scale used to select the x-ray focal plane can be attached to the x-ray table. An x-ray table with a tomographic attachment will produce acceptable linear tomographic images. Unfortunately, linear tomography will always exhibit linear parasitical streaks. (See Fig. 7-3.)

Radiographic Accessories

The use of radiographic accessories is dependent upon the skill and attitude of the radiographer. Some common radiographic accessories include:

1 *Compression band.* A compression band made of cloth or nylon (about 10 in. in width) is used to restrain the patient on a radiographic table. It is linked to the table from side to side, usually across the patient's abdomen. A tightening mechanism can be used to compress the abdomen to an overall even thickness.

An air-filled rubber bladder can be used beneath a compression band to compress the ureters during intravenous pyelography. Iodinated contrast media is held in the kidneys and upper ureters, improving the visualization of the renal collecting system. When compression is released, the contrast material drains from the kidneys into the lower ureters and bladder.

2 *Radiolucent foam rubber positioning aids.* Radiolucent foam rubber sponges (circles, squares, rectangles, and wedges of varying angles) help in the positioning of a patient. The angled wedges are used to duplicate comparison positions. The patient is also made comfortable, lessening the chance for motion unsharpness. (See Chapter 11.)

IMPORTANT: Foam rubber sponges can absorb impurities such as barium and iodine, producing opaque artifacts on the processed radiograph.

3 *Body immobilizers (restraining devices).* Pediatric and adult immobilizing devices are used to restrain uncooperative patients.

4 *Cassette holders.* Cassette holders or tunnels can be placed beneath a patient who cannot be moved to a radiographic table. These tunnels are also used in the operating room for hip pinnings, cholangiograms, and so on. Cassette holders, with or without grids, can be used for horizontal beam projection techniques. (See Figs. 5-18, 5-19.)

5 *Radiographic viewboxes.* An important radiographic accessory is the x-ray viewbox. Optical density can be influenced by the intensity of the light from the viewbox. The formula for radiographic density (see Chapter

13) assumes that the light source incident to the film is calibrated and constant. Often, an image viewed and accepted at the processor when viewed on another viewbox may seem either overexposed or underexposed owing to variations in viewbox light output. If the light output of both viewboxes were measured, a significant difference might exist. Viewboxes with different types of fluorescent lights will produce "different looks." A photographic light meter can be used to evaluate the amount of light being transmitted by individual viewboxes and to ensure that all viewbox light emissions are balanced. Periodic clean-ing of the glass on the viewboxes should be a part of the QA program.

6 *Emergency equipment.* A radiology depart-ment is not without its share of emergencies, some of which may be triggered by the pro-cedures or the use of iodinated contrast ma-terial. Radiographers should be familiar with cardiopulmonary resuscitation (CPR) tech-niques) and the location of emergency sup-plies, including oxygen and suction. Emer-gency code telephone numbers and departmental emergency guidelines should be posted in a prominent location.

4   The X-Ray Tube

THE x-ray tube is an important link in the x-ray equipment chain. It consists of a filament (cathode), a target (anode), a highly evacuated (vacuum) glass envelope, and an oil-filled, lead-lined tube housing (casing).

A high positive potential is applied to the anode of the x-ray tube. When a high negative potential is applied to the cathode, the electrons (−) are emitted from the cathode and are attracted to the anode (+) side of the tube. As the electrons strike the metal surface of the anode, they are stopped abruptly. This interaction produces both x-radiation (see Chapter 1) as well as considerable heat (a major, yet undesirable by-product). Less than 1% of the total energy produced is converted into x-radiation. Increasing the kilovoltage increases the speed at which the electrons are pulled across the tube and decreases the wavelength (penetrating ability) of the resultant x-ray beam. (See Chapter 11.)

_____

IMPORTANT: Careful consideration must be given to the production of heat. Tube rating charts and related terminology will be discussed in this chapter.

Basic Components of an X-Ray Tube

The filament, the source of "free" electrons in the x-ray tube, is a small coil (helix) of tungsten wire, mounted in a metal shield (focusing cup) (Figs. 4-1 and 4-2). Filaments used in radiographic tubes are relatively thin and, when heated to very high temperatures, can evaporate. This evaporation can be a gradual process; therefore, continuous high milliamperage settings, which can produce evaporation of the filament, should be avoided.

As the filament is heated within the vacuum of the glass tube, "free electrons" are produced. The higher the temperature of the filament, the greater the rate of the electron emission. The heat of the filament is controlled by the milliampere setting on the control panel. (See Fig. 2-7.) The electrons "boil-off" (thermionic emission) from the filament surface as an electron cloud and produce a "space charge" effect in the vicinity of the filament. This cloud of negative charges prevents other electrons from being emitted from the filament until a higher potential difference (kVp) is applied to the tube to overcome the force of the space charge.

The focusing cup, used as a support for the filament, also has a negative charge applied to it and is used to "focus" the negative electrons by the repulsion of like charges. The electrons, focused as a controlled stream from the filament, strike an area of the target known as the *actual focal spot*, producing x-radiation and heat. The size of the electron stream is related to filament size. The smaller the electron stream, the smaller the actual focal spot, therefore, the smaller the effective focal spot (Fig. 4-2, *top*).

The projected x-ray beam exits from the tube to the area being radiographed. A quality assurance (QA) tool known as a *slit camera* can be used to measure the size of the projected focal spot in a specific direction. This measurement is known as the *effective focal spot*.

Line Focus Effect

The area of the angled target surface bombarded by the electron stream, known as the *actual focal spot*, is larger in size than the effective focal spot. The larger actual focal spot helps to dissipate heat over a greater area of the target.

The "line focus effect," produced by the projection of the x-ray beam to the area being radiographed, results in an almost square effective focal spot, even though the electron stream strikes an area on the target (actual focal spot) that is rectangular in shape (Fig. 4-2).

Heel Effect

The intensity of the x-radiation across the long axis of the tube is not uniform. This variation in x-ray intensity is called the *heel effect* (Fig. 4-3A).

On the anode side of the tube, the radiation is less intense than on the cathode side owing to the absorption of the x-rays within the anode. The changes in beam intensity are significant only on the peripheral edges of the beam (extreme cathode and extreme anode). Since the intensity of the beam nearest the central ray is more uniform, the heel effect is less noticeable when an increased focal film distance or a smaller field size is used.

The thickest area of the part under study should be positioned beneath the cathode side of the x-ray tube to take advantage of the heel effect (Fig. 4-4).

Differences in sharpness across the field, cathode to anode, are also related to the heel effect. At the anode end of the tube, the focal spot is smaller than the effective focal spot measured at central ray. The difference in sharpness produced from the anode heel ef-

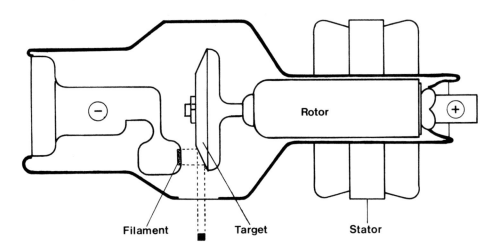

Filament   Target   Stator   Rotor   (−)   (+)

Figure 4-1   The Basic Components of an X-Ray Tube   *A basic component of a radiographic tube is the filament (source of electrons) at the cathode end of the tube. The cathode (a high negative potential) includes the focusing cup, which has a negative charge applied to it to "focus" the stream of electrons by the repulsion of like charges. The anode (high positive potential) serves as a target for the focused electron stream.*

By means of a stator (induction motor) rotor system, the anode is made to rotate at extremely high speed (usually 3000 rpm or 10,000 rpm).

A glass envelope (Pyrex) that houses the cathode and rotating anode is placed in an oil-filled lead-lined housing. (See Fig. 4-9.)

fect can be perceived on a radiograph (Fig. 4-3*B*). (See Chapter 11.)

Types of X-Ray Tubes

There are two basic types of x-ray tubes: stationary anode and rotating anode tubes.

The term *stationary anode* is self-descriptive. Probably the only experience that the reader will have with a stationary anode tube is when operating a dental unit or a low-powered mobile device. (See Chapter 3.)

A stationary anode is composed of a tungsten target embedded in a copper stem (Fig.

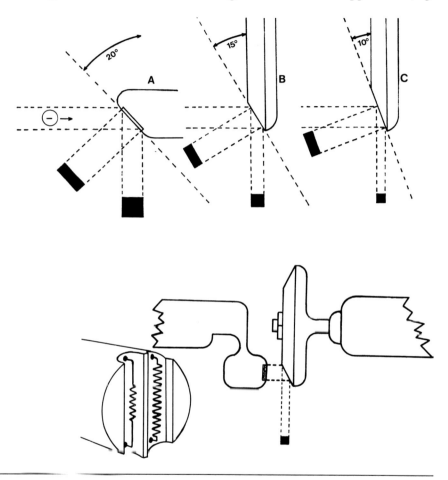

Figure 4-2 *Focal Spot Size*

The area of the angled (beveled) target surface bombarded by the electron stream is known as the actual focal spot *(top). It is larger in size than the effective focal spot. This is due to the "line focus effect." The actual focal spot is rectangular in shape, whereas the effective focal spot is projected in an almost square configuration.*

Whether the anode is stationary (A) or rotating (B, C), the line focus effect is the same.

Note the change in the effective focal spot size owing to different target angles; 20 degrees (A), 15 degrees (B), and 10 degrees (C). As the target

angle becomes steeper, the effective focal spot becomes smaller, even though the electron stream (used for A, B, and C) is the same size. The focal spots (actual and effective) would be further reduced in size if a smaller filament were used to produce the electron stream (bottom, left).

Cathode Assembly: A typical cathode has a small and a large filament. The smaller filament produces a smaller electron stream on the anode (actual focal spot) when a potential difference (kilovoltage) is applied to the x-ray tube. Most x-ray tubes use side-by-side filament mountings in dual focusing cups (bottom, left).

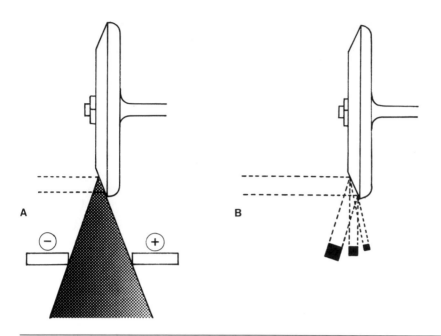

Figure 4-3 Heel Effect/Intensity of X-Ray Beam *The intensity of the x-radiation along the long axis of the tube (from cathode to anode) is not uniform. The radiation is less intense on the anode (+) side of the tube than on the cathode (−) side owing to the absorption of x-rays within the anode (A).*

Sharpness differences can occur from cathode to anode as a result of the heel effect. The focal spot measured at central ray is known as the effective focal spot. As the x-ray beam diverges along the long axis of the tube, the focal spot becomes larger toward the cathode end and smaller toward the anode end because of the line focus effect (B).

4-2*A, top*). These two metals are used for specific reasons: Tungsten has a high melting point (3700° C) and an atomic number of 74, which increases the efficiency of bremsstrahlung production in the medical x-ray range. (See Chapter 1.) Copper is selected because it is a good conductor of heat.

As in the stationary anode tube, the basic components of a rotating anode tube include cathode; anode; envelope; and oil-filled, lead lined tube housing (casing). Additional components of the rotating anode tube assembly include:

1 Induction motor used to rotate the anode

2 Rotor and bearings

As the anode rotates, unbombarded, cooler metal is made available (brought into the path of the electron stream) (Figs. 4-1, 4-5, and 4-6).

Cathode

Radiographic tubes have two filaments, usually mounted side by side to produce small and large focal spots. They are made of tungsten wires slightly greater than 0.008 in. in diameter (Fig. 4-2, *bottom*). Some manufacturers mount these filaments in focusing cups, one above the other rather than side by side.

Standby Illumination of the Filament

When the x-ray unit is "on," the filament is illuminated at a low level (standby illumination). When the anode is "boosted" to its proper number of revolutions per minute, the temperature of the filament is raised to the milliamperage selected for the study. If a delay occurs in the making of an exposure, prolonged rotation of the anode can produce excessive heat and may cause damage to the x-ray tube. When there is a delay in the making of an exposure, one should drop back to "standby illumination" by de-energizing the rotation of the anode. Prolonged rotation at high speed also produces strain on the bearings of the rotating anode.

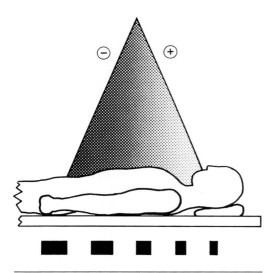

Figure 4-4 Heel Effect/Positioning Approach
Since the cathode (−) portion of the x-ray beam is more intense as opposed to the anode (+), thicker portions of the body should be positioned beneath the cathode end of the x-ray tube. There is some loss of sharpness toward the cathode side.

Rotating Anode

A tungsten disc, rotating about 3000 revolutions per minute (rpm) is a major component of the rotating anode tube. When a rotating anode is used, a focal track (circular area) is formed. The electron stream is delivered along the lateral margins of the actual focal spot as two separate sources, protecting the center of the actual focal spot (Fig. 4-5).

The intense heat moves away from the focal track and is dissipated by radiation and conduction by means of the large metal anode.

Most rotating anodes vary in diameter from 3 in. to 5 in. When using a radiographic tube with a 4-in. diameter target instead of a 3-in. diameter target, a 30% increase in the mA setting is possible. The larger the diameter or the greater the thickness of the anode, the greater the anode thermal capacity of a specific tube (Fig. 4-6).

When two anodes of the same diameter but different thickness are compared, the thicker anode will have a greater heat storage capability (anode heat storage capacity). Although the thicker anode has increased heat storage capacity, its load capability (instantaneous load) is not improved, because both anodes are of the same diameter (Fig. 4-6B).

Modern rotating anode x-ray tubes use an anode composed of either solid tungsten or

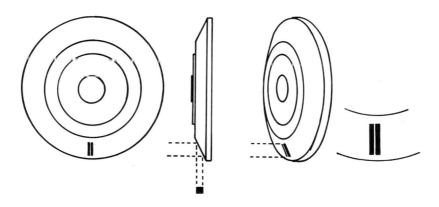

Figure 4-5 Electron Stream Bombardment of the Rotating Anode *The electrons emitted from the cathode bombard the beveled rotating anode (target) to produce x-rays and heat. As the anode rotates, the intense heat is moved away from the tube by conduction and heat radiation. The electron stream from the cathode strikes the actual focal spot as two separate energy sources to protect the center of the focal spot (right).*

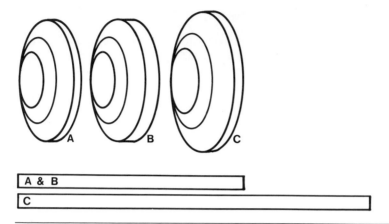

Figure 4-6 Rotating Anode Characteristics
The diameter and thickness of a rotating anode influence both the instantaneous and heat storage potential of an x-ray tube. The periphery of the target serves as its focal track. The greater the diameter of the target, the longer the focal track. The anodes represented by A and B are equal in diameter and therefore have focal tracks of equal length. The total mass of the anode determines its anode heat storage capacity; therefore, B, which is two times thicker than A, has greater heat storage capacity. Note: Since the diameter of the anode has not changed, both A and B have the same instantaneous load capacity. The larger diameter anode (C) has a longer focal track; therefore, instantaneous load capability is improved over A and B. It is possible that the total mass of C may be less than B, depending upon the anode design. If this is so, B will have a greater heat storage capacity but a lessened instantaneous load capability.

molybdenum coated with a rhenium tungsten alloy. Rhenium is used to improve the thermal stress resistance of the relatively brittle tungsten. The use of a rhenium tungsten alloy results in an anode that is more resistant to surface roughening (pitting). A thin molybdenum stem joins the anode to the rotor system, which drives the anode in a circular motion.

An induction motor is used to rotate the anode. The stator of the induction motor surrounds the tube on the external surface of the glass envelope. The rotor of the induction motor is held in place by bearings within the glass envelope (vacuum tube; Fig. 4-1). Special lubricants (a thin layer of soft metal, silver, or lead) are used with the ball bearings to facilitate high-speed rotation. The rotating anode dissipates the heat generated in the production of x-radiation over the surface area of the target (Fig. 4-6).

High-speed rotors, which permit anode rotation up to 10,000 rpm, result in a significant increase in instantaneous load ratings and permit the use of extremely short exposures. When a high-speed rotor is used, an electrical braking apparatus reduces the speed from 10,000 rpm to 3,000 rpm almost immediately after the completion of the exposure.

Focal Spot Size

The National Electrical Manufacturers Association (NEMA) lists several definitions with regard to acceptable tolerance of x-ray tube focal spot sizes (Publication XR-5-1984).

The actual focal spot is defined by NEMA as the section on which the anode of the x-ray tube intersects with the electron beam.

The projected focal spot is the projection of the actual focal spot along the central ray, perpendicular to the x-ray port plane and passing through the center of the focal spot. This is often referred to as the focal spot (see Fig. 4-2).

The effective focal spot (see Fig. 4-2) is the size of the projected focal spot in a specified direction, measured with the slit camera method. The smaller the effective focal spot, the greater the potential for radiographic sharpness. (See Chapter 11.)

Focal spots are described in terms of their nominal size, for example, a typical x-ray tube with a 1.0-mm focal spot is rated as a nominal projected focal spot measuring 1.0 mm × 1.0 mm. The projected or effective focal spot may differ from its nominal size from 30% to 50% depending on the focal spot size under consideration, according to tolerances published in NEMA Standard Publication XR-5-1974.

Most modern x-ray machines are equipped with a rotating anode tube having 0.6-mm (small) and 1.0-mm (large) focal spots (Table 4-1). Focal spots as small as 0.1 mm and as large as 2.0 mm are commercially available.

As focal spot size decreases, tube rating restrictions increase. The high temperatures (high milliampere values) required to heat the filament can cause an increase in the size of the focal spot (blooming). Low kilovoltage values can similarly affect focal spot size. Unfortunately, longer exposure times may be required because of the lower milliampere values necessitated by the use of a smaller focal spot. In some examinations, motion may become a problem. (See Chapter 11.) The selection of any technical factor is always a compromise.

"Blooming" of the focal spot is described in NEMA Standard Publication XR-5-1984 as the change in values (usually increased) in the focal spot dimensions when appropriate focal spot measurements are made. The specifications for making these measurements are outlined in this NEMA publication.

Some focal spots can increase (bloom) up to 100% in size. In theory, a 0.6-mm focal spot could approach the dimensions of a 1.2-mm focal spot. This can be discouraging to the radiographer if a small focal spot was selected with attention to radiographic detail, yet the image produced does not reflect the anticipated quality.

IMPORTANT: Every effort should be made to ensure the integrity of the focal spot. One should avoid a combination of technical factors (such as high mA/low kVp technique) that may contribute to focal spot blooming.

TABLE 4-1. Milliampere Settings/ Focal Spot Comparisons

mA	Older Tube	Modern Tube
100	Small 1.0 mm	Small 0.6 mm
200	Large 2.0 mm	Small 0.6 mm
300	Large 2.0 mm	Small 0.6 mm
500	Large 2.0 mm	Large 1.0 mm or 1.2 mm
1000	Not available	Large 1.0 mm or 1.2 mm

Up to 200 mA can be used with a modern fractional focal spot tube (0.3 mm or less at 10,000 rpm). See Table 8-1 for increased film blackening effect owing to rare-earth screen film combinations.

One must be especially concerned with blooming when performing direct roentgen enlargement techniques (see Chapter 7) using a 0.3-mm or smaller focal spot. Most of the tubes used with magnification techniques are limited to less than 200 mA. This may appear to be a low mA value, but enlargement techniques do not require the use of a grid or Bucky. (See Chapter 7.) Film blackening effect may be thought of as three to five times greater, depending upon the grid ratio needed for a conventional study of the same body part. For example, a fractional focal spot tube set at 100 mA in a magnification study would produce a "film blackening" effect similar to the 300 mA to 500 mA value required for a conventional (grid) study. (See Table 5-1.)

IMPORTANT: Angiographic technologists often use high milliampere values and short exposure times to minimize motion and increase the number of frames per second. (See Chapter 9.) The lowering of a milliampere value from its maximum and the use of moderate kilovoltage (approximately 70 kVp or higher) helps to preserve the integrity of the focal spot by minimizing the blooming effect.

The effective focal spot size also depends, in part, upon the angle of the anode. The smaller the angle of the anode, the smaller the effective focal spot. With the use of a smaller filament and a "steep angle" anode to produce a smaller actual focal spot, a correspondingly smaller effective focal spot is produced (Fig. 4-2).

"Steep Angle" Anode

The outer edge of the face of the anode is beveled toward the electron stream emanating from the filament. The angle of the anode is measured from a 90-degree angle (Figs. 4-2 and 4-5). The beveled outer edge of an anode can be manufactured with varying angles (from 10 to 17 degrees).

The use of a "steep angle" anode permits an increase in instantaneous loading when compared to a conventional tube angle. A benefit of the steep angle target is improved radiographic detail owing to the smaller effective focal spot produced. (See Chapter 11.) Early steep angle tubes (10-degree targets) were limited to field size coverage of 14 in. × 14 in. at a 40-in. focal film distance. Twelve-degree angle targets will cover a 14 in. × 17 in. field at a 40 in. FFD. An option is the use of a 10-degree angle target with a slight increase in FFD (approximately 45 in.) to cover a 14 in. × 17 in. field.

IMPORTANT: The smaller (steeper) the target angle, the smaller the field coverage, the smaller the effective focal spot, but the greater the instantaneous load capability.

When an x-ray tube is selected for undertable fluoroscopic use, the steepest target angle that will permit coverage of the input phosphor of the image intensifier (see Chapter 6) and the largest radiographic film that will be used in the spot film device should be considered.

IMPORTANT: The variation in intensity from cathode to anode (heel effect) is accentuated when using a steep angle target tube (Figs. 4-3A and 4-4).

The Effect of Tube Vibration on Focal Spot Size

Minor vibrations in the x-ray tube during an exposure can diminish the integrity of the focal spot. An improperly balanced tube or unstable tubestand or tubecrane can add to vibration, with a corresponding degradation of the focal spot. Often a last minute, frequently unnecessary, adjustment of the x-ray tube can produce an almost imperceptible vibration,

resulting in diminished sharpness in the image. (See Chapter 11.)

Housing

All x-ray tubes are enclosed in shock-proof containers (housings). The tube insert is grounded and surrounded by oil, insulating it from its metal shield. The x-ray housing, which acts as a mounting for the tube insert, is lined with lead for radiation shielding. Leakage radiation from the housing should not exceed 100 mR/ hour when measured 1 m from the source when the unit is operating at its maximal output.

A "window" in the housing permits radiation to exit from the tube.

Unfortunately, less than 1% of the energy used to produce x-rays is converted to x-radiation. More than 99% of the energy becomes heat, which is dissipated rapidly from the anode into the oil-filled housing. The heat is then dissipated from the housing into the surrounding room air. Some tubes use air circulators to facilitate housing cooling. Heavy-duty special purpose tubes may require heat exchangers for faster heat dissipation.

Tube life can be extended if a radiographic tube is operated at a lower than maximal heat capacity. The anode cools quickly; therefore, short time delays between x-ray exposures can be beneficial.

If the tube is equipped with a heat sensor, it will operate up to approximately 80% of its anode thermal capacity before the sensor will prevent the radiographer from making an additional exposure.

The oil used to cool the tube housing provides high voltage insulation.

Tube Rating Charts

Tube rating charts are guides supplied by tube manufacturers to indicate tube heating and cooling characteristics, expressed in heat units or load ratings.

IMPORTANT: When radiographers work together, studies are often quickly completed. Heat units accumulate rapidly in these situations, with a greater potential for tube damage. Portable or mobile units are often limited in their tube ratings. (See Chapter 3.)

Heat Units in Single-Phase and Three-Phase Equipment

In the United States, almost all electrical energy is supplied at 60 cycles (60 Hz)/second. The electron flow (current) is reversed (alternating current) 60 times/second. When three overlapping waves (separate currents) are used in a single circuit, three-phase current is generated. (See Fig. 2-1.)

A heat unit (HU) is defined as the energy produced in the form of heat by one kVp and one mA for one second, utilizing single-phase, full-wave rectified radiographic equipment. (See Chapter 2.) Multiphase radiographic equipment utilizes 6-pulse or 12-pulse current. (See Chapter 2.) To determine heat units when using three-phase equipment (6-pulse rectification), multiply the single-phase factors by 1.35; for three-phase 12-pulse rectification, multiply the single-phase factors by 1.41. To determine total heat units for a series of exposures, multiply the above factors by the number of exposures made in the series. (See Chapter 13.)

Three-phase generators produce higher intensity x-radiation than single-phase generators at the same kV and mA settings. For a similar film blackening effect, the three-phase 6-pulse generator needs approximately two thirds of the exposure of the single-phase equipment. The 12-pulse generator needs half the single-phase exposure for a similar film blackening effect. For example, a single-phase 80 kVp, 100 mA, 1-second exposure will generate 8,000 HU. With 6-pulse, three-phase current, one must multiply this factor by 1.35 to determine HU (10,800). In actuality, only 0.67 second would be used with a three-phase 6-pulse generator to produce the same film blackening effect as the previously described single-phase exposure. The heat units generated (6-pulse, three-pulse current) at 0.67 second would be 7,236. A similar film blackening effect would be achieved with a three-phase, 12-pulse system using a time value of 0.5 second, producing a total of 5,640 HU (Table 4-2).

IMPORTANT: There is less loading of heat upon the anode with three-phase generators than with single-phase generators if one wishes to produce a similar film blackening effect at the same kilovoltage.

There are three types of tube rating charts.
1. *Instantaneous load.* This chart indicates the maximal kVp and mA values that can be used for a given length of time for a single exposure (Fig. 4-7).
   Factors that determine the instantaneous load capacity (the heating effect of a single exposure) include:
   a. *Focal spot dimensions,* as determined by the size of the filament (small vs.

TABLE 4-2. Calculations of Heat Units With Compensation In Exposure Length For Three-Phase Equipment

Type	Heat	Compensating Factors (to approximate the film blackening effect of single-phase, full-wave exposure factors)
Single-phase, full-wave rectification (8000 HU)	80 kVp × 100 mA × 1 sec	
Three-phase, 6-pulse rectification	8000 HU × 1.35 (10,800 HU)	80 kVp × 100 mA × 0.67 sec × 1.35 (7,236 HU)
Three-phase, 12-pulse rectification	8000 HU × 1.41 (11,280 HU)	80 kVp × 100 mA × 0.5 sec × 1.41 (5,640 HU)

To achieve the same film blackening effect with three-phase equipment, approximately two thirds the time factor (or mAs) is needed for three-phase, 6-pulse equipment. For three-phase, 12-pulse equipment, the time factor (or mAs) can be reduced to approximately one half.

large) or the angle of the anode (steep vs. conventional; Fig. 4-2).

b. *Diameter of the anode.* A larger diameter anode improves instantaneous loading as well as heat storage capacity. As the diameter of the anode increases, more metal (increased mass) is available for heat storage. If a thicker anode (increased mass) is used (without an increase in diame-

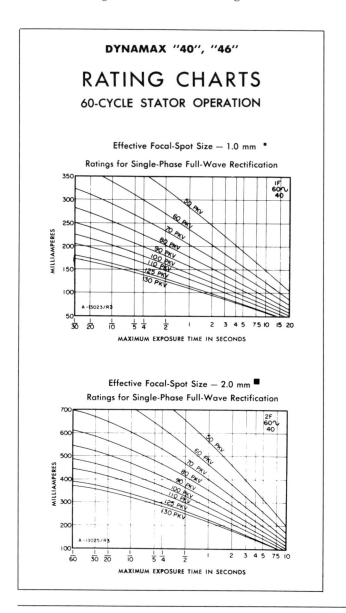

Figure 4-7 Tube Rating Charts
The small effective focal spot (1.0 mm; top) is compared with a large effective focal spot (2.0 mm; bottom). Tube ratings become more restrictive as high milliampere values are used with a given kilovoltage level. Specific tubes have their own rating charts. Do not substitute one manufacturer's chart for another, because they are not interchangeable. The tube rating chart used in this illustration is designed for a single-phase unit. (Courtesy of Machlett Laboratories, Stamford, Connecticut)

ter), the heat storage capacity increases, but instantaneous load ratings remain unchanged (Fig. 4-6).

IMPORTANT: As the diameter of the disc increases, the focal track increases in length, resulting in a dual benefit: instantaneous load improvement and increased heat storage capacity (Fig. 4-6).

    c. *Rotation speed of the anode.* If the speed of the anode can be increased from 3000 rpm to 10,000 rpm, instantaneous load capacity will be significantly increased. Exposure times can be shortened, and the use of a large focal spot can be avoided.

2. *Anode cooling chart.* This chart documents the anode thermal capacity of the tube and is used to determine the time required for the anode to cool either to zero heat units or to a level at which additional exposures are permissible (Fig. 4-8).

3. *Housing cooling chart.* This chart is used to indicate the heat unit capacity as well as cooling characteristics of the housing (Fig. 4-8).

IMPORTANT: Each specific tube or piece of equipment has its own rating charts. Do not substitute one manufacturer's chart for another; they are not interchangable.

Kilowatt Ratings of X-ray Tubes

A watt is a measure of a current of 1 ampere under an electrical pressure of 1 volt. A kilowatt is equal to 1000 watts.

Radiographic tubes have specific kilowatt ratings. As focal spot size increases, higher kilowatt ratings are obtained. Kilowatt ratings vary with different milliampere settings. See Chapter 13 for kilowatt formula.

Higher milliamperage values with short exposure times are often needed for angiographic studies to stop motion or to increase the number of frames per second recorded with a film or cassette changer. (See Chapter 9.) This is a technical compromise, since the use of a small focal spot (greater potential for improved radiographic detail) would require lower mA values and longer exposure times. The use of a rare-earth screen film combination should be considered to augment film blackening, particularly with a low kilowatt–rated x-ray tube (See Table 8-1).

Falling Load

The "falling load" generator can be used with or without an automatic exposure device (AED) to protect the tube from overloading (instantaneous load). High mA values are automatically applied to the x-ray tube; the mA is reduced (falls) during the exposure to avoid overheating of the anode. The shortest possible exposure time is achieved. This may not always be the ideal technical choice, since focal spots tend to bloom at higher mA settings. Minimal response time difficulties may occur with chest radiography or thin body parts when using an AED. (See Chapter 2.)

Grid-Controlled X-ray Tubes

Conventional x-ray exposures begin and end when the sinewave is at zero point. (See Fig. 2-1.) The shortest possible single-phase exposure is usually 1/120 second. In addition to the cathode and anode, the grid-controlled tube has another component called a "grid" (not to be confused with the grid used for scatter control). (See Chapter 2.) The grid-controlled focusing cup is electrically isolated from the filament. During the operation of the x-ray tube, a negative (bias) voltage is applied to the focusing cup (grid), making it negative with respect to the filament. As previously noted, the focusing cup is always negative to restrict the electrons to an appropriate electron stream to form the actual focal spot. In a grid bias tube, a negative electrostatic field is set up, which acts as a gate to stop the electron flow to the anode by repelling the negatively charged electrons. A large enough voltage will completely cut off the tube current; no electrons will flow from cathode to anode. When this high voltage (bias) is removed, the electrons flow to the anode to produce x-rays. Extremely short exposure times are possible with grid-controlled tubes.

With a grid-controlled x-ray tube, exposures do not have to begin or end at the zero point of the wave. Exposures can be synchronized to a particular portion of the sinewave. Often the middle third (the peak) of a single pulse (1/120th second) is used, resulting in a 1/360th-second exposure. Since only the por-

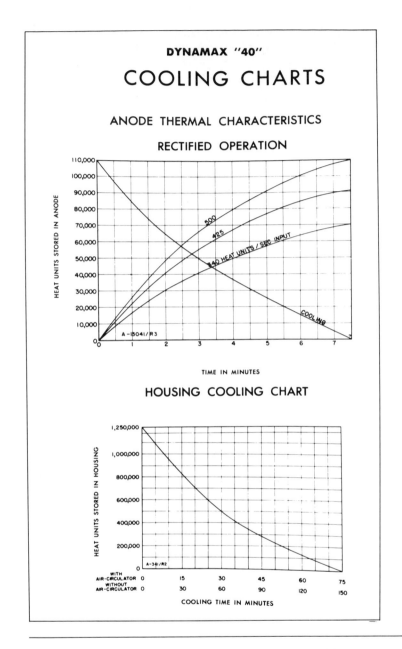

Figure 4-8 Cooling Charts
When serial radiographic studies such as tomography are performed, the anode thermal characteristic cooling chart should be consulted prior to the examination (top). Even though an individual exposure (instantaneous load) can be tolerated by a tube, the accumulation of heat units due to the serial exposures can damage the tube.

Housing cooling is rarely a problem with conventional radiographic procedures because of the high heat storage capacity of modern tube housings (bottom). (Courtesy of Machlett Laboratories, Stamford, Connecticut)

tion of the wave that produces high-energy photons is used, absorbed dosage from low-energy photons is reduced.

Grid-controlled tubes are used to advantage for cinefluorography and are synchronized to the cine camera shutters. Exposure to the patient occurs only when the camera shutter is open. (See Chapter 6.)

Radiographic Tube Damage

Radiographer error is responsible for most x-ray tube damage.

Tube damage can be attributed to the following:

1 *Evaporation of the filament.* When an x-ray unit is turned on, the filament is illuminated to a standby level of heating. As the anode is rotated to maximal revolutions per second, the filament is boosted to a predetermined heat level, and "free electrons" are released (boiled-off). Minute particles of tungsten can evaporate from the filament and be deposited on the glass envelope of the tube. Cracking of the glass envelope is possible owing to high voltage arcing between the cathode, by way of the glass envelope and the anode. When tungsten buildup occurs, the use of higher kilovoltage increases the possibility of arcing.

IMPORTANT: A prime cause of filament evaporation is the holding or delaying of the exposure after the filament has been heated to incandescence. Filament evap-

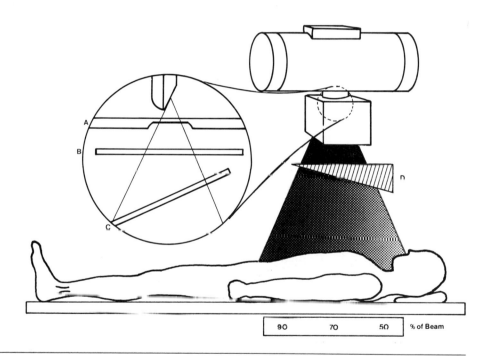

Figure 4-9   Filtration
Inherent filtration includes the glass window (A) of the x-ray tube as well as the insulation oil of the housing. Added filtration includes filters installed at the tube port (B) in compliance with federal, state, or local regulations. The mirror (C) in the collimator is considered part of the added filtration. The combination of inherent and added filtration is known as total filtration.

On occasion, a compensatory filter (D) can be added to the collimator to overcome variations in anatomical size or tissue density.

The filter shown (D) is wedge-shaped and absorbs more primary radiation at its thicker end. Note the variation in x-ray intensity from the thinner to the thicker end (90%–50%) accomplished by the filter used in this illustration.

A compensatory filter at port is recommended as opposed to underpart filters. (See Chapters 5 and 9.) The disadvantage of underpart filters is that the part being examined receives the full x-ray exposure.

oration is accentuated by high miliampere values. Occasionally, tungsten can also be vaporized from the surface of an over-heated anode.

2 *Anode damage.* Pitting of the anode can occur with high instantaneous exposure. Thermal stress (too much x-ray, too quickly) can cause the anode to warp, crack, or excessively erode.

A heat load on a cold target may also cause the target to crack, although the same heat load or multiple exposures on a properly warmed-up x-ray tube should not cause anode damage. Multiple exposures on a cold anode may produce cracks in the anode.

IMPORTANT: Manufacturers' warm-up procedures for heating the x-ray target to ductile temperatures without overstressing the anode must be rigidly followed.

3 *Damage to the bearings of the x-ray tube.* Conventional anodes rotate at approximately 3,000 rpm as opposed to high-speed anodes (10,000 rpm). This increased speed helps to

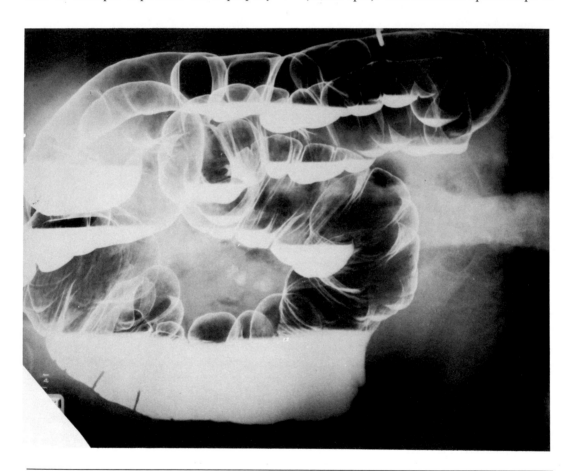

Figure 4-10   Lead Acrylic Wedge Filter for Lateral Decubitus Radiography *Often, severe differences in radiographic density occur when a patient is placed in the lateral decubitus position. There is a tendency for the dependent portion of the anatomy to be thicker than the remaining tissue. With double-contrast studies of the colon, an* additional problem may occur. Barium may puddle in the dependent segments of the colon while air may be trapped in upper portions. A more overall uniform radiographic density is obtained with a compensatory filter. (Courtesy of Victoreen Nuclear Associates, Carle Place, New York)

dissipate heat from the anode. Unfortunately, x-ray tube bearings deteriorate more rapidly at high speeds. Overheating of the x-ray tube can affect the rotor and rotor bearings. When the anode thermal capacity is exceeded, considerable heat is conducted to the rotor and rotor-bearing structure. This can shorten the life of an x-ray tube.

_____

IMPORTANT: Do not stand in a control booth rotating the anode at maximal speed while attempting to communicate with a difficult patient.

Two of the most common problems relating to heat production and therefore potential

tube damage occur simultaneously. The filament of the tube is heated to maximal incandescence while the anode of the tube is rotating at maximal speed. Some simple rules to extend tube life include:

1 Follow the manufacturers recommended warm-up procedures and consult tube rating and cooling charts. Whenever possible, allow cooling time between exposures or a series of exposures.

2 Do not operate the filament at maximal incandescence for any longer than needed. Energize the high-speed rotor immediately prior to an exposure. Drop back to standby illumination if an exposure is delayed.

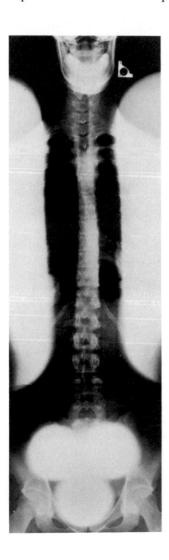

Figure 4-11 Scoliosis Evaluation of the Full Vertebral Column *It is impossible to uniformly expose the full vertebral column with a single exposure when evaluating the spine. The cervical spine is relatively thin as opposed to the remaining vertebral column. The thoracic area is easy to overexpose because of the radiolucent nature of the lungs; the lumbar vertebrae require increased exposure.*

By using a compensatory filter that (1) holds back a considerable portion of the x-ray to the cervical area, (2) holds back half or more of the exposure to the thoracic area, and (3) permits the full exposure to reach the lumbar area, proper radiographic density can be achieved throughout the entire spinal column. The compensatory filter selectively attenuates the x-ray beam, reducing patient dosage. Note the presence of a gonadal shield (See Fig. 5-7.) as well as the shielding of the breast of this young female patient.

The use of high-speed rare earth screen film technology combined with breast and gonadal shielding and compensatory filtration significantly reduces dosage to the patient. When breast shields are not available for AP imaging, the patient can be radiographed in the PA position, avoiding unattenuated primary radiation to the breasts. Since the vertebral column is further away from the cassette (increased OFD), image sharpness will be lessened. This is not a problem because the examination is being done primarily for vertebral alignment. If vertebral enlargement is a problem, an increased FFD can be used to overcome the effect of the increased OFD. (Courtesy of Victoreen Nuclear Associates, Carle Place, New York)

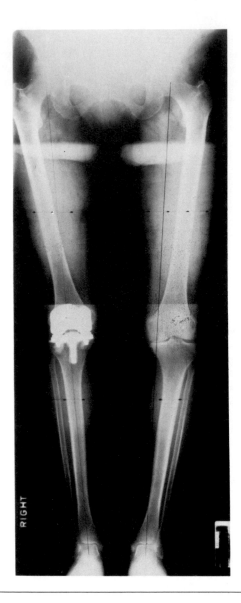

Figure 4-12 Full-Length Radiography of the Legs *Selective attenuation of the x-ray beam with compensatory filters achieves of uniform density from the hip to the ankle with a single exposure. This radiograph was made with the patient in the weight-bearing position. (Courtesy of Victoreen Nuclear Associates, Carle Place, New York)*

3 Use lower milliampere–second values whenever possible.

4 Do not abruptly change the direction of the x-ray tube while the high-speed rotor is energized. The anode can snap from its stem.

5 Do not adjust the x-ray tube either by bumping or striking it with your hand; do not bump the tube against the tabletop or wall.

6 Whenever possible, use high-speed, rare-earth screen film technology. (See Table 8-1.)

Diagnostic X-Ray Filters

Any obstacle through which x-rays pass on their way from the focal spot to the object under study is called a *filter*. Filtration removes low-energy quanta (photons) from the x-ray beam (Fig. 4-9).

Three types of filtration are of interest. They are inherent filtration, added filtration, and total filtration.

Inherent filtration includes the glass envelope of the tube (window) and the insulation (oil) of the housing.

Additional (added) filtration increases the hardness of the x-ray beam, improving beam quality by removing the portion of the x-ray beam that consists of soft x-rays (long wavelengths). (See Chapter 1.) These soft x-rays do not contribute to the information on the radiograph, because they are not of sufficient strength to penetrate the part and are mostly absorbed by the patient. Unless these soft x-rays are absorbed by added filtration, they contribute to patient dosage. Added filtration should be inserted as close to the tube as possible in order to blur out any impurities. that the filter may contain (Fig. 4-9).

The most common material used for added filtration in diagnostic radiology is aluminum. Federal, state, and local regulations determine the amount of filtration necessary for specific equipment. Total filtration is the combination of inherent and added filtration. When using a light beam collimator, the mirror must be considered as part of the total filtration (Fig. 4-9). (See Fig. 5-7.) Tungsten evaporation from either the filament or the anode, deposited on the window of the tube, can add to the total filtration.

Half-Value Layer

Filtration can also be described in terms of half-value layer (HVL). This refers to the thickness of aluminum that would be needed to reduce the intensity of the original x-ray beam to one half.

Any filtration material may be specified as aluminum equivalent (equal to the thickness of aluminum that would produce the same filtering effect).

IMPORTANT: A filter should be installed in a permanent or semi-permanent way so that it cannot be inadvertently removed.

Variable Thickness or Compensating Filters

Compensating filters are used to overcome variations in patient anatomy, providing a more uniform density across the radiographic image. Image quality is improved as a result of overall uniform film density (Fig. 4-9).

Some compensatory filtration materials in use include barium-impregnated clay, opaque plastic, aluminum, copper, and lead acrylic.

Over- or underpenetration of segments of the radiograph is reduced. Severe variations in patient thickness can be imaged with a single exposure (Figs. 4-10, 4-11, and 4-12).

Full-length vascular studies of the abdomen and lower extremities benefit from compensatory filtration. (See Chapter 9.)

Underpart filters (compensatory) such as sandbags or bags filled with cornmeal, flour, or rice are used in angiography or tomography to balance densities by restricting undercutting of the image. (See Fig. 5-5.) The disadvantage of underpart filters is that the part being examined receives the full x-ray exposure. The use of a compensatory filter at tube port is recommended as opposed to underpart filters.

5 The Production and Control of Scatter Radiation

SCATTER radiation is a supplemental density that produces a foglike image on a processed radiograph. All foglike densities that appear on a radiograph should not be attributed to scatter radiation. Some of these densities may be caused by careless handling or improper storage of x-ray film, use of incorrect safelights, as well as other film processing difficulties. (See Chapter 10.)

A descriptive word for scatter is "spatial." More oblique in nature than primary radiation, scatter diffuses in all directions (spatial) and often travels through longer paths in the body than does primary radiation (Fig. 5-1).

Production of Scatter Radiation

Interaction of X-rays With Matter

The production of a radiographic image is influenced by the interactions of x-ray photons with matter. The x-rays may be absorbed totally or partially (photoelectric effect) or may interact with the subject and create characteristic or secondary radiation (Compton effect). (See Figs. 1-7 and 1-8.) As patient thickness and tissue density (mass) increase, x-rays in-

teract with more tissue, and an increase in scatter radiation occurs.

In addition to patient thickness and tissue density, the size of the area being radiographed has a considerable effect on the production of scatter radiation. The greater the area being exposed to radiation, the greater the amount of scatter radiation produced (Fig. 5-2). In a full field (14 in. × 17 in.) radiographic study of the pelvis, 50% or greater of the total number of x-ray photons exiting from the patient consists of scattered radiation.

The x-ray photons passing through the subject exposing the image detector and the Compton interactions that produce scatter radiation form the remnant beam, which produces the radiographic image. When x-ray energy (kilovoltage) is increased, the percentage of Compton interaction (scatter) increases and the percentage of photoelectric interactions (absorption) rapidly decreases. (See Chapter 1.) Minor increases in kilovoltage provide an increased amount of x-ray photons to the image detector, with a corresponding reduction of absorbed photons. As kilovoltage is increased, however, scatter radiation is also intensified, resulting in a corresponding decrease in radiographic contrast. (See Chapter 11.)

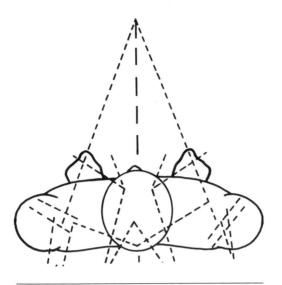

Figure 5-1 Schematic Representation of Scatter Radiation *Scatter radiation, caused by the interaction of x-rays with matter, is more oblique in nature, can travel through longer paths in the body than primary radiation, and is given off from the object under study in all directions (spatial).*

Other Forms of Scatter

Another supplemental density, "backscatter," arises from the back of the cassette, tabletop, or wall.

Since the primary beam does not correspond to the contour of the part under study, scatter from the tabletop may cause "undercutting" of the image, greatly reducing image quality. This is a particular problem in cerebral angiography or skull radiography as well as in full-field intravenous urography (Figs. 5-3 and 5-4).

Control of Scatter Radiation

The best way to control scatter radiation is to reduce its production. One way to accomplish this is to limit the area being exposed to the primary beam.

The effects of controlling scatter are two-fold: (1) reduction of dosage to patient and operators, and (2) improvement of image quality. As patient thickness increases, scatter radiation also increases. (See Chapter 11.) When examining the abdomen in the prone

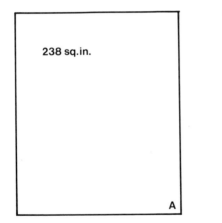

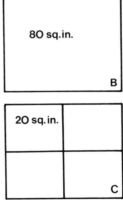

Figure 5-2 The Effect of Collimation on Scatter Radiation *Patient thickness (density) affects the amount of scatter radiation generated in a given examination. The size of the area being radiographed also has an effect on the production of scatter. The greater the area exposed to radiation, the more scatter radiation produced.*

A 14 in. × 17 in. film (A) images approximately three times more patient area than an 8 in. × 10 in. film (B). A typical fluoroscopic spot film (four on one) using 1/4 of one 8 in. × 10 in. film, 4 in. × 5 in., (C) images 1/12th the field size of the full frame study (A).

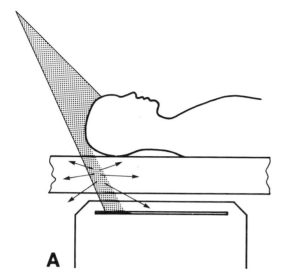

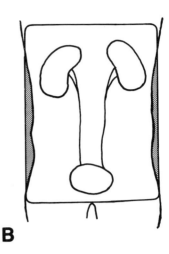

Figure 5-3   *Primary Beam Leak*
When an unattenuated primary beam strikes the tabletop, scatter radiation is produced. Scatter is given off in all directions; therefore, an undercutting of the radiographic image occurs (A).

A similar effect occurs with intravenous urography (B) or other abdominal studies where the body configuration does not match the shutter pattern.

position, patient thickness decreases; therefore, less scatter is generated. Compression devices can be used with similar results in the supine position.

Scattered rays (Compton effect) produced by the object under study or from backscatter are of no value in the making of a radiographic image. Unfortunately, these rays contribute to the overall density of the image while diminishing contrast. (See Chapter 11.) Lead rubber-masking, sandbags, cornmeal, water, rice, or flour bags placed on the tabletop rather than on the cassette or serial film changer help eliminate the undercutting effect generated by a primary beam leak (Fig. 5-5).

Backscatter, arising from the back of the cassette, the tabletop, or adjoining wall (when a wall-mounted upright cassette holder or Bucky is used) is lessened by the use of lead foil backing in the cassette. (See Fig. 8-13.)

The kilovoltage values selected for a specific examination should be considered in terms of the part under study. Kilovoltage must be adequate to produce x-rays capable of penetrating the part. X-rays of insufficient penetrating ability result in absorption of the rays by the patient. (See Chapter 11.) Almost all contrast media studies require low or moderate kilovoltage values. (See Chapter 12.) Exceptions are barium studies or examinations that require a direct placement of an iodinated contrast medium into the organ under study.

__IMPORTANT:__ Lowering the kilovoltage to lessen scatter while raising the mAs is not an acceptable substitute for beam restriction and a proper ratio grid.

Beam Limiting Devices

Over the years, a variety of beam restricting devices (Fig. 5-6) have been developed, including:

1 Primary source aperture diaphragms

2 Conventional cones

3 Telescopic cones

4 External lead apertures, including keyhole diaphragms

5 Light beam collimators, including positive beam limiting (PBLs) devices

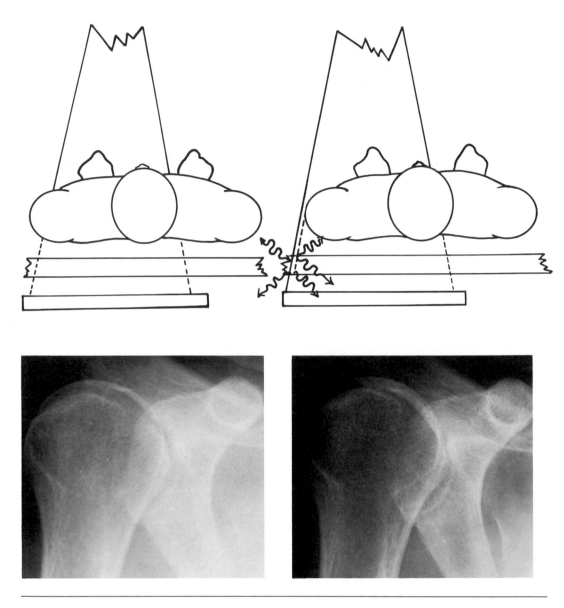

Figure 5-4 The Effect of a Primary Beam Leak *The primary beam should be restricted to the part under study* (top, left). *Scatter from the tabletop owing to a primary beam leak will undercut the radiographic image* (top, right). *Representative radiographs are shown. Note the density of the image with the primary beam confined to the shoulder* (bottom, left). *Compare the increase in density caused by the primary beam leak* (bottom, right).

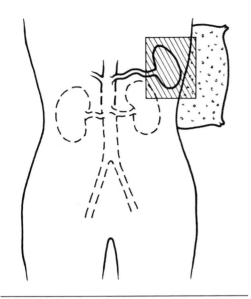

Figure 5-5 Control of Image Undercutting *The use of a filter material on the tabletop rather than on the cassette or film changer will minimize undercutting of the radiographic image by attenuating a portion of the primary beam.*

Sand, cornmeal, water, rice, or flour bags or lead rubber masking can be placed on the tabletop to filter the primary ray and minimize the undercutting effect.

These beam limiting accessories restrict the area under study to a predetermined field size. Restriction of the primary ray as close to source as possible is also important. A single diaphragm at source can be more effective than an extension cone or cylinder with a diaphragm some distance from source (Fig. 5-6A).

Collimators

Radiographic collimators simultaneously adjust several pairs of lead shutters (synchronously with a beam defining light) to restrict the primary beam. A high intensity light source, coupled with a reflection mirror, projects a light field, which matches the x-ray field size, onto the part under study. The mirror is part of the inherent filtration of the x-ray tube. (See Fig. 4-9.) The alignment of the light field to the x-ray field (Fig. 5-7)

should be checked regularly by quality assurance (QA) personnel.

With a PBL device, shutter patterns are automatically determined by the size of the cassette being used. Changes in the focal film distance automatically adjust the beam configuration to the cassette size.

Extension Cones and Diaphragms

When extension cones or diaphragms are used in the external tracks of a collimator, attention must be given to the position of the internal collimator shutters. It is easy to add an accessory such as a cone, diaphragm, or keyhole diaphragm and produce an acceptable light beam pattern on the part under study, even if the internal shutters of the collimator are open to maximum. In this situation, the light beam and not the x-ray beam is being restricted in size (Fig. 5-6). Scatter control is not maximized.

The Air Gap

Since the patient is the major source of scatter radiation and since scatter is disseminated in all directions, it would be ideal if the film could be moved some distance from the patient to take advantage of the spatial effect of scatter radiation. When the patient is moved away from the cassette, less scatter radiation will reach the film. This approach is known as the *air-gap technique*. Since the scatter emanating from the patient is at acute angles to the primary beam, much of the scatter misses the detector because of the increased OFD (Fig. 5-8). (See Chapter 7.) Some of the scatter reaching the film is reduced in intensity because of the Inverse Square Law principle. (See Chapters 11 and 13.) Air gap techniques are often used as a substitute for a grid or Bucky for the lateral cervical spine, chest (see Chapter 15), and direct roentgen enlargement studies. (See Fig. 7-14.)

Off-Focus Radiation

Ill-defined radiographic details extending beyond the preselected collimated field are often produced by off-focus (extra-focal) radiation. This supplemental image can be controlled by lead shutters or a lead iris in the collimator as close to source as possible. Since off-focus

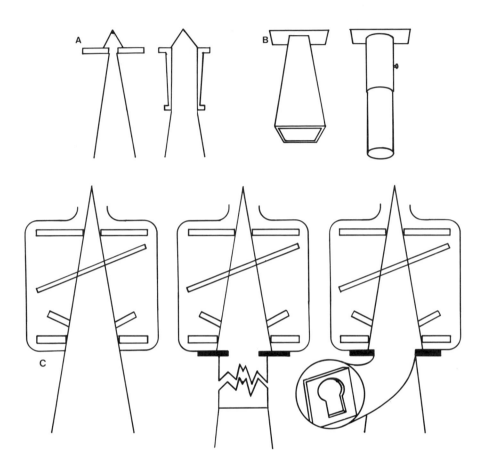

Figure 5-6 Primary Ray Restricting Devices
A primary source aperture diaphragm restricts the x-ray beam as close to source as possible. An aperture diaphragm of this type can be more effective than a conventional cone or extension cone that does not restrict the primary beam at source (A).

Conventional radiographic cones can be either square, rectangular, or circular in shape. A specific cone is usually used to match a specific cassette size (B). The rectangular cone is preferred to the round cone because it more closely matches cassette configuration; therefore, only the patient area being examined is exposed to radiation. An extension cone can be used for tight primary ray restriction.

A light beam collimator uses multiple sets of lead diaphragms mounted at several levels within its housing (C). A mirror coupled with a light source *is used to outline the shutter pattern on the part being examined. The mirror is considered added filtration. (See Fig. 4-9.) An extension cone (C, center) or a keyhole aperture diaphragm (C, right) can be added to the collimator. Note the position of the internal shutters in relation to the primary x-ray beam. Both of these devices are installed incorrectly in this illustration. The primary diaphragm of the extension cone or the keyhole aperture is smaller in size than the exit beam formed by the internal collimator shutters. The internal shutters should be reduced in size to conform to the openings in the external aperture. If a keyhole is used and the internal shutters are left completely opened, an acceptable light pattern will appear on the object to be examined. Although the light beam has been restricted, the x-ray beam has not been collimated. The effect of collimation has been minimized.*

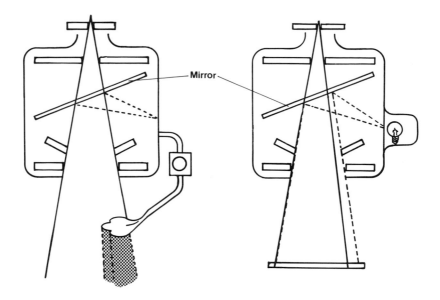

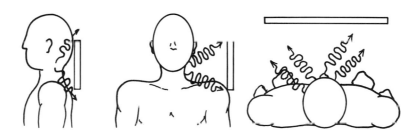

Figure 5-7 Gonadal Shielding Collimator Attachment: Primary Beam/Light Beam Alignment *A gonadal shield can be externally attached to a radiographic collimator (left). The shield shown is positioned within the light beam. The shaded area represents a reduction in primary radiation; therefore, when the shield is properly positioned, a lower gonadal dosage occurs.*

A light source is shown in position on the outside of the collimator (right). Image "cutoff" can occur if one of the internal shutters of the collimator is out of alignment (right). The first set of shutters within the collimator are shown out of alignment. The x-ray beam, therefore, is smaller than the projected light beam (represented as a dotted pattern). When this occurs, particularly with tight field collimation, the radiograph could exhibit collimator shutter cutoff because of the misalignment of the internal shutters to the light beam.

Figure 5-8 The Use of an "Air Gap" to Reduce Scatter Radiation *When the major source of scatter radiation (patient) is separated from the cassette (increased OFD), the effect of scatter radiation on the image is minimized. This technique is used without a grid or Bucky. In the AP position of the cervical spine (left), a grid is required since the cassette is in close contact with the part being examined. When the lateral projection is made, an air gap is formed owing to the placement of the cassette approximately 8 in. to 10 in. from the cervical spine (center).*

Much of the scatter from the patient is given off at acute angles to the primary beam and misses the detector. Some of the scatter is reduced in intensity owing to the Inverse Square Law. (See Chapter 13.) Because of the increased OFD, an extended FFD (72 in.) is required to overcome magnification of the part.

Another use for the air gap technique (right) is for chest radiography. The patient is positioned 10 in. to 12 in. (OFD) from the cassette with the tube positioned 10 ft. to 12 ft. (FFD) from the cassette to overcome cardiac enlargement.

radiation exists at a variety of angles from the x-ray tube, it is important that primary beam collimation begin as close to the source of x-radiation as possible (Figs. 5-9 and 5-10).

Grids

The grid and the Bucky (Potter-Bucky diaphragm) are radiographic accessories designed to minimize the effect of scatter radiation. The use of a grid (stationary or moving) is recommended for the clean-up of scatter radiation generated by large or dense body parts. A general rule to follow is that a grid or Bucky be used for any part that is 10 cm or more in thickness. The major exception to this rule is the adult chest. (See Chapter 14.)

Grids—Stationary or Moving

Gustav Bucky, M.D., developed a cross-hatch stationary grid in 1913 to assist in the clean-up of scatter radiation. In 1920, Hollis Potter,

M.D., redesigned Dr. Bucky's grid so that all the grid lines were aligned in the same direction (linear). Potter was then able to move the grid back and forth during the x-ray exposure.

MOVING GRID (POTTER-BUCKY DIAPHRAGM)

A grid is moved during an x-ray exposure to blur out grid lines as well as impurities in grid design. A grid can be made to move continuously during the x-ray exposure. Moving grids can be designed to move in one direction (single-stroke), or they can be driven back and forth, 1 cm to 3 cm (reciprocating). Some grids move forward faster and slower on return (catapult) or can move in a slow almost imperceptible circular motion (oscillating). Regardless of the type of movement used, the intent is to blur out lead strips while moving the grid in synchrony with the pulses of the x-ray generator. As the grid moves back and forth, a form of "lateral decentering" occurs with a loss of as much as 20% of the primary beam.

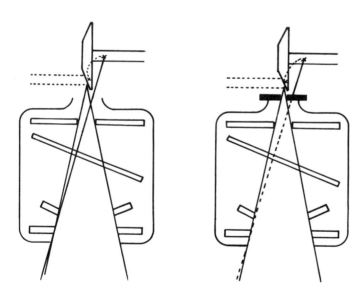

Figure 5-9 Off-Focus Radiation
An additional source of radiation is generated when electrons rebound from the target and strike metallic areas other than the actual focal spot.

Most off-focus (extra focal) radiation arises from areas of the anode other than the actual focal spot. For the purposes of this illustration,

off-focus radiation is shown emanating from the stem of the anode.

Note radiation emanating as a solid line from the stem of the anode (left). The placement of a lead diaphragm (or lead iris) as close to source as possible (right) restricts a considerable portion of the off-focus radiation.

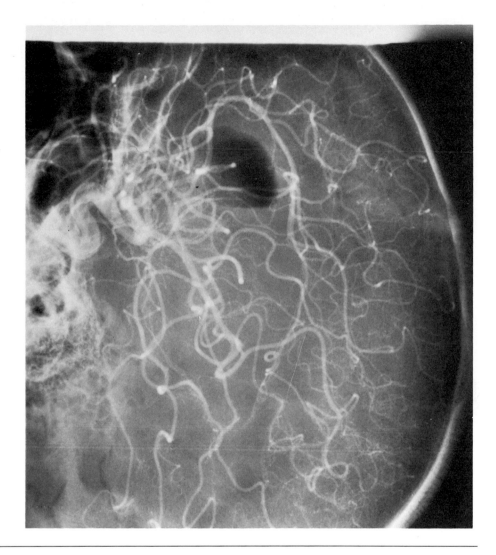

Figure 5-10   Off-Focus Radiation
Supine lateral cerebral arteriogram. Radiographic details (poorly defined soft tissue structures) are seen as a result of off-focus (extra-focal) radiation outside the restricted shutter pattern of the collimator. Note air in the ventricles (brow up position) owing to a recent pneumoencephalogram.

Although the term *Bucky* is used to represent the Potter-Bucky diaphragm moving grid, in actuality, the stationary (cross-hatch grid) was invented by Bucky, and the moving linear grid was designed by Potter.

Basic Grid Design

Grid design has not changed dramatically since its modification from cross-hatch to linear by Potter. Most grids are manufactured with lead lines aligned in the same direction (linear) and separated by organic or inorganic interspacing materials. The lead strips are relatively thin (0.05 mm); whereas the radiolucent interspaces are relatively thick (0.33 mm). Recent improvements in grid design (up to 200 lines/inch) alter this relationship. The radiolucent materials that separate the lead lines permit the passage of the x-ray beam (Fig. 5-11).

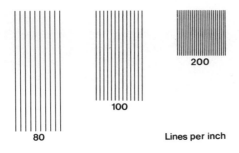

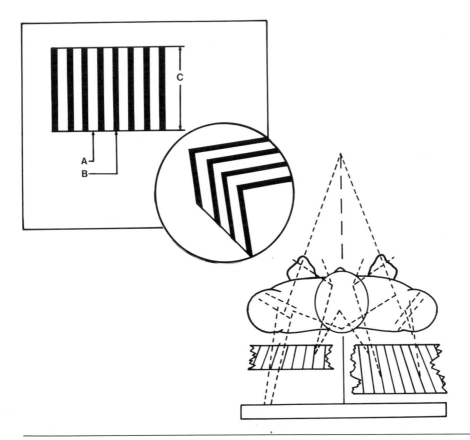

Figure 5-11   Basic Grid Design

Linear grids are designed with their lead lines aligned in the same direction but separated by a radiolucent interspacing material to permit the passage of the primary beam. The interspaces permit the passage of the primary beam; the lead lines absorb most of the scatter radiation.

The interspacing material (center, A) separates the lead lines (B). Grid ratio is determined by the height of the lead lines (C) compared with the distance between each lead strip (A). A low ratio grid (bottom, left) does not absorb as much scat-

ter radiation as does a higher ratio grid (bottom, right).

Most grids are manufactured with 100 or more lead lines per inch. When grids are made with an increased number of lines per inch (up to 200 lines), the lead strips must be made narrower. If the grid ratio is to be maintained, the grid lines must be decreased in height. This results in a thinner grid. These extra-fine grid lines are virtually invisible on the processed radiograph, eliminating the need to move the grid to obliterate the grid pattern.

The interspacing material may be organic (paper, cardboard, plastic, fiber) or inorganic (aluminum). Inorganic material absorbs more x-radiation at lower kilovoltage than do organic materials. The benefit of aluminum interspacing compared with organic material is that aluminum does not absorb moisture (nonhygroscopic) and will not warp.

GRID RATIO

Grid ratio is defined as the height of the lead lines compared to the distance between each lead strip. As grid ratio increases, the height of the lead lines increases, but the distance between the lead strips remains the same (Fig. 5-11). The higher the ratio of the grid, the more restrictive its focal range (Table 5-1).

A table such as Table 5-1 is designed to aid in the conversion of a non-grid technique to a grid or Bucky study. In actual practice, a radiographer would rarely have an occasion to make this type of conversion. This table can serve as a guide when converting from one grid ratio to another. (See Chapter 13.)

IMPORTANT: The cross-hatch grid must be used in the stationary mode, since the grid lines running in the direction of the grid motion will not blur out.

If a non-grid chest examination (80 kVp at 5 mAs) were to be converted to a grid technique (12:1 ratio) using Table 5-1, an increase in the original mAs value 5× would result in 25 mAs to overcome the absorption of the grid.

The change in contrast produced by the high ratio grid would result in short-scale contrast (abrupt black and white). When examining the chest, the lung fields would appear very dark, whereas the mediastinum would be chalk-like in appearance.

A more contemporary approach would be to raise the 80 kVp value to 120 kVp or greater, with a corresponding adjustment in mAs. Several benefits occur. The osseous structures of the thorax would be made less visible (less likely to obscure underlying pulmonary structures) by the use of the higher energy value. Contrast between the bones, soft tissues, and aerated lungs would be lessened. Retrocardiac structures would be better visualized. (See Chapters 11, 12, and 14.) Tube angle techniques are not possible with cross-hatch grids.

LINES PER INCH

Most grids are manufactured with 100 or more lead lines per inch, although many older grids made with 60 or 80 lines/inch are still in use. When grids are made with an increased number of lines per inch (up to 200 lines), the lead strips are made narrower. If a grid ratio is to be maintained, there must be a decrease in the height of the lead lines. With these fine-line grids, the grid lines are virtually invisible, even when the grid is used in the stationary mode. No movement is required to obliterate the fine lead-line pattern (Fig. 5-11).

IMPORTANT: The ratio of the grid as well as the amount of lead in the grid are good indicators of the contrast improvement capability of the grid (its ability to remove scatter radiation).

Types of Grids

Grids may be either linear or cross-hatch in design (Fig. 5-12).

TABLE 5-1. Technical Compensation For Grid Conversions

Type	Ratio	Focal Range (in.)	Maximum kVp	+ mAs	+ kVp
Non-grid				1×	
Linear	5:1	28–72	85	2×	+8
Linear	6:1	28–72	85	3×	+8
Linear	8:1	34–44	95	3×–4×	+15
Linear	12:1	36–40	110	5×	+20–+25
Linear	16:1	40	125	6×	+20–+25
Cross-hatch	12:1	28–72	110>	5×	+20–+25
Cross-hatch	16:1	34–44	125>	6×	+20–+25

LINEAR GRIDS

Most grids are designed with their lead lines arranged in linear fashion (aligned in the same direction). Linear grids can be either parallel or focused.

PARALLEL GRIDS

The lead strips of a parallel grid are positioned vertically across the entire width of a linear grid. Parallel grids (usually low ratio) are useful when positioning is difficult owing to limitations imposed by focal film distances (see Chapter 11) and large field sizes. Geometric cutoff can result on both sides of the image when using a parallel grid, particularly at shortened focal film distances. The parallel grid is acceptable with smaller size cassettes, since the central portion of the x-ray beam is virtually parallel to the parallel grid lines. With larger field sizes, the divergent beam will bilaterally intercept the parallel grid lines, and significant bilateral grid cutoff will occur (Fig. 5-12).

FOCUSED GRIDS

The lead strips of a linear focused grid are aligned with all the strips tilted toward an imaginary predetermined centering point in space. Grid focus or radius is determined when an imaginary line is drawn from the outer aspects of the width of the grid and intersects at this imaginary point. The manufacturing process of inclining the grid lines uniformly and bilaterally is known as *canting*.

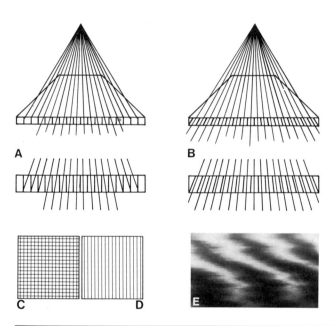

Figure 5-12 Types of Grids

Linear grids can be designed with their lead lines aligned in either parallel fashion (A) or focused (B). The lead strips of a parallel grid (A) are positioned vertically across the width of the entire grid. Geometric cutoff can result on both sides of the image with a parallel grid.

The lead lines of the focused grid (B) are tilted uniformly and bilaterally to a predetermined focus film distance. This process of manufacturing a grid and inclining its lead lines to a prefixed focus film distance is known as canting.

A linear grid is seen from above in D. When two linear grids are crossed at right angles (crosshatch) to one another (C), maximal scatter cleanup occurs. Note: Tube angle techniques are possible only if the tube is angled so that central ray is projected in the direction of the linear lead pattern. When grids are cross-hatched, tube angle techniques are not possible because grid lines run in two directions.

If two grids are inadvertently positioned with their lead lines running in the same direction, a "moiré" artifact is produced (E).

IMPORTANT: A focused grid, if positioned correctly, is preferable to a parallel grid over a wider range of focal film distances and for full field radiography if one wishes to minimize bilateral grid cutoff (Fig. 5-12).

CROSS-HATCH GRIDS

Two linear grids (parallel or focused) superimposed at right angles to each other for maximal scatter clean-up are called *cross-hatch grids*. A high grid ratio effect can be achieved if two low-ratio grids are used in a cross-hatch configuration (Fig. 5-12). A cross-hatch grid exhibits a slightly greater improvement in contrast than a comparable ratio linear grid. The combination of two linear grids (cross-hatch) is more efficient in scatter cleanup than a linear grid of a similar ratio.

IMPORTANT: Remember that the higher the ratio of the grid, the more restrictive its focal range. The highest ratio grid used in a cross-hatch combination determines the focal range of the cross-hatch grid (Table 5-1). A cross-hatch grid must be carefully aligned to central ray (Fig. 5-13). Tube angle techniques are prohibited.

Related Grid Terminology

Lead content. The amount of lead in a grid as well as its design determines the ability of a grid to clean up scatter and improve radiographic contrast.

Selectivity. The percentage of primary radiation that passes through the grid is known as *primary transmission*. In an ideal situation, a grid would transmit 100% of the primary radiation generated for the procedure. Unfortunately, some primary (as well as scatter) is absorbed by the grid. (See Chapter 13.) The ratio of transmitted primary radiation to transmitted scatter radiation is called grid selectivity. Although selectivity is related to grid ratio, the lead content of the grid also has an effect on selectivity.

Contrast improvement factor. The ratio of the radiographic contrast measured in a study using a grid as compared to the contrast in a non-grid procedure (all other factors unchanged) is known as the contrast improvement factor. (See Chapter 13.)

Grid cassette. When a grid technique is needed for a special projection such as a horizontal beam study (e.g., lateral hip, decubitus barium enema, bedside or operating room radiography), cassettes can be purchased with a built-in grid substituted for the cassette front. When a grid cassette is not available, most radiographers use a stationary grid taped to the front of a conventional cassette for these procedures.

Grid frames can also be temporarily attached to most existing cassettes. This can be particularly helpful at the bedside when a considerable number of cassettes are in use.

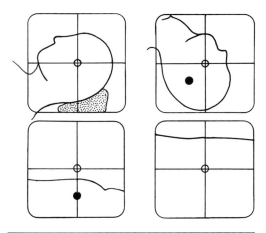

Figure 5-13 The Use of a Cross-Hatch Grid for Angiography *Central ray must be centered to the exact center of a cross-hatch grid to avoid grid cutoff. An open circle is used to represent the center of both grids. A patient is shown positioned for a lateral skull radiograph with central ray bisecting the intersection of the centers of both grids. Both grids will therefore be in focus (top, left).*

A patient is shown in the base position for a lateral study. Note: Central ray (closed circle) is positioned to the area of interest. The central ray is off-center to both the horizontal and vertical grids (top, right).

A cross-hatch grid is shown for an abdominal study (bottom). A small patient is positioned (bottom, left) with the x-ray beam (closed circle) centered to the abdomen, approximately 4 in. off-center to the horizontal segment of the grid. A larger patient (bottom, right), who in theory should be more difficult to examine, is positioned correctly, with central ray bisecting both grids in the cross-hatch configuration.

Inverted Kodak X-Omatic Cassette as a Grid Substitute. Richard J. Sweeney, in his paper "The Use Of An Inverted Kodak X-Omatic Cassette As An Improvised Grid", Radiol Technol 49: 257–261, 1977, described the difficulties encountered with proper centering and distance relationships between the x-ray source and the grid. Sweeney suggested the use of a Kodak X-Omatic cassette in the inverted position (tube side down) as a grid substitute. This cassette has a thin sheet of lead foil mounted behind the posterior intensifying screen to absorb backscatter. (See Fig. 8-13.)

When used as an improvised grid, below 80 kVp, the lead foil back requires an approx-imate 30% increase in mAs over a conventional non-grid technique. Sweeney believes that the inverted cassette functions in a manner similar to a 5:1 ratio grid without grid focus difficulties. In the higher kilovoltage ranges (up to 120 kVp), Sweeney used a stationary grid with the inverted cassette, taking advantage of the increased technical latitude of higher kilovoltage. He stated that no change in exposure is required over the normal grid technique.

IMPORTANT: See Figure 8-16 for patient identification problems that can occur when using an inverted cassette.

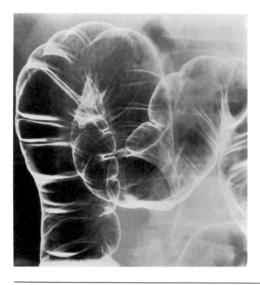 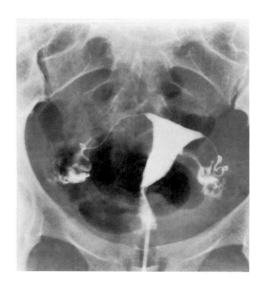

Figure 5-14   *The Use of a Grid in the Spot Film Tunnel: Small Focal Spot Combined With Cross-Hatch Grid* *Because of the variability of the focal object distance, grid focus must be considered when using a fluoroscopic spot film tunnel. A low-ratio grid with an extended focus film length is usually installed in a fluoroscopic spot film tunnel.*

If a higher grid ratio is required, two linear grids can be used in a cross-hatch configuration to overcome the focal range limitations of higher ratio linear grids (Table 5-1). A fluoroscopic grid (linear) helps to control scatter in the larger patient. A second linear grid can be brought into position at a right angle to the first grid for spot film radiography.

For pediatric fluoroscopy, the fluoroscopic grid can be removed from the fluoro field. A single low-ratio linear grid can be used for pediatric spot film studies, if needed.

Unsharpness associated with fluoroscopic spot filming resulting from the shortened focal object distance can be minimized with the use of a small focal spot (0.6 mm). When the small focal spot is used with a cross-hatch grid, fluoroscopic spot films resemble conventional Bucky radiographs. An erect spot film of the hepatic flexure (double contrast study; left) and a supine salpingogram (right) are shown. Both radiographs are fluoroscopic spot films but resemble Bucky quality radiographs. The increased film "blackening" gained by the use of a high-speed rare earth screen film combination permits the use of low or moderate milliampere values. (Courtesy of Eastman Kodak Company, Rochester, New York)

Use of a Grid in a Fluoroscopic Spot Film Tunnel

The size of the part under study affects the focal film distance during fluoroscopic procedures. Although the radiographic tube is in a fixed (predetermined) position, the fluoroscopic spot film tunnel changes position with the part being examined. For example, there is a significant difference in the size of an infant in the supine position compared with an adult in the lateral position. Lower ratio grids are usually used in fluoroscopic spot film tunnels to avoid grid cutoff (Table 5-1).

Since higher kilovoltage values are often used for studies such as barium procedures, a higher ratio grid is needed for adequate removal of the scatter radiation. The use of a cross-hatch grid in the fluoroscopic tunnel (two 6:1 or two 8:1 linear grids) provides the cleanup needed for higher kilovoltage techniques while allowing for significant variations in the focal ranges. A steep angle target x-ray tube (see Fig. 4-2) combined with a cross-hatch grid and small focal spot (0.6 mm or less) produces Bucky-like radiographs (Fig. 5-14 and Table 5-1).

The development of high-speed rare-earth intensifying screen film combinations makes the use of higher ratio grids possible for fluoroscopic spot films. (See Table 8-1 and Chapter 12.)

Grid Artifacts

When high milliampere seconds are used in conjunction with high-speed rare-earth screen film combinations, a new problem can occur. Short exposures can "capture" the grid in motion, accentuating grid imperfections. A widening or banding of the grid lines may be seen (Fig. 5-15). Some types of grid defects never fully "erase" at short exposure times when used in a Potter-Bucky diaphragm (moving grid).

A fine-line aluminum interspaced stationary grid is an appropriate substitute for a moving grid. Damage to the grid can produce uneven density patterns on a radiograph (Fig. 5-15).

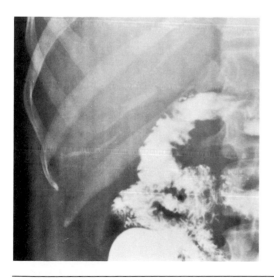 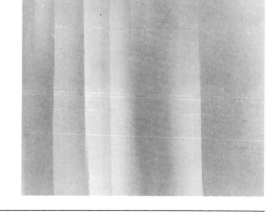

Figure 5-15   Grid Artifacts
A Bucky (moving grid) must be in motion before and after the x-ray exposure.

A moving grid can be "captured" in motion by the use of short exposure times. A widening or banding of the grid lines is seen. This corduroy pattern represents not only widening of the grid lines but also accentuated grid defects (left).

A damaged aluminum interspaced grid can exhibit low-density patterns (banding) throughout the grid (right). These uneven density patterns can be detrimental to image quality. Defects of this nature are generally caused by careless handling of the grid.

IMPORTANT: When an aluminum inter-spaced grid is purchased, it should be radiographed for uneven density patterns whether it is intended to be used as a fixed or moving grid (Bucky). A low exposure (1 mAs to 5 mAs; 40 kVp to 50 kVp, depending upon the screen film combination used) produces an acceptable density (approximately 1.0 density) to evaluate an aluminum interspaced grid. If the radiographic density is too great, grid imperfections may be masked.

Grid Cutoff

When the lead lines of the grid are not focused to the primary radiation, grid cutoff occurs. Lead strips can be projected radiographically as wider images with a significant absorption of the primary beam (Fig. 5-16).

Some of the more common causes of grid cutoff are due to:

1 Lateral decentering of the grid
2 Grid focus distance centering (improper FFD)
3 A combination of the above
4 The use of a focused grid upside down (a rare occurrence).

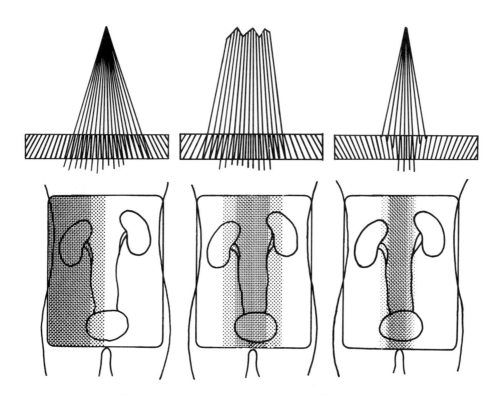

Figure 5-16 Grid Cutoff
If the tube is positioned off-center in relation to the focused grid, severe differences in radiographic density can be noted from one side to the other on the radiograph (left).

When an improper focal film range is used, for example, a 72-in. FFD with a grid focused at 40-in. FFD, there is a loss of density bilaterally. One-to 2-in. segments on both lateral aspects of the radiograph can appear underexposed (center).

When a grid is used in the reverse position, only x-rays parallel to the center of the grid reach the detector (right).

The higher the grid ratio, the more pronounced these defects will be.

Grid Lines

Unwanted grid lines on a radiograph can be due to the following:

1 Improper centering of the x-ray tube to the grid. The higher the grid ratio, the more critical the problem (Fig. 5-16).

2 An increase or decrease in focal film distance. This can produce a widening of the grid lines on the lateral aspects of the radiograph, causing a corresponding bilateral decrease in radiographic density (Fig. 5-16).

3 Capture of the grid in motion owing to the use of too short an exposure time (Fig. 5-15). This is a particularly troublesome problem with pediatric techniques.

4 Poor synchronization of the moving grid to the x-ray exposure. The grid must be in motion before and after the exposure (Fig. 5-15).

5 Shifting the radiographic tube for a stereo technique (see Chapter 7) across the grid lines rather than lengthwise with the grid lines (Fig. 5-16, *left*).

6 Misalignment of a cross-hatch grid. An artifact ("moiré" pattern) may occur when a linear grid is placed on top of a second linear grid or grid cassette with the grid lines overlapping rather than positioned at right angles to each other (Fig. 5-12*E*).

7 Pressure on the grid. The weight of the patient can cause a moving grid (Bucky) to rub against the front of the cassette. A thick lead identification marker or a marker covered with extra layers of adhesive tape (used to fasten the marker to the cassette) can catch on to the moving grid, producing grid striping artifacts. The catching of the tape on the moving grid can also cause the cassette to move during the exposure (Fig. 5-17).

Grid Focus And Grid Ratio Markings

Most grids are appropriately labeled as to distance (FFD) recommendations as well as to grid ratio. If the decal listing this information becomes unreadable or is missing from a grid, the grid ratio, focus, and serial number can usually be found embossed on an edge of the front or back of the metal covering.

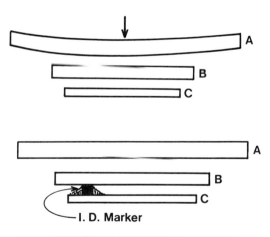

Figure 5-17 Common Causes of Moving Grid Artifacts *Occasionally, an overweight patient, particularly when placed in the lateral position, can cause the tabletop (A) to bend (top). The pressure of the tabletop against the grid (B) may cause the grid to move erratically, producing a grid artifact.*
Thick adhesive or masking tape used to fasten a lead marker to a cassette (C) can cause grid synchronization difficulties (bottom). The taped lead marker can rub against the moving grid (B) causing the cassette (C) to move during the exposure, resulting in a corduroy stripping effect. (See Fig. 5-15. left.)

Grid Line Placement for Horizontal Beam Studies

A unique grid positioning technique can be helpful with horizontal beam studies. Traditionally, the x-ray beam is centered to the cassette with the grid lines in a horizontal position (grid lines parallel to the floor). When the grid lines are positioned parallel to the floor, the part being examined must be centered to the grid cassette, regardless of the size of the patient. By positioning the grid cassette with its grid lines perpendicular to the floor, increased positioning latitude is gained. Grid cutoff is avoided unless the tube is shifted off-center (right or left) (Figs. 5-18 and 5-19).

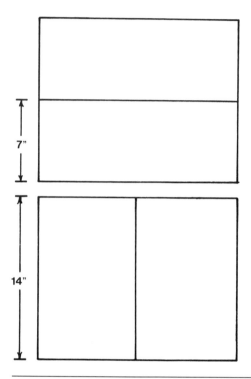

Figure 5-18 **Use of a Grid With a Horizontal Beam Technique** *When a stationary grid is used for horizontal beam radiography, the size of the patient does not always correspond to the center of the grid cassette. The middle of the cassette and grid may be perfectly aligned to a large patient, but a smaller patient may require off-centering of the beam toward the inferior portion of the cassette.*

If the grid lines are positioned with the lead lines perpendicular to the floor, regardless of the size of the patient, tight beam collimation is possible without concern for grid cutoff.

A problem occurs using a 14 in. × 17 in. field for lateral decubitus imaging of the chest, abdomen, or air contrast studies of the colon. When the grid is placed with the lead lines running parallel to the tabletop (top), we must assume that to avoid grid focus difficulties, the center of every patient must be exactly 7 in. from the tabletop. This is rarely true. Therefore, if a grid were used with the lead lines placed in the short dimmension (14 in.) of the cassette, one could center anywhere from 0 in. to 14 in. from the tabletop and produce a radiograph without grid cutoff.

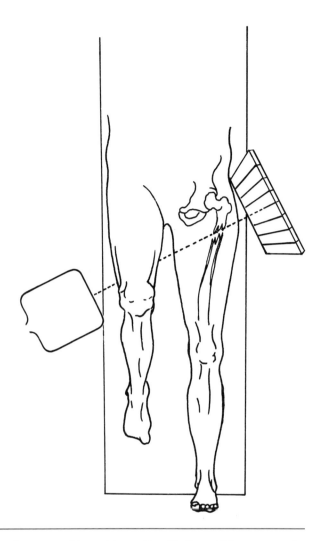

Figure 5-19 Lateral Projection of the Hip; Grid Line Placement The use of a grid for the lateral projection of the hip often results in grid cutoff. Since patients vary in size, it is unlikely that the center of a typical 10 in. × 12 in. grid positioned parallel to the table would be aligned to every patient to be examined. By positioning the grid or grid cassette with the grid lines perpendicular to the tabletop or floor (12 in. × 10 in.), the central ray can be raised or lowered for large or small patients.

A similar positioning approach can be used with cross-table myelography.

6 Electronic Imaging Equipment and Techniques

THE image intensifier is the best known electronic imaging device. Some of the newer electronic imaging technologies will be introduced in this chapter, and their recording media will be addressed in Chapter 9.

Image Intensifiers

Conventional fluoroscopic techniques require dark adaptation of the eyes. (See Chapter 3.) Fluoroscopists must wear adaptation goggles (dark red lenses) for up to 20 minutes prior to a fluoroscopic examination to accommodate the eyes to the low light level of the fluoroscopic image.

The rods and cones of the eye are visual receptors that are highly sensitive to light stimulation. Rod vision is most sensitive to low light levels. The electron fluoroscope (image intensifiers), available since the late 1940s, when linked to a mirror optic system stimulates the rods in the retina of the eyes. Visual acuity (keeness or sharpness in visual perception) uses cone vision, which is stimulated only by bright light. With the advent of television systems, cone vision of the eyes could be used to advantage.

The first image intensifiers had a brightness gain approximately 100 times greater than a conventional fluoroscopic screen. An image intensifier and television system increase light levels as much as 10,000 times. Television monitors also permit more than one person to view the fluoroscopic image. The intensification factor of a fluoroscopic screen was originally judged against the Patterson type B-2 fluoroscopic screen. Prior to the introduction of the image intensifier, this screen was an industry standard for measurement of fluoroscopic light output. More precise light gain measurement techniques have been developed, and intensifier gain is now evaluated in terms of light output per unit area per given amount of x-ray.

An image viewed on a fluoroscopic screen (conventional or image intensified) is reversed compared with that of a radiographic image (i.e., bone and barium are seen as black).

Components and Principles of Operation

The image intensifier consists of a large vacuum tube with an input phosphor fluoroscopic screen, generally composed of cessium iodide (CsI) crystals laminated to a photocathode (thin transparent photoemissive surface).

CsI crystals, which are hygroscopic (absorb water), can be used within the vacuum of an image intensifier but are not suitable for intensifying screens.

The CsI input screen is designed with more crystals packed together (increased packing density) compared with the zinc cadium sulfide phosphors used in early image intensifiers. Over twice the x-ray quanta for the same amount of x-ray exposure is absorbed by the CsI phosphor compared with the zinc cadmium sulfide phosphor. This improves the quantum detection efficiency (QDE) of the intensifier, which is a measurement of how well x-radiation is detected. Since CsI has about double the packing density of zinc cadmium sulfide, only one half the CsI crystals are needed. The thinner CsI input phosphor coatings improve spatial resolution.

As x-ray from the fluoroscopic tube passes through the patient, representative tissue attenuation is displayed as a fluoroscopic image. The fluoroscopic image is simultaneously converted to an electron pattern on the photocathode.

The input phosphor is usually 6 in. or 9 in. in diameter. Some newer image intensifiers have an input phosphor as large as 15 in. in diameter. In theory, the smaller the input phosphor, the finer the spatial resolution. The smaller (6 in.) diameter, high-resolution, input phosphor is preferred for studies such as cinecoronary angiography.

Some intensifiers have multiple scanning fields, and less than the entire input phosphor is used. When the virtually distortion-free center portion of an input phosphor is used, not only is sharpness improved, but the vignetting often associated with the peripheral portions of the fluoroscopic image is minimized.

Electrostatic lenses within the intensifier focus the electron pattern, reducing it in size to the configuration of the output phosphor. The electron pattern is then attracted to the output phosphor by high voltage (25 kVp or greater).

The output phosphor, made of fine-grain zinc cadmium sulfide crystals, situated at the opposite end of the vacuum tube is smaller in size than the input phosphor. Since the output phosphor is smaller in size (1/2 in. and 1 in. on most image intensifiers), even if the electrons were not accelerated by high kilo-

voltage, there would still be a gain in intensification. The electronic gain resulting from the high kilovoltage adds to the total light gain of the system.

The entire system is housed in a glass tube and operates in a vacuum. The image from the output phosphor is transmitted to a mirror viewer on some type of television readout (Fig. 6-1).

As with all radiographic images, one must be concerned about quantum mottle, contrast, resolution, and distortion.

Image intensifier resolution is measured by a line pairs per millimeter (lp/mm) test object. Most CsI tubes will resolve between 4 lp/mm and 6 lp/mm. Earlier zinc cadmium sulfide screens could only resolve 1 lp/mm to 2 lp/mm.

Small image intensifiers with a 6 in. diameter input phosphor can be mounted directly on a conventional fluoroscopic spot film tunnel. (See Fig. 3-9.) The larger intensifiers, particularly those that have dual or trimode viewing fields, require counterbalanced ceiling mounts.

Image Distributor

Mirror viewers, television monitors, cine cameras, and single-or multiframe photographic cameras can be linked to the image intensifier. A beam splitter, placed in close proximity to the output phosphor of an image intensifier, provides optical channels for diverse imaging techniques (Fig. 6-2).

The image distributor (beam splitter) reflects a predominant percentage of the light from the output phosphor in one direction for photographic recording while transmitting a lesser percentage of light to the mirror or television viewing system. Fiber optics are sometimes used to couple the output phosphor to an optical system. The collimating lens (set in relationship to the output phosphor) must be focused at infinity, and the beam splitting mirror (Fig. 6-2) must be in proper alignment. Suboptimal contrast and brightness adjustments of the television monitor can degrade the image.

Television Viewing Systems

Three types of television cameras—the vidicon, plumicon, and orthicon—can be used with image intensifiers. The vidicon camera

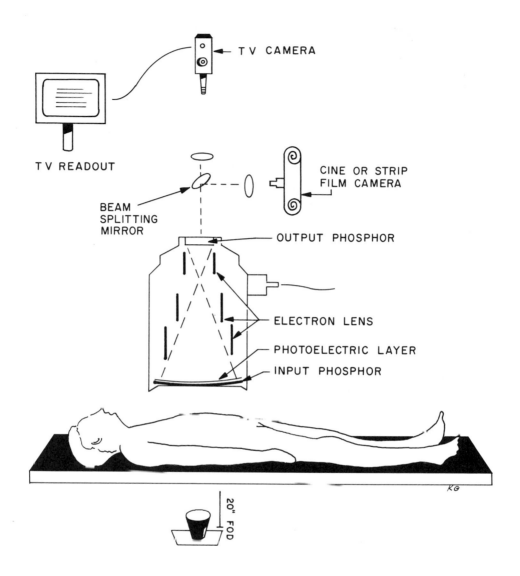

TV CAMERA

TV READOUT

CINE OR STRIP FILM CAMERA

BEAM SPLITTING MIRROR

OUTPUT PHOSPHOR

ELECTRON LENS

PHOTOELECTRIC LAYER

INPUT PHOSPHOR

20" FOD

KG

Figure 6-1 Representation of Components of an Image Intensifier System *The image intensifier is an electronically enhanced fluoroscope. As with conventional fluoroscopy, the patient is placed between the x-ray tube and the fluoroscopic screen (input phosphor) of the image intensifier. Note the shortened focal object distance (approximately 20 in.), which enlarges anatomical details when compared with the 40 in. FFD used in radiography.*

Remnant radiation as well as scatter radiation strikes the input phosphor. A fluorescent image is generated and converted into an electronic image on the photoelectric layer of the intensifier. Elec-trons are accelerated to the output phosphor of the intensifier by the application of high kilovoltage. The electron pattern is focused by electron lenses to conform to the smaller size of the output phosphor. A beam splitter (see Fig. 6-2) is used to transmit some of the light to a television camera. The remaining light is used for motion picture, strip film, or cut film imaging.

The size of the input phosphor (from 6 in.–15 in.) determines the viewing field.

Television readout is not essential for image-intensified viewing. A mirror optic system can be substituted for television.

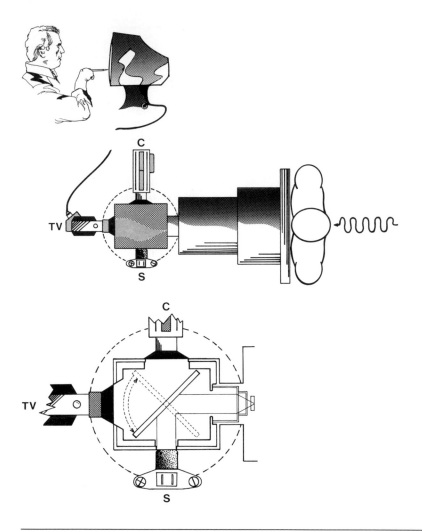

Figure 6-2 Image Distributor for Use With an Image Intensifier The image distributor (beam splitter) is placed in close proximity to the output phosphor of the image intensifier (center). Several channels are available for diverse imaging techniques (bottom). The image distributor reflects a predominant percentage of the light from the output phosphor in one direction for photographic recording and transmits a lesser percentage to a television viewing or mirror optic system. A series of lenses and mirrors within the beam distributor are used to channel light to the appropriate camera. A 16-mm or 35-mm cine camera can be linked to the beam distributor for cineradiography (C). Seventy millimeter to 105 mm roll film cameras (S) can be used for either single-spot filming or multiframe imaging. A 4 in. × 4 in. (100 mm) cut film is also available for single or multiframe imaging.

Regardless of the type of television camera (vidicon, plumicon, or orthicon) used, the light image is converted from the output phosphor into thousands of picture elements by means of a scanning beam and is usually displayed on a 525-line television monitor.

The television monitor provides an ideal teaching tool compared to the mirror optic system, where only one person at a time can view the fluoroscopic image. Some mirror optic units have dual mirror viewing capability. The advantage of the television viewing system is that one or more interested parties can share in the examination. The fluoroscopist, while remaining in a fixed position, can move the image intensifier while observing the image on the television screen.

tube is relatively inexpensive but requires a large amount of light from the output phosphor for operation. The plumicon camera tube is somewhat more sensitive; the orthicon camera tube is most sensitive to light.

A video signal is usually transmitted from the television camera to a television monitor by means of closed circuit (Figs. 6-1 and 6-2). The camera tube converts the light image from the output phosphor into a series of electrical impulses (video signal) and usually transmits the image as a 525 scan line pattern on a television monitor. High-resolution monitors (1024 or 2048 lines), although available, are not in common use.

Video Recording Systems

The transmitted signal can be transferred directly to videotape by a videotape recorder. Advantages of video recording include lower radiation dosage, no need for processing, instant playback, stop motion capability, and reusable tapes. Resolution, however, does not equal that of cineradiographic images.

Video disk scanners use a rigid disk (magnetic or optical) recording medium rather than a flexible tape. The video disk scanner can freeze a single television frame for image comparison or subtraction techniques; can display an image at normal, slow, or reverse speeds; and can provide stop motion studies. Video disks, used to store thousands of individual frames, will become a major part of the electronic file room of the future.

Multiple television monitors are required when more than one video image must be simultaneously evaluated.

Image Intensifier Geometry

As with conventional fluoroscopy, the distance between the x-ray tube and the patient (FOD) is shortened (Fig. 6-1). Image unsharpness can be reduced by using a smaller focal spot (0.3 mm or 0.6 mm) for fluoroscopic spot film imaging. (See Fig. 5-14.)

IMPORTANT: When an undertable image intensifier is used with an overtable x-ray tube, there can be a significant increase in radiation dosage to the fluoroscopist and attending radiographer. Lead shielding should be extended from the over-table tube to the tabletop to minimize exposure to the upper portion of the body of the operator (Fig. 6-3).

Automatic Brightness Control

An automatic brightness control (ABC) is a type of automatic exposure device (AED). (See Chapter 2.) An ABC senses the light output of the image intensifier and adjusts kVp or mA or both to produce a predetermined fluoroscopic density. The introduction of a contrast agent, differences in patient thickness, or any abrupt density change in the area under study, that is, from the base of the right lung (radiolucent) to the liver (radiodense) is compensated for by the ABC.

Cineradiography

Physiologic events that occur too rapidly for normal fluoroscopic viewing can be recorded by cineradiography. Most cineradiographic units use grid-controlled x-ray tubes (see Chapter 4) with a third electrode in the cathode assembly. This third electrode controls the flow of electrons across the x-ray tube, permitting extremely accurate short exposure times. The cathode focusing cup acts as a *grid*. A "bias" voltage applied to the cathode stops the continuous flow of electrons across the x-ray tube from cathode to anode. This occurs even though the filament is heated to thermionic emission levels. When the voltage level at the cathode is dropped to zero, electrons flow across the tube. The current that ordinarily would be flowing through the x-ray tube is stopped by a process (on and off) called *pulsing.* This "gating" effect makes it possible to synchronize the x-ray exposure with the shutters of the motion picture camera.

Sixteen millimeter or 35 mm cine cameras are used for cineradiography. Motion picture cameras typically operate as slow as 8 frames/second or as fast as 60 frames/second. When slow motion studies are desired, the frame per second rate of the camera is increased to record more frames per second. If 24 frames/second are made and projected at 24 frames/second, a normal rate of motion would be seen. If higher frame rates, for example, 60 frames/second, are taken but projected at 24 frames/second, it takes approximately 2 1/2 times longer to view the study, resulting in a slow motion effect. If only 12 frames/second were made and shown at 24 frames/second, motion would seem to occur twice as fast.

Two different sizes of motion picture film are available for cineradiography: 16-mm film (40 frames/foot) or 35-mm film (16 frames/foot). (See Fig. 9-12.)

Cineradiographic framing concepts vary from exact framing of the image to total overframing. (See Fig. 9-13.)

Special cineradiographic rating charts, designed for individual systems, must be consulted to prevent tube damage.

Cineradiographic film is discussed in Chapter 9.

Strip or Cut Film Imaging

Seventy-millimeter to 105-mm roll film cameras or a 4 in. × 4 in. (100 mm) cut film camera can be used for single- or multiframe imaging from the output phosphor. The cameras used for these techniques require special magazines that can be preloaded with strip or cut film. Self-threading take-up magazines permit the processing of individual roll film studies between examinations.

Static photographic images made from the output phosphor of an image intensifier require less radiation (about 1/20th or less) than a screen film radiograph, with a saving in film cost as well as examination time.

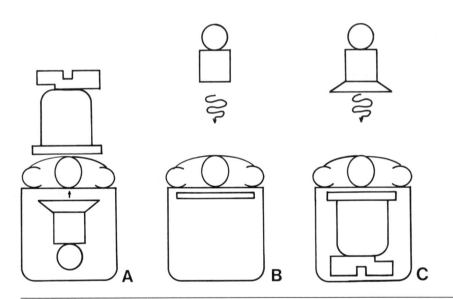

Figure 6-3 Overtable vs. Undertable Image Intensifier Comparison A conventional fluoroscopic configuration is shown (A) compared to a standard 40 in. FFD table Bucky imaging arrangement (B). Note the decreased FOD (approximately 20 in.) associated with the fluoroscope.

According to a report entitled *Statement from the 1985 Paris Meeting of the International Commission on Radiological Protection, Radiology, Sept. 1985,* when an image intensifier is mounted underneath the table (C) and an overtable tube is used for fluoroscopy, substantial x-ray exposure to the operator can occur compared to a conventional fluoroscopic configuration (A).

With the operator wearing a protective apron and standing beside the patient, the dose from an overtable tube compared with that from an undertable tube can be 250 times higher to the hands, 100 times higher to the eyes, and 35 times higher to the whole body.

Lead shielding extended from the collimator to the patient can reduce scatter. A surface shield taped to the side of the patient during an intraventional procedure can reduce scatter radiation up to 75% according to Amplatz et al: *Surface Shield: Device to Reduce Personnel Radiation Exposure, Radiology, 159:3, June 1986.*

One of the disadvantages of the strip or cut film camera is frame size when compared with a screen film study. (See Fig. 9-12.) The strip or cut film images are small and are usually mounted in clear plastic holders for viewing and storage.

Mobile Image Intensifier

Mobile radiographic/fluoroscopic units can be used in the emergency room, intensive care unit, coronary care unit, operating room, or fracture rooms. A C arm fluoroscope with a television attachment enables a physician to view the fluoroscopic image in "real time."

An x-ray tube is mounted at one end of the C frame in alignment with an image intensifier, and a television camera is mounted at the opposite end. The C arm can be rotated around a fixed axis in many directions to avoid moving of the patient (Fig. 6-4). Fracture reduction, needle biopsy, catheter placement, or hip pinning studies are often performed using a mobile fluoro unit.

When high-detail radiographic images are required, a screen film study can be made. Legal documentation of the procedure can be accomplished by conventional radiography, which also serves as a baseline for follow-up examinations.

Digital Subtraction

An elaborate contrast enhancement system with subtraction capability can be linked to an image intensifier. Images can be quickly subtracted electronically with a digital subtraction unit. Electronic subtraction eliminates the need for time-consuming frame-by-frame screen film subtraction of images. (See Fig. 9-17.) The contrast enhancement capability of the computer permits the visualization of small amounts of diluted contrast material, which would be barely visible with screen film radiography. The injection of iodinated contrast material intravenously to avoid arterial intervention was one of the original purposes of digital subtraction techniques. As digital subtraction angiography (DSA) became more widely used, selective arterial injections often replaced the intravenous method, in which

all the vessels under study were simultaneously filled.

Although the resolution of the image intensifier does not equal screen film imaging, excellent quality digital subtraction images are possible (Fig. 6-5).

Images can be viewed and recorded in their normal mode or can be reversed electronically.

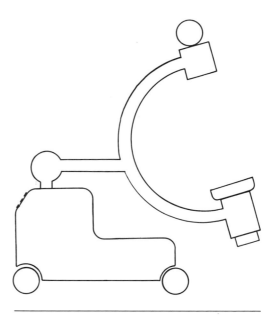

Figure 6-4 "C" Arm Mounted Image Intensifier *A mobile image intensifier is available with a "C" arm configuration. The C arm is designed with an intensifier and television camera on one end and the x-ray tube on the opposing end. The C arm can be rotated around a fixed axis in many directions, avoiding moving of the patient. Note the image intensifier positioned so that the x-ray beam is perpendicular to the input phosphor. As the C arm is rotated, the relationship between central ray and the input phosphor is maintained. With the C arm intensifier and television camera, a fluoroscopic image can be viewed in "real" time.*

The C arm configuration is not limited to mobile units. Some angiographic and fluoroscopic equipment is designed with a C arm permanently installed in radiographic/fluoroscopic rooms. When the C arm is mounted to a ceiling crane, the flexibility of the unit is increased.

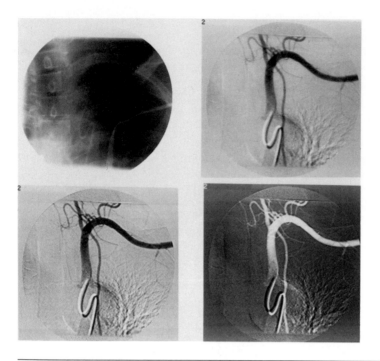

Figure 6-5 Digital Subtraction Angiography
Conventional angiographic subtraction techniques can be time consuming. Electronically enhanced angiographic images can be produced with a digital subtraction angiographic unit (DSA). With a DSA unit, multiple images can be rapidly subtracted electronically, frame to frame, if needed and recorded with a multiformat camera or laser printer. While the resolution of the image intensifier does not equal conventional screen film imaging, excellent quality subtraction studies are possible. The computer-enhanced DSA unit permits intravenous injection of iodinated contrast material for certain procedures, whereas conventional angiographic studies usually require arterial injections. Although the computer enhancement feature of the DSA unit produces superb image contrast of the intravenously injected (diluted) opaque medium, many angiographers use arterial injections for digital subtraction angiographic procedures.

Superimposition (register) difficulties can be caused by patient or vessel motion during the procedure. Some DSA units use "gated" techniques so that individual fluoroscopic frames are exposed when vascular pulsation is at a minimum. The patient is linked to cardiographic leads to determine when vascular relaxation occurs. At this point, the exposure is made. Electronic "filtering" systems can also be used to "smooth" the DSA image, minimizing the blur often associated with subtraction register difficulties.

Images of the left subclavian artery illustrate an electronic digital mask image (top, left), *an electronically subtracted image.* (top, right), *an electronically subtracted image using a filter program to smooth the image* (bottom, left), *and an electronic reversal of the subtracted image* (bottom, right).

The catheter is not subtracted because of misregistration caused by a slight whipping of the catheter during the injection. (Courtesy of The Genesee Hospital, Department of Diagnostic Radiology, Rochester, New York)

Electronic Radiography

An electronic radiograph has many of the characteristics of a conventional radiograph, with some additional benefits. The electronic image can be manipulated by a computer to enhance contrast, extend image latitude, electronically reverse the image, be stored and retrieved, and be printed as hard copy.

Two types of electronic enhancement techniques use a laser scanner for their operation. The first uses a pair of conventional intensifying screens in a cassette and an "extended" latitude radiographic film. The radiograph exhibits an extended long-scale contrast with subtle differences in density and must be scanned by a laser. Data are displayed on a video monitor for interpretation or computer manipulation. Multiformat cameras or laser printers can be used to produce hard copy.

A second method of electronic radiography requires a reusable phosphor-coated plate. The plate is housed in a conventional cassette. Intensifying screens are not needed. After exposure to x-radiation, changes in the phosphor are "read" by a laser scanner. The image can be computer manipulated (enhanced) for interpretation and reproduced as hard copy.

A distinct advantage of both electronic ra-diographic systems is that a wide variation in technical factors can produce acceptable images. The image can be manipulated to change density, contrast, and/or latitude. Underexposed radiographs can be manipulated to an acceptable density level; overexposed images can be reduced in density to a diagnostic level. Portions of the image can be selectively adjusted to enhance an area of interest. For example, an anteroposterior (AP) radiograph of the thoracic spine can be manipulated to visualize the ribs or the lung fields. The image can be reversed electronically so that white areas appear black. In theory, repeat examinations as a result of over- or underexposure should no longer be required.

Digitized information can be stored on videotapes or video disks and transmitted by

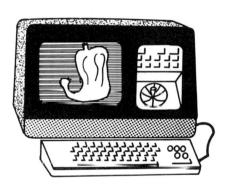

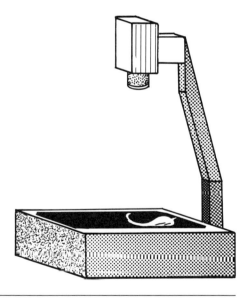

Figure 6-6 Picture Archiving and Communication Systems With a picture archiving and communication system (PACS), a conventional radiograph or other medical image can be displayed on a television screen, digitized, and transmitted to interested parties at remote locations. Medical images can be sent by either telephone, fiber optics, coaxial cable, or microwave transmission. The medical images are placed on a viewbox and transmitted by means of a television camera to a television screen adjacent to the viewbox. A television viewbox and camera (right), and a television monitor with a desk-top computer (left) are shown. A radiograph or other medical image, when digitized, can be electronically manipulated to enhance certain anatomical features. (See Fig. 6-7.) Images can be stored on standard computer disks for viewing at a later time.

An image can be transmitted to a radiologist for interpretation or to another radiology department for consultation. A radiologist could be used for emergency call at a number of facilities.

Electronic storage and retrieval may represent the file room of the future.

means of television for interpretation or consultation.

Picture Archiving and Communication Systems

Picture archiving and communication systems (PACS) can image conventional radiographs and other medical images on a television screen. These images can be digitized, manipulated, and transmitted to remote locations by telephone, fiber optics, coaxial cable, or microwave systems (Figs. 6-6 and 6-7). Video monitors, as opposed to radiographic viewboxes, are used for interpretation. Silver halide films (radiography or multiformat images photographed from cathode ray tubes) used for hard copy are currently stored and filed in paper envelopes. This manual filing process is labor intensive, requiring considerable filing space.

Images comprised of electronic signals can be stored electronically. Image archiving and retrieval may eliminate conventional storage and retrieval practices.

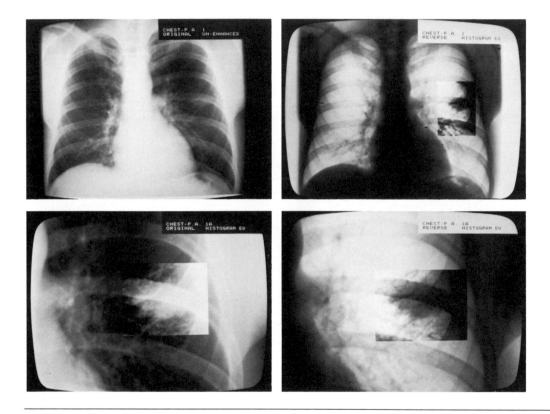

Figure 6-7 Electronically Manipulated Radiographic Images *Representative images recorded from the television screen of a picture archiving and communication system (see Fig. 6-6) are shown.*

A digitized representation of a PA chest radiograph (top, left) is compared with a "black bone" (reversed image) with a segment of the left lung enhanced (top, right). A soft tissue lesion is seen in the lung superimposed on a rib. This portion of the left lung can be enlarged by the operator by means of the television zoom feature. Further enhancement of the lesion is achieved by computer manipulation (bottom, left). A "black bone" presentation helps to further define the boundaries of the lesion and its relationship to the adjacent rib (bottom, right). (See Fig. 6-6 for a description of the PACS equipment used to generate these images.) (Courtesy of Eastman Kodak Company, Rochester, New York)

Other Medical Imaging Procedures

Other types of diagnostic medical imaging procedures are listed in the order of their development or acceptance.

Because many of these procedures are performed in departments of diagnostic medical imaging, an introduction is appropriate. A detailed description of these modalities is beyond the intent of this textbook.

Nuclear Medicine Imaging

After an injection or oral administration of a radioactive compound, organs or osseous structures can be evaluated with a gamma camera or other nuclear medicine scanning equipment. These radioactive substances have an affinity to specific areas within the body. The absorbed radionuclides are detected by the scanning equipment and are imaged directly on film or a CRT from which hard copy can be made (Figs. 6-8 and 6-9).

Depending upon the radioactive substance and the body part being evaluated, the study can be used to locate a disease process; plan chemotherapy treatment; and indicate normal activity, hypoactivity, or hyperactivity of an organ.

Many of the radionuclides used for nuclear imaging have a short half-life and must be prepared in a laboratory in the Nuclear Medicine department.

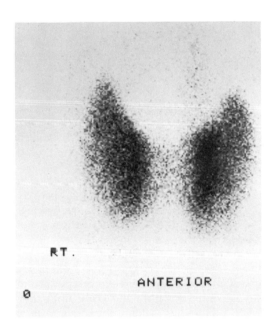
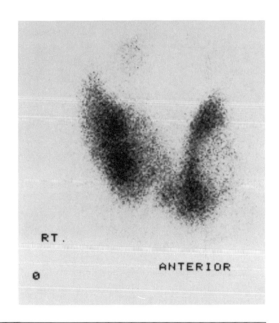

Figure 6-8 Nuclear Medicine Imaging of the Thyroid Gland   *In nuclear medicine imaging, an administration of a radioactive compound is used to evaluate organs or osseous structures.*

When the patients are scanned with a Gamma camera or other type of radionuclide scanning equipment, radioactive substances that have an affinity to specific body parts can be detected and imaged.

The thyroid gland is shown (left) with an uptake of Tc 99m, demonstrating the classic thinning "butterfly" appearance of a normal thyroid gland. Note the pyramidal lobe arising from the left side of the thyroid gland.

A single cold nodule is noted in the left lobe of a diseased thyroid gland (right). (Courtesy of The Genesee Hospital, Department of Nuclear Medicine Imaging, Rochester, New York)

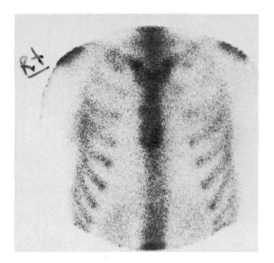 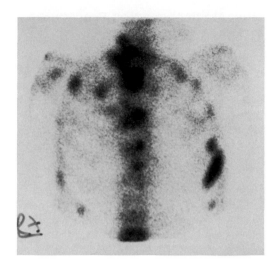

Figure 6-9 Nuclear Medicine Imaging of the Osseous Structures of the Chest *A normal scan of the osseous structures of the chest (left) compared with a chest exhibiting metastatic changes (right) is shown. Note the increase in uptake of the radionuclide Tc 99 MDP by this disease. Bone scans can detect early changes in bone density. (Courtesy of The Genesee Hospital, Department of Nuclear Medicine Imaging, Rochester, New York)*

Medical Thermography

All objects having a temperature above absolute zero (see Chapter 13) emit infrared radiation, which can be detected by heat-sensing equipment.

The naturally emitted heat patterns of the body can be detected and displayed on a CRT (Fig. 6-10). No ionizing radiation is required for or produced by this technique, which evolved from heat-sensing detectors used by the military in World War II.

Because of its lack of specificity, medical thermography has not been well accepted as a primary diagnostic tool and is often used in conjunction with another imaging modality or with physical examination.

Although medical thermography is most commonly used for evaluation of the breasts in conjunction with mammography, thermography has also been used to detect inflammatory or compromised vascular conditions. Changes in vascular patterns in gangrenous extremities as well as evaluation of graft sites in severely burned patients are some of the other uses for medical thermography.

Ultrasonography

Sound wave technology (ultrasound) evolved from sonar equipment used during World War II to locate naval vessels.

Ultrasound (sonography) is a non-ionizing form of diagnostic imaging. It is especially useful for obstetric and gynecologic evaluations, in which the use of x-radiation is not advisable.

Ultrasound equipment utilizes a transducer, which emits short pulses of ultrasonic waves in a forward direction. The sound waves continue within the body until they reach a boundary where the density of a structure changes. When boundaries of different densities are encountered, some of the sound waves are reflected backward to the transducer, which is also used to receive the reflected echoes.

The images are usually viewed "live" on a CRT and recorded on single emulsion film with a multiformat camera or laser printer (Fig. 6-11). Instant photography (a reflective image) is sometimes used, particularly with mobile ultrasonographic units.

(Text continues on page 99)

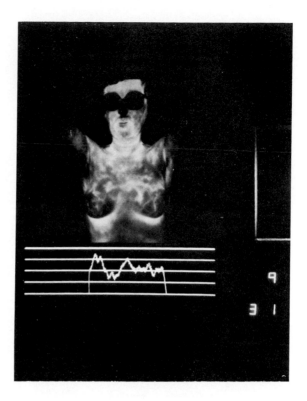

Figure 6-10 Thermographic Representation of the Breasts *A pictorial representation of the infrared heat patterns of the skin is the basis for medical thermography.*

Medical thermography, rarely a primary diagnostic tool, is usually used in conjunction with some other imaging modality or physical examination. No ionizing radiation is required for or produced with this technique.

Any object with a temperature of above absolute zero will emit infrared radiation, which can be detected by heat-sensing equipment and converted into a visual image on a CRT. Infrared rays lying just beyond the visual end of the visible spectrum (see Fig. 1-3) are converted into visible light on a cathode ray tube. Liquid nitrogen, an odorless, colorless, tasteless gas (temperature of −320°F) is used to cool the detector cell in a thermographic unit.

The patient should be cooled and examined in a room maintained at 68° to 70° F. Drafts that will cause uneven patient cooling artifacts must be avoided.

The study in this illustration was made to evaluate the breasts. Prior to the examination, the patient was disrobed to the waist. The arms were elevated for at least 5 minutes to dissipate the heat trapped in the axillae.

The heat pattern can be electronically presented on a CRT as either a white or black format.

In this image, heat is represented as white, and cooler structure as black. Note the white halo effect (a normal heat accumulation) beneath the folds of the breasts at the chest well. Venous patterns are seen as prominent vascular structures distributed throughout the breasts. A "hot" thermographic pattern can represent benign as well as malignant diseases. For example, an abscess may cause a thermogram to appear "hot."

Note the fluctuating scale beneath the breast image that is used to measure and compare temperatures from one side of the image to the other. Thermographic equipment can also detect and measure temperature changes within specific areas of the breast.

The patient in this illustration is wearing glasses, which are displayed as having a lower temperature than the adjacent skin surfaces. The surface temperature of the nose is also lower than that of the face and is seen as a darkened area on the image. (Courtesy of Wende W. Logan, M.D., Rochester, New York)

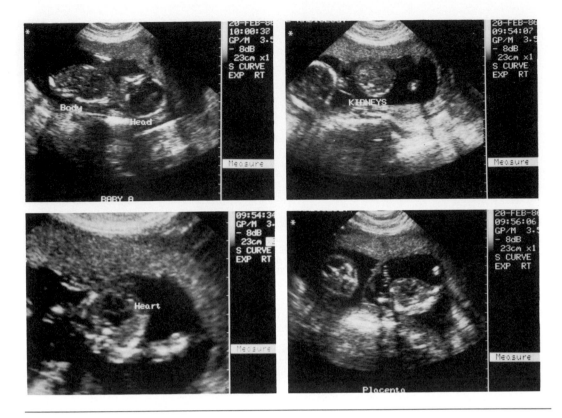

Figure 6-11 Ultrasonographic Images

Medical sonographic equipment emits short pulses of ultrasonic waves from a transducer. These sound waves are used to demonstrate boundaries of tissue where the density of a structure changes. The transducer also receives the backward reflected sound waves that are converted to ultrasonic images on a CRT and are usually recorded on single emulsion photographic film with a multiformat camera or laser printer. Instant photography (reflective paper prints) can also be used to make hard copy. Since ionizing radiation is not required for ultrasound studies, this procedure is routinely used for obstetric and gynecologic studies.

The images shown demonstrate a mature fetal skeleton (top, left). Adequate measurement of the size of the fetus and gestation dating can be determined. Often, the kidneys (top, right) and the heart of the fetus (bottom, left) can be imaged, and the position and size of the placenta (bottom, right) can be determined. Subsequent images in this examination demonstrated a second fetus. (Courtesy of Ide Radiology, Rochester, New York)

Computed Tomography

Computed tomography (CT) is used to image cross-sectional anatomy, which, when displayed on a CRT, can be reconstructed in several planes (transverse, coronal, and lateral).

These studies differ from screen film radiography in that density and contrast can be computer manipulated to distinguish minute differences between and within tissues. For example, gray and white matter densities within the brain can be imaged. The tomographic feature helps to overcome the superimposition of organs or structures associated with conventional radiography. Multiple scans (thin sections) are required to image an anatomical area in its entirety.

The equipment used for CT differs from conventional tomographic equipment (see Chapter 7) in that after the x-ray beam traverses the body, the remnant x-ray beam strikes multiple detectors that sense degrees of x-ray attenuation. This information is sent to a computer, which rapidly evaluates the data. Digital information is reconstructed by complex computer algorithms and is displayed as an image on a CRT monitor. The information is stored electronically and can be retrieved for review as needed. Hard copies are made for diagnostic interpretation (Fig. 6-12).

Magnetic Resonance Imaging

Magnetic resonance imaging (MRI) equipment generates images based on the electromagnetic properties of certain nuclei of body tissues (most commonly hydrogen). While the mass of a structure (mass per tissue volume) is a primary consideration in conventional imaging, MRI detects small changes in radiofrequency perturbed hydrogen nuclei within the magnetized tissue samples. Signal strength, therefore, is particularly dependent upon hydrogen density.

A comprehensive description of the physics associated with MRI is beyond the scope or intent of this textbook. A series of three articles by Nelson, Ritenour, and Davis, "Magnetic Resonance Imaging: The Basic Physical And Clinical Concepts," Radiol Technol 56:6, 1985; 57:1, 1986; 57:2, 1986, is recommended for readers interested in a thorough explanation of MRI.

Patients are placed on an examining table that slides into and out of the magnet within the gantry. Magnetic resonance equipment containing powerful magnets is used to alter the normal spinning action of the hydrogen nuclei within the atoms of tissue. In a nonmagnetized state, the spinning action (precession) of the nuclei is random. Within a magnetized field, the nuclei will attempt to align themselves with or against the applied magnetic force field. By introducing a radiofrequency pulse, the spinning nuclei within the tissues absorb energy and change their angle of rotation to the main magnetic field. The frequency of the precessional motion is proportional to the strength of the main magnetic field.

When the radiofrequency waves are turned off, the excited nuclei produce radiofrequency energy that can be detected, measured, and computer manipulated to produce an image that is displayed on a CRT.

By varying the MRI pulsing sequence and slice orientation (Figs. 6-13 and 6-14), it is possible to produce clear details of soft tissue structures and obtain useful information about these tissues.

Since cortical bone emits little or no magnetic resonance signals, structures obscured by bony tissue on other imaging modalities can be well demonstrated by MRI. For example, the brain, nervous system, and spinal cord can be evaluated by MRI (Fig. 6-13). Cardiac muscles, valves, and blood chambers can be easily demonstrated.

A patient with a pacemaker, ferromagnetic aneurysm clips, or a metallic foreign body in the eye should not be scanned with MRI equipment. A large metal prosthesis can create image artifacts if it is in the field of view. Small metal objects and tools can be strongly attracted to the gantry by the force field, and injury to patients or personnel can occur if safety precautions are not followed.

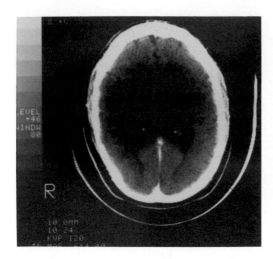 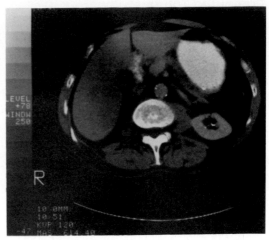

Figure 6-12 Computed Tomography

Since only transverse or axial sections could be made with early computed tomographic units, this imaging technology was introduced as computerized axial tomography (CAT). Complex computer algorithims can now be used to reconstruct transverse anatomy in additional planes, including coronal and lateral. Computed tomography (CT) is now the accepted designation for this procedure.

Although the resolution of the computer generated image does not match the resolution associated with screen film technology, density and contrast manipulations made possible by the computer more than compensate for this limitation. Computer manipulation can be used to display minute differences between and within tissues. Densities from bone to air can be separated, enhanced, and displayed on a CRT. Differences between gray and white matter of the brain as well as intracranial space-taking lesions can be distinguished. Subdural, epidural, or intracranial bleeding can also be demonstrated. Ventricular patterns can be evaluated for abnormality without the introduction of air into the ventricles (pneumoencephalography or ventriculography). Sinus cavities and the structures of the inner ear and eye can be seen.

Since the procedure is tomographic in nature, anatomy can be demonstrated free of superimposed organs or structures. Multiple scans (sections) are needed to image an area or organ under study in its entirety. Transparent hard copy is usually made.

A CT study of the head is shown (left). Note that the ventricular system appears black owing to the computer-enhanced subject contrast between the fluid-filled ventricles and the brain. Calcifications are seen bilaterally in the choroid plexuses. There is a linear opacity (falx) seen posteriorly dividing the brain. At the superior portion of this image, the sulci pattern of the external surface of the brain is demonstrated just beneath the bony vault of the skull.

A section of the upper abdomen is also shown (right), with excellent demonstration of the lumbar vertebrae and surrounding muscular shadows. The liver is seen on the right side of the abdomen. A lucent circular shadow, adjacent to the undersurface of the liver represents a sectional cut of the gall bladder. Medial and superior to the gall bladder but below the separation of the main body of the liver and its left lobe is an opacity, which is radiographic contrast media in the duodenum. The stomach is filled with a diluted opaque contrast medium, and an air–fluid level in the stomach is seen. Since the patient is supine, air rises to the superior portion of the stomach. Note above the lumbar vertebrae, slightly off center to the left, a circular object with peripheral calcific flecks (calcifications within the aorta). On the left side, the kidney can be seen with contrast medium in the renal collecting system and fat within the renal sinus. (Courtesy of Ide Radiology, Rochester, New York)

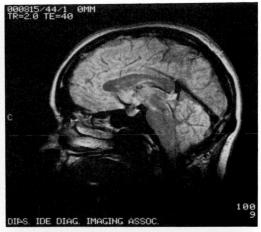

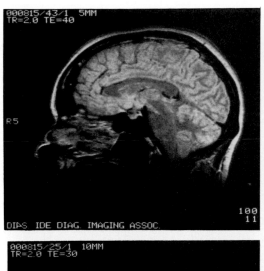

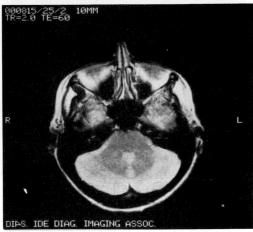

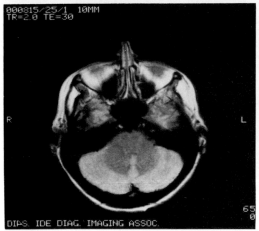

Figure 6-13 Magnetic Resonance Imaging of the Head *Ionizing radiation is not required for or produced by magnetic resonance imaging (MRI).*

At first glance, MR images seem to resemble CT images. Note, however, the absence of cortical bone, which would be well demonstrated on CT images. Direct imaging in the sagittal plane is usually not possible with CT, whereas it is always possible with MRI.

Midsagittal spin echo images of the head (top, left, right) are shown. These scans were made with a 2-second repetition time (TR) and an echo delay

time (TE) of 40 milliseconds. The slice orientation was varied. The right slice was at the 5-mm level (from right of the machine center); the left at 0.0-mm (machine center). Gray and white matter can be seen within the cerebellum.

A transaxial spin echo of the head (bottom, left, right) at the level of the internal auditory canals demonstrates the differences between images produced with first and second echos (30 msec and 60 msec TE). These images were obtained using dedicated head coils. (Courtesy of Diasonics MRI, Ide Diagnostic Imaging Associates, Rochester, New York)

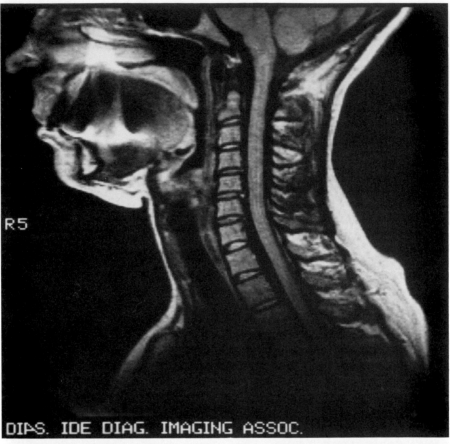

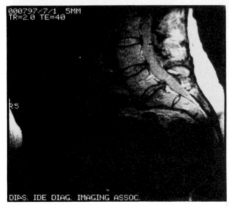
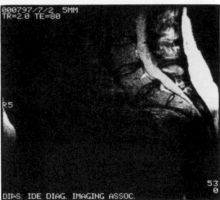

Figure 6-14 Magnetic Resonance Imaging of the Spine *An image of the cervical region was obtained using "Send-Receive" magnetic resonance coils (top). There is excellent visualization of the spinal cord and intervertebral spaces.*

A metal-induced artifact arising from the teeth can be seen overlying the facial structures.

The images of the lumbosacral region obtained using surface coils were produced with echo delay times (TE) of 40 milliseconds (bottom, left) and 80 milliseconds (bottom, right) and repetition times (TR) of 2 seconds. These images are of the same body section; therefore, they vary slightly (e.g., note CSF is white on the 80-millisecond image). (Courtesy of Diasonics MRI, Ide Diagnostic Imaging Associates, Rochester, New York)

7 Special Radiographic Equipment and Techniques

THE procedures described in this chapter—tomography, mammography (screen film and electrostatic imaging), and direct roentgen enlargement—can be labeled *specialized techniques*, although they are in common use in many facilities.

Tomography

Tomography is the generic term selected by the International Commission of Units and Standards to designate all systems of body section radiography. The term *tomography* is derived from the Greek word *tomos*, meaning a cut or section. Planigraphy, stratigraphy, and laminography are other terms used to signify the use of radiographic equipment to blur out superimposed body structures on a radiograph. This type of sectional radiography should not be confused with computed tomography (CT).

The technical aspects of tomography, whether linear or pluridirectional, can be complex.

A typical tomographic unit is connected mechanically to an adjustable fulcrum. This permits levels of the body to be selected for tomographic evaluation. Newer electronic systems using microcomputer principles eliminate the need for mechanical linkage.

The fulcrum can be adjusted to a predetermined level (focal plane) prior to the making of an exposure. The tube moves in opposing directions to the x-ray film.

Terminology

In order to discuss tomography, the terms commonly used as imaging parameters are described.

Tube Film Trajectory: Several tube film movements (trajectories) are possible (Fig. 7–1). The moving of the x-ray tube and cassette in opposite directions blurs superimposed anatomical details above and below the focal plane (Fig. 7–2). The anatomical structure to be imaged determines the type of tube film motion. Any structure that is positioned parallel to the motion of the tube and film is difficult to blur out. All tube film patterns produce some type of phantom imaging (artifact). As complex tube patterns such as hypocycloidal are used, the probability of phantom imaging is reduced, but never completely eliminated.

Linear Motion: When the tube and film move in parallel lines, the trajectory is known

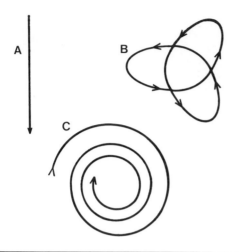

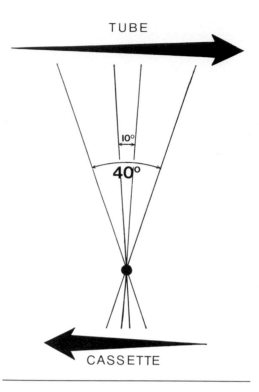

Figure 7-1 Tube Cassette Movements
Several types of tube cassette travel patterns are available for tomography, the most popular being linear (A). The radiographic tube is made to move in a linear direction, and the cassette is made to move in the opposing direction about a pivot point or fulcrum. As with all tube cassette patterns, the x-ray tube and the cassette must be in motion throughout the entire exposure. The descending spiral pattern (B) is an elongated motion that provides increased exposure angle with improved separating capacity (cleanliness of cut).

The first complex pluridirectional device used the hypocycloidal movement (C). This motion is an asymmetrical cloverleaf trajectory. It is about five times greater than the linear route. The more complex the tube cassette trajectory, the better the separating capacity.

Some other types of tube cassette patterns include eliptical, circular, and sinusoidal motions.

Figure 7-2 Basic Concept of Linear Tomography *The x-ray tube and radiographic cassette move in opposing directions in linear tomography. The darkened circle in this illustration represents the pivot point or fulcrum of the x-ray beam. The position of this fulcrum determines the focal plane. The exposure angle determines the thickness or thinness of cut. An increased exposure angle (40 degrees) represents a thin cut, approximately 1 mm to 2 mm in thickness. The narrow exposure angle (10 degrees) represents a thicker cut, approximately 1 cm in thickness.*

Tomographic exposure angles, 10 degrees or less, result in zonograms. With the linear tube cassette movement, striations or linear streakings may occur on the image. The tube and cassette move in straight parallel lines; therefore, shadows of rodlike objects parallel to the direction of the tube motion may not be completely erased. Rodlike structures above or below the focal plane will produce parasitical linear streaks. (See Fig. 7-4, center, top.) Streaking can be minimized if the tube/cassette motion crosses the long axis of the structure at a right angle or in some tangential fashion.

---

as linear motion (Fig. 7–2). As the tube and film move in parallel lines, anatomical structures in this path will not blur out, and striations or linear artifacts may appear in the tomographic image. Even structures out of the focal plane may not be completely erased. When using the linear tomographic unit, the body part should be positioned so that its long axis is not parallel to tube film motion. The tube film motion should cross the long axis of the area under study at a right angle or at least in some tangential fashion (Fig. 7–3 and 7–4).

Circular Motion: A circular motion is used

to improve separating capacity (less phantom imaging). Occasionally, a small circular anatomical structure within the patient will appear as a larger circular shadow (phantom image) on the radiograph.

Pluridirectional Motions: Pluridirectional motions (complex obscuring patterns) produce a better blur effect (separating capacity with less phantom imaging) compared with linear tomography. Some of these motions include circular, eliptical, spiral, and hypocycloidal. Long exposure times (from 6 seconds to 9 seconds) are required for complex tube film patterns (Fig. 7–1). Pluridirectional tomographic units also have linear capability.

Objective Plane: This is the plane in which all points of a radiographic image or section will be sharply imaged by the image receptor. It is the plane of maximal focus in a tomogram (Fig. 7-5).

Focus Plane Distance: This is the distance between the x-ray source and objective plane, also known as the source plane distance.

IMPORTANT: This plane should not be confused with the term focus object distance, since the focus plane of interest could be at any depth within the object.

Plane Film Distance (plane image receptor distance): The difference between the objective plane and the detector as determined by the position of the fulcrum and the image receptor is the plane film distance.

Separating Capacity: The more complex the tube film pattern, the greater the probability of reduced phantom imaging (Fig. 7–1). Elaborate tube film trajectories, while influencing the thinness of cut, are of greater value for their effect on the cleanliness (separating ca-

(Text continues on p. 108.)

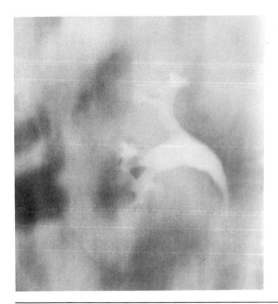 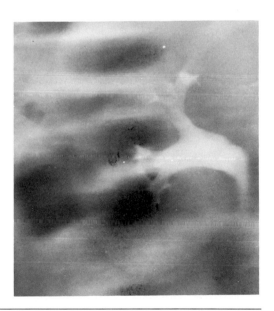

Figure 7-3 Streaking Artifacts Associated With Linear Tomography *With the patient in the supine position, a linear tomographic section was made with the x-ray tube and cassette running lengthwise (top to bottom) to the kidney. The structures above and below the focal plane, particularly those parallel to the tube cassette motion can never be completely obliterated* (A). *The pa-* *tient was repositioned so that the linear tube cassette motion would cross the kidney (medial to lateral aspect of the patient). Linear streaking is again demonstrated paralleling the tube cassette trajectory. Poor separating capacity often occurs with linear tomograph. Complex pluridirectional motions minimize phantom imaging, improving separating capacity. (See Fig. 7-4,* center, bottom.*)*

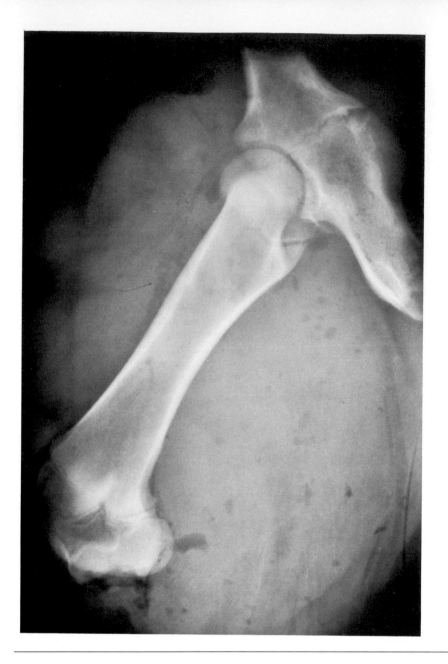

Figure 7-4 Linear and Complex Pluridirectional Tomographic Comparison When evaluating tomographic motions for thinness or cleanliness of cut (separating capacity) or both, a suitable phantom must be found. A phantom composed of dried bones encased in plastic will produce adequate images with regard to resolution and sectional thickness. Unfortunately, little scatter radiation is generated with some of these phantoms. The phantom used in this illustration is the thigh of an animal (bone, flesh, muscle, and other scatter-producing tissue). The femur measured approximately 12 in. in length, and the overall specimen weighed about 20 lb and was easy to handle; it was a processed ham. A conventional radiograph of the ham was made (above), exhibiting good bony detail. Tomographic studies using different tube cassette motions are shown. A linear study of the thigh in abduction shows the relationship of the head of the femur to the acetabulum. Note the parasitical streaking through the shaft of the "out of focus" femur (opposite, top left). The femur was then adducted so that it paralleled the tube cassette motion pattern (top right). It appears that the shaft of the femur is now in plane; however, this is not true. Since the femur is positioned in the direction of the tube cassette motion, good blur is not possible. When linear structure parallels the tube cassette movement, the radiographer may believe that the

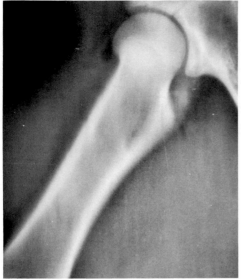

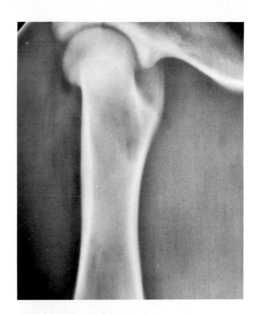

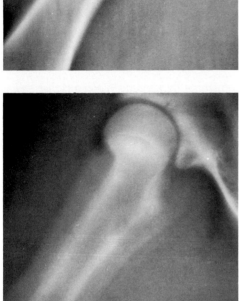

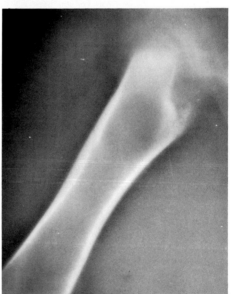

proper focal plane has been selected, yet the details in the original conventional image that lead to tomography may not be visible in the tomographic section. Whenever a linear anatomical structure is visualized running parallel to the tube cassette motion, an accurate focal plane cannot be guaranteed. A tomographic study should be repeated with the tube cassette motion crossing the long axis of the structure at a right angle or at least in some tangential fashion.

A complex tube cassette pattern (hypocycloidal) was used for the remaining sections. With the focal plane still at the same level, a section was made (bottom left). A phantom image (doubling effect) of the shaft of the femur is seen because the femur is out of plane. This is an artifact associated with hypocycloidal or other complex tube cassette trajectories.

The focal plane was readjusted to a higher level in an attempt to place the shaft of the femur in sharp focus (bottom right). Note the sharp cortex, the artifact free medulla, and the absence of the head of the femur owing to the excellent separating capacity of the hypocycloidal movement. The head of the femur appears to have been surgically excised.

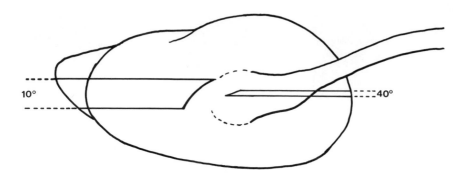

10°   40°

Figure 7-5 Objective Plane; Extended Angle Tomography (40 degrees) vs. Zonography (10 degrees) *An extended angle tomographic study produces a relatively thin objective plane or section. This thinner cut sectioning is used for definitive tomography (analysis). The thicker cut is used to lift out thick layers of anatomy from their surroundings. (See Fig. 7-10.) The increased amplitude used with extended angle tomography produces a thin objective plane with good blur above and below the area being examined. With linear tomography, the extended tube angle produces se-rious parasitical streaking. The zonographic cut (10 degrees or less) yields a relatively thick section, approximately 1 cm. With linear zonography, the narrow angle study results in less parasitical streaking than the thicker section and a higher degree of radiographic contrast since less tissue is being exposed to x-radiation. When an extended angle tomographic study is made, the x-ray beam enters the body at an increased angle, transversing through significantly more tissue than the zonographic section. (See Fig. 7-7.)*

---

pacity) of the sections. (See Fig. 8-4.) Individual cuts are more artifact-free with less phantom imaging.

Thickness of Section: The position of the fulcrum determines the layer to be sectioned. The thickness of the section is controlled primarily by amplitude. Amplitude can be described as the distance that the x-ray tube travels during the actual radiographic exposure.

IMPORTANT: The x-ray tube must be in motion before and after the exposure. Only the time that exposure is being made is considered amplitude. The longer the travel of the x-ray tube (during exposure), the thinner the tomographic section (Fig. 7–6).

Extended angle tomography (exposure angle, 40 degrees to 50 degrees) and narrow angle tomography (10 degrees or less) can be used to advantage in specific examinations (Fig. 7–7 and 7–8). The thicker cut (zonography, 10 degrees or less) can be used to radiographically lift out thick layers of anatomy from their surroundings (Fig. 7–9). The thinner cut (extended exposure angle) is used for definitive tomography (Figs. 7–10 and 7–11).

If one were to tomographically evaluate the kidneys, the zonographic cut would produce a layer thickness of approximately 1 cm (a gross radiographic specimen). The extended angle cut would produce a layer of approximately 1 mm (a radiographic biopsy; Fig. 7–5).

Focal Film Distance: Focal film distance, the distance between the x-ray source and the detector, can also influence the thickness of a tomographic section. In practice, the focal film distance is rarely changed. If the focal film distance were to be decreased, exposure angle would increase (Fig. 7–6).

Basic Technical Considerations

Dosage Consideration: Since tomographic studies can require increased radiation exposures, the use of rare-earth imaging systems (400 speed or greater) must be considered. (See Chapter 8.)

When examining the skull, particularly in

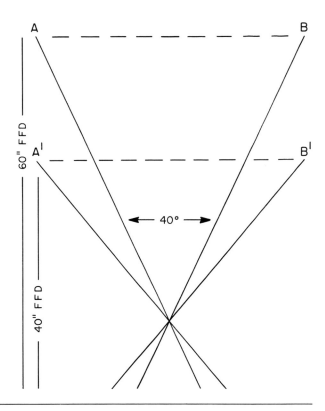

Figure 7-6 Thickness of Section Determination *The thickness of a tomographic section is controlled primarily by amplitude. Amplitude describes the distance that the x-ray tube travels during the actual radiographic exposure (from A to B, at a 60 in. FFD; and from A' to B', at a 40 in. FFD). The greater the amplitude, the thinner the cut; the lesser the amplitude, the thicker the cut.*

Note that tube travel in both examples at both focal film distances is exactly the same; A to B or A' to B'. When the focal film distance is lowered, even though the same amplitude is used, the exposure angle is extended. Increased amplitude and decreased focal film distance results in the thinnest possible cut.

the anteroposterior (AP) position, the possibility of a cataractogenic radiation dose to the cornea must be considered. Tight beam collimation will lessen the dosage to surrounding tissues. The use of an eye lens shield will reduce dosage but may result in pronounced parasitical streaks on a linear tomographic study. Placing the patient in the prone position reduces dosage to the lens of the eye, since primary radiation enters the posterior portion of the skull and remnant radiation exits through the eye. The use of the posteroanterior (PA) projection approximates the dosage to the lens of the eye attained when the AP projection is used with lens shielding.

Image Sharpness: Contrast and resolution are affected by tomography, particularly extended angle tomography. Tight beam collimation can minimize the effect of scatter radiation on radiographic contrast. Motion in the mechanical linkage or patient motion (voluntary and involuntary) can affect recorded image detail. (See Chapter 11.)

Cassette Selection: When multiple consecutive exposures are made, the same screen film combination in the same type of cassette should be used. Screens can be mounted within cassettes at slightly different levels, creating a focal plane problem for thin section tomography. Cassette fronts can also vary in

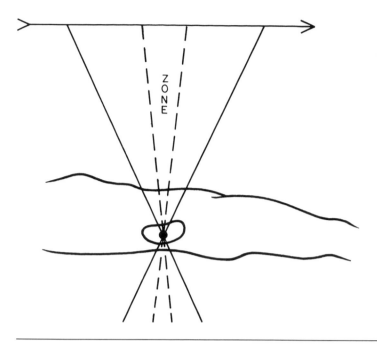

Figure 7-7 Extended Angle Tomography vs. Zonography *The extended angle tomographic section is represented as a solid line. With this increased amplitude, an increased exposure angle occurs and thinness of cut is maximized. (See Fig. 7-6.) When a narrow angle tomographic section,* *represented as a dotted line, is made, a thicker tomographic section results. The zonographic area is represented by dotted lines. A clinical example of extended angle vs. narrow angle tomography is shown in Figure 7-9, petrous ridge tomography.*

absorption, producing corresponding variations in radiographic densities. (See Chapter 8.)

Multilevel Cassettes: Multiscreen (book) cassettes are used for simultaneous multilevel tomographic studies. Book cassettes hold from three to seven pairs of intensifying screens to simultaneously expose three to seven sheets of x-ray film with a single exposure. With kilovoltage remaining the same, a seven level book cassette requires about two and one half times the milliampere second value of a single section. These images are of marginal quality, and this technique has not been well accepted.

A special book cassette with four sets of intensifying screens (spaced approximately 1 mm apart) is known as a *plesiocassette*. The exact 1-mm spacing of the intensifying screen pairs in the plesiocassette produces four equidistant radiographic images with one exposure.

Intensifying screens used in the book cassettes are carefully balanced to produce comparable densities. For example, the first screen pair is very slow, and the last screen pair is very fast. This variation in screen speed is not a problem with calcium tungstate screens. Newer rare-earth screens, with their high absorption/conversion potential (see Fig. 8-7), are not practical for book cassette tomography. The first pair of intensifying screens often absorbs much of the primary beam, leaving little or no radiation available for the remaining screen pairs. (See Chapter 8.)

Direct Roentgen Enlargement

Direct roentgen enlargement (magnification) should not be confused with photographic enlargement when a photographic negative of a radiographic image is optically enlarged. Ra-

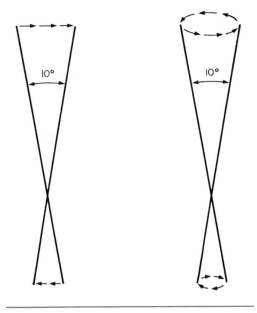

Figure 7-8 Zonographic Tube Cassette Motion *Zonography is not a type of tube cassette motion but is simply narrow angle tomography. A small angle circular movement* (right) *is available on some units for zonographic studies. Regardless of the type of film cassette motion, whether linear* (left) *or circular* (right), *zonography is accomplished with an exposure angle of 10 degrees or less. With the narrow exposure angle, a thicker layer is lifted from the body. Areas such as the facial bones or mandible can benefit from zonography. With linear zonography, there is a reduction in the parasitical streaking. The striations are shorter in length than those generated with extended angle linear tomography. Zonography will exhibit better radiographic contrast when compared to extended angle tomography. Less tissue is exposed to primary radiation with the narrow exposure angle, so less scatter radiation is generated.*

diographic enlargement occurs when the radiographic image is projected to an image receptor some distance from the part under study (increased OFD) (Figs. 7–12 and 7–13).

For a conventional 2× linear (4× area) magnification study, the part must be equidistant between the tube and detector. For 3× linear (9× area) magnification, the part is approximately one third the distance (TOD) from the tube and two thirds the distance

(OFD) from the detector (Fig. 7–14). (See Chapter 13.)

Be separating the image detector from the object under study (air gap), a grid-like scatter cleanup occurs. If the image detector is not in close contact with the part under study, most of the scatter radiation generated during an exposure will not reach the film. A high percentage of the scatter, because of its oblique nature, misses the detector. (See Fig. 5–8.)

Different parts of the human body are at various distances from the screen film combination, even when a fixed FFD or OFD is used (Fig. 7–15). For example, when the patient is positioned equidistant from the focal spot between the tube and the detector in the lateral skull position, the vessels to be studied (right or left side) will not be magnified equally. Regardless of the side injected (right or left), the anterior cerebral arteries, being midline, will be enlarged approximately to the same degree. With the patient in the left lateral position, the middle cerebral artery (left-sided injection) is closer to the detector; the middle cerebral artery (right-sided injection) is further from the detector and closer to the x-ray source. The right middle cerebral artery will therefore appear larger in size than the left middle cerebral artery.

The primary beam should also be restricted to the part under study. If a primary beam leak occurs, undercutting of the image can result. (See Figs. 5–3 and 5–4.)

X-ray tubes with ''fractional'' focal spots (0.3 mm or less) have been used for direct roentgen enlargement techniques for more than three decades. Early fractional focus x-ray tubes had severe rating restrictions, and their use was limited to enlargement of thin body parts. New steep angle targets (see Fig. 4–2) have made magnification studies of thicker body parts possible.

Focal Spot Size and Penumbra

IMPORTANT: Small focal spots (0.5 mm or 0.6 mm) are not acceptable for direct roentgen enlargement studies.

The 0.3-mm focal spot (usually rated less than 200 mA) is universally accepted as the minimal focal spot permissible for direct roentgen enlargement studies. Some radiographic tubes have a 0.1-mm capability with reduced milliampere ratings (less than 75 mA). A stationary anode microfocus tube is available, with a focal spot corresponding to a nominal diameter of 0.09 mm (rated less than 10 mA).

Radiographic details smaller than the focal spot can "disappear" on an enlargement study. A minute radiographic detail present on a conventional radiograph may not be seen on the enlarged study if the structural detail to be enlarged is smaller than the focal spot (Fig. 7–12).

Every effort must be made to ensure the integrity of the focal spot size. Technical factors such as low kilovoltage with high milliamperage may contribute to focal spot blooming. (See Chapter 4.)

Screen Film Combinations

The use of detail screens for high-detail magnification studies are acceptable with direct roentgen enlargement technology. High-speed rare-earth technology (600 to 1200 speed) permits an increased number of frames per second for direct roentgen enlargement angiography (see Chapter 9) without compromising the instantaneous load capacity of the fractional focal spot tube. (See Chapter 4.)

The effect of quantum mottle (see Fig. 8–12) sometimes seen on high-speed rare-earth images is minimized by the magnification process. As the degree of enlargement increases, the effect of noise on the image is diminished. The quantum mottle, still visible on the processed radiograph, is not increased in size since the mottle is generated within the screen. Anatomical details increase in size, but the quantum mottle remains the same size, making the detector more efficient (Fig. 7–16).

Mammography

One in 11 American women will develop breast cancer. The smaller the cancer when

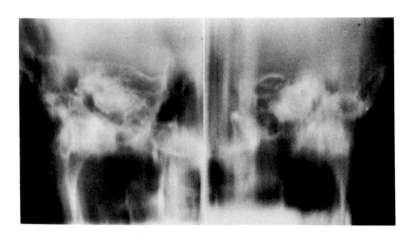

Figure 7-9   Tomography of the Petrous Ridge
Separate exposures were made of the petrous ridge to demonstrate extended angle (50-degree) vs. narrow angle (zonography, 10-degree) images.

The entire petrous ridge is almost completely disengaged from the skull in the zonographic study (left). *The petrous ridge has been radiographically removed from its surroundings. When a 50-degree exposure angle is used* (right), *a thin section approximately 1 mm is available for diag-* *nosis. The hearing structures housed within the petrous ridge are now available for evaluation. Zonography (10-degree exposure angle) looks within the skull and lifts out the petrous ridge; increased angle tomography (50-degree exposure angle) looks within the petrous ridge within the skull. Zonography represents a gross radiographic specimen; extended angle tomography results in a radiographic biopsy.*

found, the greater the likelihood that it will be localized to the breast. If the disease is localized to the breast, the 5-year survival rate can be as high as 85%. The importance of early detection of breast cancer is supported by the recommendations of The American Cancer Society and American Medical Association for periodic breast examination.

A mammogram provides information about normal anatomy as well as pathology. The types of tissue structures within the breast, represented by muscles, glands, blood vessels, and fatty tissue, differ little in radiodensity (low subject contrast).

Special dedicated mammographic equipment and techniques are needed to demonstrate these subtle differences in tissue density. Microcalcifications (50 micra to 200 micra or greater) must be imaged, and parenchymal architecture (fine vascular-like breast patterns) must be clearly seen.

Screen film mammographic techniques require short-scale, high-contrast imaging to demonstrate subtle density differences between soft tissue structures (water-like and fat). Radiographic contrast is essential to visualize subtle density differences and breast microcalcifications. Sufficient radiographic contrast is not possible with conventional x-ray equipment. When a tungsten target tube is used for screen film mammography, a beryllium window and minimal filtration are recommended. In the kilovoltage range needed for mammography, a molybdenum target tube produces a higher contrast, almost homogeneous x-ray beam, which improves radiographic contrast and helps in the visualization of minute radiographic details.

Subject contrast is related to the ratio of the x-ray intensity transmitted through one part of the breast to the intensity transmitted through a more absorbing adjacent area of the

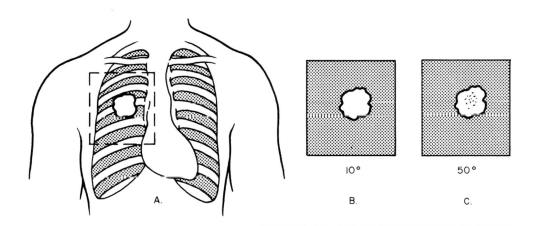

A.

10°   50°

B.   C.

Figure 7-10 Narrow Angle vs. Extended Tomography *Before beginning a tomographic examination, it is important that thick or thin cut technology determination be made.*

A chest image requiring tomography for additional diagnostic information is shown with a lesion in the right lung (A). If one intends to simply erase the image details of other structures in the path of the beam, zonography (10 degrees or less) is suggested. With zonography, the lesion is lifted out of the chest as a relatively thick cut (approximately 1 cm in thickness) (B). If the internal composition of the lesion is to be evaluated, extended angle tomography may be required (C). Note the calcific flecks in the extended angle cut (C) not *visualized in the narrow angle section (B). Remember that the zonogram yields a full centimeter of tissue, whereas the extended angle images demonstrate only a millimeter of tissue. If the chest measured 25 cm in thickness, 25 zonographic cuts would be required to visualize the entire chest; if extended angle tomography were used, it would require 250 cuts to visualize the entire chest. Often, the number of radiographs is confused with the amount of information. It is important to evaluate the conventional radiograph prior to a tomograph study in order to localize the area to be examined tomographically and to minimize dosage to the patient, examination in time, and film usage.*

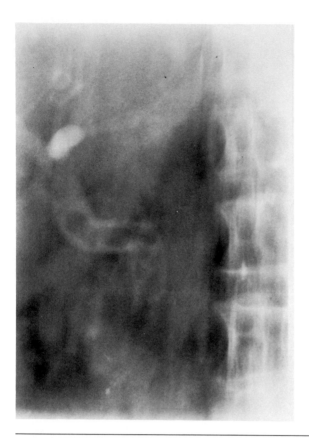

Figure 7-11 *Tomographic Section of an Intra-venous Cholangiogram* An extended angle study was made of the biliary system after intravenous injection of an opaque contrast agent. Some linear parasitical streaks can be seen. The common hepatic duct as well as the common duct are in good focus. Note the radiolucent defects within the opacified biliary system. Unfortunately, the distal end of the common duct, as it enters the ampula of Vater, is not in focus. Additional cuts must be made to visualize this portion of the anatomy. Often a radiolucent calculi will be lodged at the distal end of the common duct producing a ''check valve'' effect. Because of the lower contrast level associated with intravenous opaque media, moderate to low kilovoltage must be used with high mAs values to produce radiographic contrast. Since this is a relatively thin section, radiographic contrast is further reduced. The x-ray beam has to traverse through considerably more tissue for the extended angle tomogram when compared to conventional radiography.

breast. Absorption differences in the breast (thickness and density) as well as the radiation quality affect subject contrast. Optimal kilovoltage settings for short-scale contrast range from 45 kVp to 55 kVp for electrostatic imaging with a tungsten target tube, and from 22 kVp to 28 kVp for screen film mammography.

Dual Filter Concepts

Molybdenum filters are used with molybdenum target tubes for screen film mammography, whereas tungsten target tubes and aluminum filters are recommended for electrostatic imaging. Often, a dedicated mammographic unit will contain an alumi-

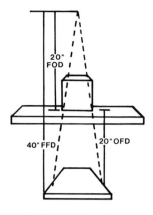 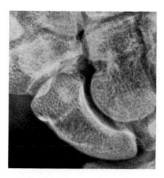 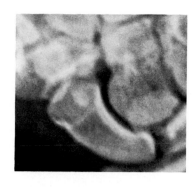

Figure 7-12 Direct Roentgen Enlargement: Focal Spot Comparison *A typical arrangement for direct roentgen enlargement is shown* (left). *A fractional focal spot tube (0.3 mm or less) is a prerequisite for this technique. The part is positioned approximately midway between the tube and image detector (20 in. FOD; 20 in. OFD). This results in a 2× linear, 4× area enlargement. (See Table 11-1.) If the part to be examined is positioned 13 in. from the tube with a 26-in. object film distance (air gap), a 3× linear, 9× area enlargement will occur. A 0.3-mm focal spot was* used for the enlargement of the scaphoid (navicular) bone (center). *Note the excellent osseous details. A 1.0-mm focal spot was used for an exact duplication of the roentgen enlargement technique, shown in the center illustration, and radiographic details are greatly diminished* (right). *This image is completely out of focus. The use of the proper focal spot is essential. A minute radiographic detail smaller than the focal spot and barely visible on a conventional image could disappear on the enlargement. (See Fig. 7-13.)*

num filter as well as a molybdenum filter. The aluminum filter can be inserted either manually or electrically if electrostatic imaging is used. If the wrong filter is moved into position, the quality of the radiographic study will deteriorate.

If a dedicated unit is not available and a tungsten target tube must be used for screen film mammography, added filtration must be removed. The mirror in the collimator is part of the filtration system. (See Fig. 4–9.)

IMPORTANT: After a mammographic study has been performed, it is essential that any filtration removed be reinserted in the collimator, prior to conventional radiography.

Because the technical parameters for mammography are so unique, quality assurance (QA) is of great importance. As with all ra-

diographic equipment, scheduled periodic checks of peak tube voltage, half value layer, timer accuracy, and focal spot size should be performed. High milliampere values can produce focal spot blooming. (See Chapter 4.)

Image Geometry

The size of the x-ray focal spot and related image geometry must be considered. Selection of a small focal spot (0.6 mm or less) is always recommended with screen film mammography when this choice is available.

Early dedicated mammographic units used very short focal film distances (less than 13 in.). Newer "long cone" units use a 30 in. or greater FFD. The long cone techniques improve image geometry. (See Chapter 11.) When the compression plate of a dedicated unit is attached to the bottom of the cone, image geometry can be compromised, because focal film distance is decreased as compression is applied.

Scatter Control

As in all medical radiography, it is important that the area to be examined be as close to the image detector as possible. The female breast is pyramidal in shape—thicker at the chest wall than at the nipple area. A compression device should not only immobilize the breast but also compress it, minimizing its conical shape so that overall breast tissue approaches even thickness. Aggressive compression of the breast brings the breast tissue closer to the image detector while lessening the production of scatter (Fig. 7–17).

Every effort should be made to gain the

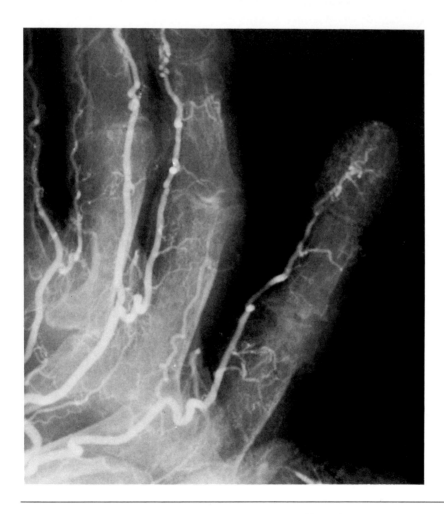

Figure 7-13 Direct Angiographic Enlargement of the Hand *This illustration represents a 3× linear, 9× area enlargement made during an angiographic serial study. Note the excellent vascular patterns except for the area of the second phalangeal joint. There is a lack of blood vessels in this region as a result of a disease process. Note: The distal vessels of the thumb are magnified but are also out of focus. These vessels are smaller than the focal spot and therefore cannot be held in focus. Image blur (penumbra) hampers resolution.*

patient's confidence and cooperation when using a compression device. Compression should be applied slowly and carefully so as not to bruise the skin (Fig. 7–18).

Some advantages of aggressive breast compression include:

1 The structures of the breast are in better contact with the image receptor—geometric blurring is reduced.

2 There is more uniform tissue thickness—less difference in radiographic density.

3 Less scatter is produced because of the compression effect.

4 There is a reduction in radiation dosage.

5 Patient motion is eliminated.

IMPORTANT: Visualization of the rib cage on the lateral view of the breast does not necessarily ensure that the entire posterior portion of the breast has been imaged (Fig. 7–19). The radiographer must gently pull the breast tissue away from the chest while applying compression so that the posterior portion of the breast will be imaged.

High-quality fine-line grids (up to 200 lines/ in.) or moving grids (Bucky) have been developed for use in mammography. Much of the scatter radiation associated with dense glandular breast architecture can be eliminated with these grids (Fig. 7–20). The grids, usually 3.5:1 in ratio, can vary in size as well as in focal range. Grid focusing distances must be considered when a grid is purchased. Stationary mammographic grids can be installed within a cassette or can be used on top of a cassette or vacuum bag. These thin fine-line grids are easily damaged.

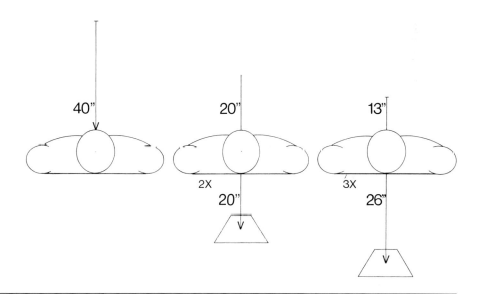

Figure 7-14 Direct Roentgen Enlargement Comparison *A patient is positioned for conventional radiography (left) using a 40-in. focal film distance. In the center panel, 2× linear, 4 × area enlargement is shown, with the patient equidistant between tube and detector. A 3× linear, 9× area study (right) is shown with a 13-in. target object distance and a 26-in. object film distance.*

(See Chapter 13 for magnification formulas.) By separating the image detector from the object under study, a grid-type cleanup effect occurs. Since the radiographic film is in direct contact with the part (left), most of the scatter radiation will strike the film. When an air gap is used (center and right), a high percentage of the scatter radiation completely misses the film. (See Fig. 5-8.)

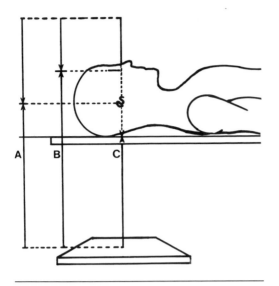

Figure 7-15 Anatomical Relationships to Tube and Detector *Different segments of anatomy enlarge to different degrees, depending upon their position within the body. For example, the posterior portion of the skull (C) is equidistant between tube and detector. A 2× area, 4× linear enlargement will occur. When different parts of the skull are to be enlarged, such as the sella turcica (A), the relationship between target, object, and film changes dramatically. There will be an increase in the size of the sella turcica greater than 2× linear. If the orbits (B) are to be examined, severely decreased target object distance occurs, with significant enlargement of the orbits. Magnification in this illustration could be up to 4× linear, 16× area and the orbits will be out of focus. The focal film distance is often changed to compensate for this difficulty, and the cassette is raised closer to the part under study. This is an error, because a 20-in. air gap is required to adequately clean up scatter when a grid or Bucky is not being used. If the orbits are to be enlarged, placing the patient prone will help to maintain a better FOD/OFD relationship. When performing direct enlargement studies, not only should geometric relationships be a concern, focal spot size must also be considered. Roentgen enlargement requires carefully measured focal spots.*

If the non-grid kilovoltage value is to be maintained, an approximate two to two and one half times increase in the milliampere second value is needed to overcome the absorptive quality of the grid. When using the same milliamperage second value, an increase in 3 kVp to 4 kVp should be adequate to duplicate non-grid densities.

Automatic Exposure Device

Many dedicated mammographic units use an automatic exposure device (AED) to control exposure time. (See Chapter 3.) As in conventional radiography, the body part (breast) must be positioned carefully over the sensor. Radiographic densities are balanced by the AED, even if significant absorption differences occur between both breasts. A change in the length of the exposures between the breasts should be brought to the attention of the radiologist.

Tube Orientation— Anode vs. Cathode

When conventional radiographic equipment was used for mammography, it was common practice to position the cathode side of the x-ray tube to the base or thicker portion of the breast to take advantage of the anode heel effect. (See Fig. 4–3.) Prior to the use of aggressive compression techniques, the increase in exposure to the thicker portion of the breast (chest wall) was of value. There may be a disadvantage, however, in the positioning of the cathode to the thicker portion of the breast, because although intensity increases at the cathode side of the tube, resolution decreases. (See Fig. 4–4.) The effective focal spot widens toward the cathode side of the tube and narrows toward the anode side. Minute calcifications, particularly those not in intimate contact with the detector, could "disappear." In dedicated mammographic units, the radiographer is not able to change the cathode/anode relationship to the breast.

Occasionally, the mammographic image near the chest wall may lack radiographic detail or density or both. "Whiteout" of the tissue near the chest wall is the result of improper compression. When a curved-edge compression device is used, breast tissue can be forced backward and upward along the chest wall, producing a "stepwedge" difference in breast thickness, with the tissue at the chest wall considerably thicker than the compressed tissue. By using straight-edge compression, the possibility of whiteout of the

(Text continues on page 122.)

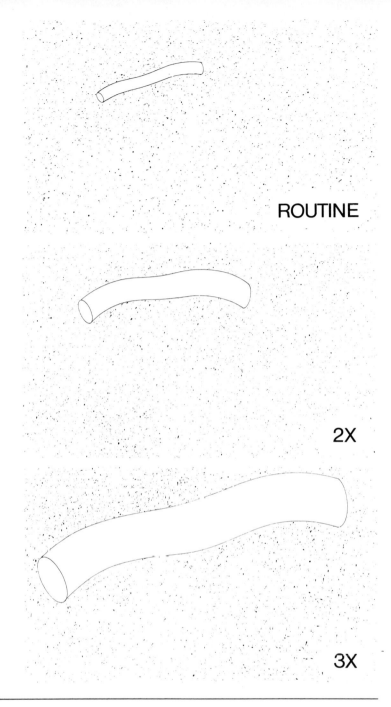

ROUTINE

2X

3X

Figure 7-16   The Effect of Quantum Mottle on Various Degrees of Enlargement *Occasionally, quantum mottle will be seen when using a high-speed screen film combination. Quantum mottle occurs in the intensifying screen and can damage resolution in the radiographic image (top). The effect of quantum mottle (see Fig. 8-12, and Chapter 11) on the image can be minimized by the direct roentgen enlargement process. When a body seg-*

ment or vessel is enlarged to 2× linear, 4× area, magnified anatomy is demonstrated (center). When a greater degree of enlargement is required (bottom), such as a 3× linear, 9× area study, the effect of quantum mottle on resolution is even further diminished. The anatomical details increase in size, but the quantum mottle remains the same size, since it occurs in the screen, making the image detector more efficient.

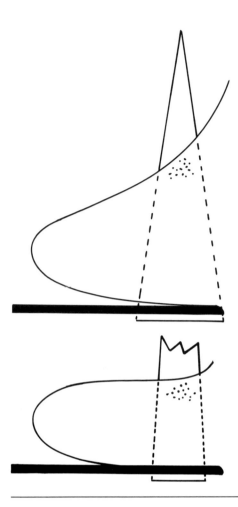

Figure 7-17 The Effect of Compression on Mammography *Because the female breast is pyramidal in shape, compression is essential for mammography. It is difficult to adequately image the breast without using breast compression, because the breast is thicker at the chest wall than in the nipple area. Aggressive compression of the breast brings the breast tissue closer to the image detector while lessening the production of scatter. The pyramidal-shaped breast (top) presents several imaging difficulties. If the proper exposure were used to image the breast tissue near the chest wall, the nipple area would be overexposed. Note the presence of calcifications in the superior portion of the breast and the distance of the calcific flecks from the detector. A widening, therefore a blurring, of these structures may occur when they are imaged. The use of a small focal spot helps to overcome this difficulty. When the breast is compressed to an even overall thickness, (bottom) calcifications are brought closer to the detector (decreased object film distance). This change in OFD should help to minimize blur. When compression techniques are combined with small focal spots, image resolution improves dramatically. Note the difference in the thickness of the breast as it is compressed (flattened) and spread over a greater area of the image detector. The decrease in the tissue thickness results in less scatter production. Compression, therefore, aids in improving image geometry as well as scatter control. Since less radiation is required for the compressed tissue, lower exposure factors can be used.*

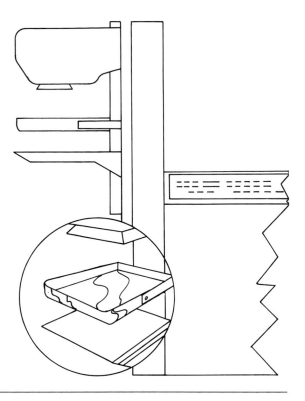

Figure 7-18 A Dedicated Mammographic Unit
Early mammograms were made with existing radiographic equipment. The collimator was removed from the unit and replaced with special
mammographic cones. Filtration was also removed because of the lower kilovoltage required
for breast examinations. Early direct exposure
technology utilized 22 kVp to 35 kVp at up to 1800
mAs (300 mA at 6 seconds). These exposure factors
were necessary to expose the fine-grain industrial
film (Eastman Kodak Type M) used for mammography. Today's new screen film mammographic
technique reduces dosage from 50 to 100 times.
Xeromammography also was developed in an effort to reduce patient dosage. Xeroradiographic
techniques with increased aluminum filtration permit the use of slightly higher kilovoltage values for
mammography.

Conventional radiographic equipment has
some limitations when used for mammography.
Calibration of kilovoltage should be a constant
concern. The collimator presents a problem. Even
when added filtration is removed, the mirror continues to function as part of the filtration system.
A buildup of tungsten on the tube window often
occurs if the unit is used regularly for other examinations. This tungsten deposit acts a a filter,
attenuating the x-ray beam.

In the later 1960s, a dedicated mammographic
unit using a molybdenum target with a 30-micra

molybdenum filter was made commercially available. This unit permitted vigorous compression
techniques. The patient for the first time was able
to be positioned, while erect, for both the cranio-
caudad and lateral projections. Prior to the introduction of this unit, the patient had to be seated
against the side of the table or a special tray for
the cranio-caudad projection and placed recumbent for the lateral or oblique projections. A typical
dedicated mammographic unit is shown with a
straight edge compression device (circular insert),
independent of the cone or collimator. Early units
had the compression paddle attached to the bottom of the cone. As the breast was compressed,
focal film distance changed producing some geometric difficulties. (See Fig. 7-17.) Some dedicated
units have a built-in Bucky for high-contrast mammography. This is particularly helpful when evaluating the dense breast. An automatic exposure
device is an option on most units. Small focal spot
tubes ensure high-resolution images. Direct roentgen enlargement techniques can be performed
with units having a fractional focal spot tube. The
breast is situated at a predetermined distance (increased OFD) from the detector to produce an
enlargement mammogram. Additional attachments are available to aid in localization techniques
prior to biopsy. The dedicated unit is recommended for screen film mammography or xeromammography.

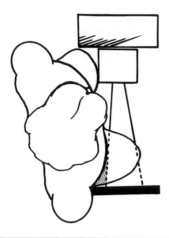

Figure 7-19 Visualization of the Chest Wall
When the rib cage is visualized on the lateral projection of the breast, it does not always indicate that all the posterior portion of the breast (shaded area) has been imaged.

The mammographer must gently pull the breast tissue forward from the chest wall while lifting the breast tissue into contact with the support tray and gently applying vigorous compression. If the patient's arm is hyperextended, it is difficult to pull the breast tissue forward. The arm should be relaxed, which in turn will relax the muscles along the chest wall. It is important to explain your intentions and the nature of the compression to the patient. Most patients are surprised by the vigorous compression and inadvertently fail to cooperate. A "whiteout" effect can occur adjacent to the chest wall if proper compression is not used. The use of an exaggerated curved edge compression device can intensify this problem. (See Figs. 7-21 and 7-22.)

image can be minimized (Figs. 7–21 and 7–22).

Film Holders for Mammography

Several types of mammographic film holders are available, including:

1 A polyvinyl chloride vacuum bag that uses an external vacuum source to exhaust air from the bag, producing screen film contact.

2 A polyethylene bag that is air evacuated in the darkroom, using a special heat-sealing vacuum unit to achieve screen film contact.

3 A screen film cassette. Because of the kilovoltage range needed, the front of a mammographic cassette must be made of a low x–ray-absorbing plastic. Maintaining screen film contact regardless of the system used is an ongoing concern.

Specific information regarding film holders for mammography can be found in Chapter 8 under the section entitled Specialty Cassettes.

Image sharpness is improved with a single intensifying screen and a single emulsion film designed with an antihalation backing to help prevent crossover of the light within the cassette. (See Fig. 8–11.)

Recent improvements in screen film design permit the use of two intensifying screens with a dual emulsion tabular grain (T-grain) mammographic film with crossover control. (See Fig. 8–3.)

Darkroom: Safelight Filters

There are two types of screen film combinations used for mammography: conventional phosphors (emitting primarily a blue light), and rare-earth phosphors (emitting primarily a green light). (See Chapter 8.) Appropriate blue or green sensitive films are matched to the screens. The use of an improper safelight with a green sensitive film will produce a fog-like supplemental density on the radiograph. Green sensitive film requires a special safelight filter (Eastman Kodak GBX). Either blue or green sensitive film can be used with the GBX safelight filter.

Automatic Processing

The manufacturer's recommendations for film processing of mammographic film regarding time, temperature, and processor maintenance must be followed. (See Chapter 10.)

Mammographic Enlargement

A fractional focal spot (0.3 mm or less) is a prerequisite for any enlargement technique, including mammography.

The image detector is placed at an increased distance from the breast (increased OFD) with a shortened FOD. The breast is approximately midway between the tube and

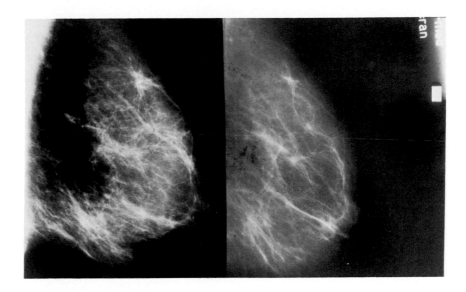

Figure 7-20 Screen Film Grid Study Compared With Direct Exposure Non-Grid Study *There is a considerable improvement in radiographic contrast on the grid or Bucky radiograph* (left) *compared with the direct exposure medium-speed industrial film mammogram* (right).

The moving grid was introduced in 1978 as part of a dedicated mammographic unit. Stationary grids with 200 lines per inch that fit inside mammographic cassettes are also available. They vary in ratio from 3.5:1 to 5:1. (See Fig. 5-11.)

Industrial film, direct exposure mammography is no longer in common use. (Courtesy of W. W. Logan, M.D. Rochester, New York)

the image receptor. This produces an enlarged radiograph (approximately 1.7×), making subtle details easier to detect.

IMPORTANT: Conventional focal spots cannot be used for direct roentgen enlargement techniques. Special stationary anode tubes with 90-micra focal spots are available for this procedure.

Electrostatic Imaging (Xeromammography)

Xeroradiography uses an electrostatic imaging process. A charged photoconductive plate made of selenium, held in a light-proof container (cassette), is used as a substitute for x-ray film or a screen film combination. The xeroradiographic process is described in Chapter 9.

Approximately 45 kVp to 55 kVp is required for xeromammography. Because of the higher kilovoltage, additional aluminum filtration must be used.

Radiation Dosage Consideration in Mammography

The dose levels of single screen/single emulsion mammographic film combinations can be up to 50 times lower than the dose levels of direct exposure film methods used in the 1960s, when patients were examined using low kilovoltage (25 kVp to 35 kVp at 1800 mAs) with direct exposure fine-grain industrial film.

The new dual screen/dual emulsion (T-grain) film mammography system is approximately two and one half times faster than single screen/single emulsion mammographic imaging products.

Mammographers should be aware of the reduction in dosage made possible by screen film and xeroradiographic techniques and

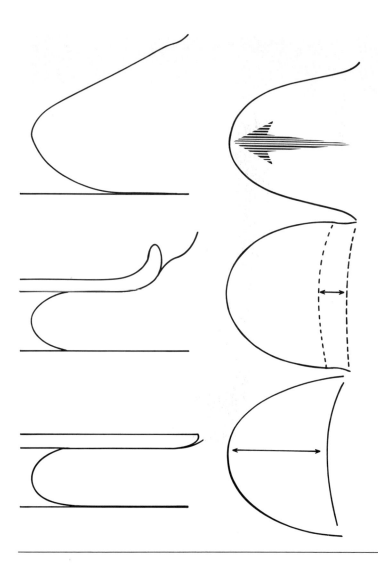

Figure 7-21. Compression Concepts for Mammography *The breast is shown with and without compression (left). Mammographic representations are also shown (right). Note the thickness of the breast at the chest wall (left, top). When an exaggerated curved compression device is used to flatten the breast tissue, note that the breast tissue moves backward and upward off the curved surface of the compression paddle (left, center). When a straight-edge compression paddle is used, an overall even tissue thickness is produced (left, bottom). The schematic representation of the breast on the right demonstrates these concepts. In the illustration (top, right), the arrow represents the difference in density from nipple to chest wall. The darkened portion of the arrow represents increased radiographic density, whereas the lightened posterior area of the arrow represents the thicker portion of the breast and decreased radiographic density. The dotted line (right, center) represents the "whiteout" often seen with poor compression. The bottom, right illustration represents visualization of all breast tissue from nipple to chest wall, achieved with vigorous straight edge compression. (See Fig. 7-22.) The radiographer, making a visual inspection prior to the exposure, can usually determine whether all breast tissue has been positioned over the image detector and is in alignment with the central ray.*

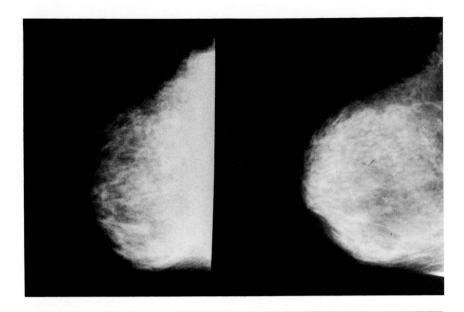

Figure 7-22 Clinical Application of Straight-Edge vs. Curved-Edge Compression *A lack of radiographic details ("whiteout") (left) adjacent to the chest wall is partially due to a portion of the breast tissue being pushed upward and backward along the chest wall by the curved edge of a plastic compression device. (See Fig. 7-21.) When vigorous straight-edge compression is used (right), more uniform compression of the breast tissue adjacent to the chest wall lessens the whiteout effect. Along with straight-edge compression, the mammographer must gently pull the breast forward while lifting the tissue onto the support tray to maximize tissue visualization. (Courtesy of W. W. Logan, MD, Rochester, New York)*

should be able to discuss these values when questioned.

Feig, in "Low Dose Mammography; Assessment Of Theoretical Risks in Breast Carcinoma; Current Diagnosis and Treatment", 1983, pp 69–76, Maisson Publishing USA, Incorporated, states that an examination with low-dosage techniques (single-emulsion) would carry a theoretical risk of about 1 excess cancer case/year/2 million women examined. The level of risk, 1 death/4 million women/year, is extremely small and can be equated with the following: 100 miles traveled by air, 15 miles traveled by car, smoking one fourth of one cigarette, one third of a minute of mountain climbing, and 5 minutes of being a man 60 years of age.

8 Conventional Recording Media

CONCURRENT with the production of x-radiation and x-ray images, the information must be recorded on x-ray film or other types of image detectors. Regardless of how carefully the image is produced, if attention is not given to the processing and handling of the recording media, a poor radiographic image will result. (See Chapter 10.)

The most commonly used recording media is x-ray film, used either in direct exposure techniques (an increasing rarity) or in conjunction with intensifying (fluorescent) screens. Intensifying screens, used to enhance the film blackening effect of x-radiation, will be described later in this chapter. Special image recording media is discussed in Chapter 9.

Composition of X-Ray Film

X-ray film consists of two major components: an emulsion (a gelatin mixture containing silver halide compounds), and a flexible support (film base) for the emulsion (Fig. 8–1). Within the film emulsion are very fine crystals or tablets of silver halide compounds (silver and bromide, chlorine, or iodine) suspended in a pure gelatin base. These compounds are sensitive to both light and x-ray. Gelatin is a very good vehicle for the silver compounds, because, in a solution, it will swell (become soft and flexible) without dissolving. Gelatin also rehardens quickly during the fixing process. (See Chapter 10.) The silver halide particles are dispersed as evenly as possible throughout the gelatin binder. The emulsion, 5 μm to 10 μm thick, is bound to the film base, approximately 180 μm thick, by an adhesive material (substratum).

The film base used to support the emulsion is made of transparent, nonflammable polyester or cellulose acetate. It must be strong, rigid, and flexible enough to be transported through all cycles of the processor. (See Chapter 10.) Polyester shrinks less when emersed in liquid, retains less moisture, and is thinner than cellulose acetate base. As a rule, radiographic film base is tinted blue to minimize the effect of ambient light passing through large unexposed areas of the radiograph. Some single emulsion medical imaging films used for procedures such as nuclear medicine imaging are coated on a clear base (Fig. 8–1C and D).

A protective coating is used over the emulsion to minimize damage resulting from handling.

By design, radiographic films are more sensitive to one part of the light spectrum than to another. Films are often described as either being panchromatic (sensitive to all colors of the light spectrum) or orthochromatic (sensitive to all colors of the light spectrum except red). Orthochromatic emulsions are sensitive to wavelengths less than 620 nm, whereas the panchromatic emulsions are sensitive to the whole visible spectrum, including the shorter wavelengths (Fig. 8–2). Prior to the early 1970s, x-ray films were primarily blue light sensitive. With the development of rare-earth intensifying screens, orthochromatic films came into common use.

Most radiographic films have emulsion on both sides of the film base (duplitized) and are used with a pair of intensifying screens so that the least amount of x-radiation can be used to produce a satisfactory radiographic density minimizing patient dosage.

Crystal Size and Shape

Silver halide crystals appear as pebble-like grains in conventional emulsions. With new silver halide technology known as *T-grain* (tabular grain), the crystals appear flat and tablet shaped. The tabular grains can be dispersed more evenly throughout the emulsion, resulting in better silver coverage, with less tendency to form film grain (Fig. 8–3).

The Effect of Light and X-Ray on Film

There are considerable bromide ions in silver halide crystals. When silver halide crystals absorb light or x-ray energy, a physical change occurs, which becomes apparent when the film is developed. When the proper level of energy strikes the bromide ions, they emit electrons. These electrons move to a sensitivity center in the halide crystal. The electrons

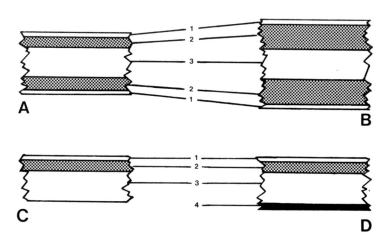

Figure 8-1   Cross Section of Types of Radiographic Films   *Most radiographic emulsions are coated on a blue tinted film base (2). Duplitized medical radiographic film (A and B) has emulsion coated on both sides of the base (2). A protective coating (1) covers the emulsion to minimize damage from handling.*

Medical screen x-ray film (dual emulsion; A) is used with intensifying screens. The emulsion is designed to respond primarily to the light of the intensifying screen. Nonscreen radiographic film emulsions (B) respond primarily to the direct effect of x-ray and are considerably thicker than the emulsions used for screen-type radiographic film. Single-emulsion radiographic films (C and D) are generally used with a single high-detail intensifying screen for extremity radiograph or mammography or in multiformat cameras for cathode ray tube (CRT) imaging. These films, similar to photographic film, are usually designed with an antihalation backing (D) to minimize the effect of "crossover" of light within the cassette.

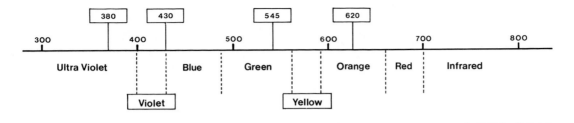

Figure 8-2 Electromagnetic Spectrum *The electromagnetic spectrum is illustrated from 300 nm to 800 nm. Ultraviolet, blue, and green sensitivity ranges are shown. Film is designed to respond to specific emissivity ranges of the phosphors used in the intensifying screens.*

(negatively charged) attract the silver ions (positively charged). The electron and sensitivity speck interaction causes the silver halide crystal to be converted into atoms of metallic silver.

The degree of absorption of light or x-ray energy by the crystals produces a latent image, which is converted into a visible image (the presence of black metallic silver) by chemical processing.

Characteristics of X-Ray Film

Medical x-ray film must possess the following characteristics:

1 *Speed* (sensitivity). The emulsion must possess the ability to respond to both light and x-ray. Radiographic film is often referred to as being of standard, medium, or fast speed. This type of rating is no longer appropriate with new intensifying screen film combinations. In the past, film could be rated independently of the intensifying screens. If 100-speed intensifying screens were matched to 100-speed radiographic film, the system speed would be rated at 100. In many rare-earth combinations, faster screens may be used with a slower film. Rather than labeling a screen or a film individually as to speed, screen film combination speed should be considered.

2 *Latitude.* Latitude can be described in two ways: (a) *Film latitude*: the emulsion must be able to record a relatively long range of densities, from the blackest black (gas or air) to the whitest white (dense osseous structures or barium-filled organs), with all shades in between. (b) *Exposure latitude*: the margin for exposure error with any given technique. (See Chapters 11 and 12.)

3 *Contrast.* The capability of a film to record differences in density. Film contrast is directly related to latitude. A film possessing long-scale contrast will exhibit increased exposure latitude. (See Chapters 11 and 12.)

Sensitometry

Quantitative measurements of the response of the film to exposure and development, known as sensitometry, can be made.

A sensitometer is used to expose a step-wedge of photographic densities on an unexposed radiographic film. To avoid variations in light intensities, a high quality light source and timer is incorporated into this unit (Fig. 8–4, *top*).

The film, exposed with a sensitometer to a predetermined level, produces a stepwedge of densities from clear (white) to black after processing. (See Fig. 11–2). The sharply demarcated density variations are then evaluated (read) with a densitometer (instrument used to measure various degrees of blackening on the processed radiograph; Fig. 8–4, bottom).

A sensitometer and densitometer are prerequisites for a quality assurance (QA) program. These devices are also used to monitor the automatic processor. (See Chapter 10.)

Density variations can be displayed on a meter or electronic readout and recorded on graph paper. These readings are used to gen-

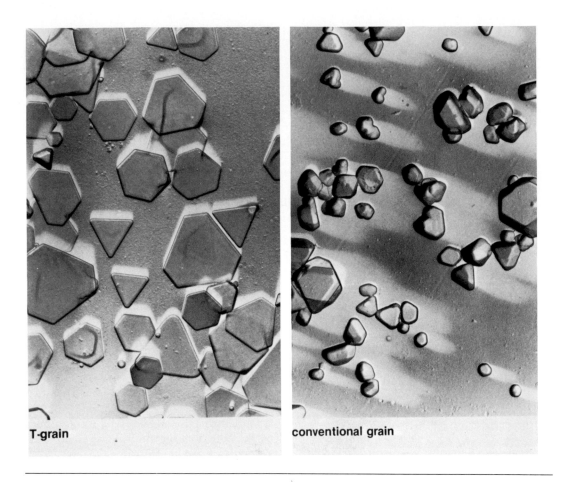

T-grain

conventional grain

Figure 8-3 T-Grain Emulsion (Tabular Grain) *Silver halide crystals can be described as pebble-like grains in conventional radiographic film emulsions. T-grain crystals found in new film emulsion technology are tabular shaped. These flat grains can be dispersed more evenly throughout the emulsion. Better silver coverage occurs with the flat tablet-like grains. A dye is used in the film emulsion in T-grain technology to minimize light crossover within the cassette during an x-ray exposure. (See Fig. 8-11.) with a significant improvement in image sharpness. (Courtesy of Eastman Kodak Company, Rochester, New York)*

erate a sensitometric curve (characteristic curve or H & D curve, after Hurter and Driffield). The characteristic curve was first described by Hurter and Driffield, students of photography in Great Britain, in 1890. The curve is a graphic representation between the exposure received by the film and the densities produced after processing (Fig. 8–5). A logarithmic scale is necessary to confine the graph to a reasonable size. (See Fig. 11-4). A relationship can be expressed between the logarithm of exposure and the radiographic density. (See Chapter 11.)

A typical characteristic curve consists of a toe, a straight line portion, and a shoulder (Fig. 8–5, *left*).

The toe or lower portion of the curve is measured after an adjustment has been made for base density (inherent in every radiographic film) and base plus fog density.

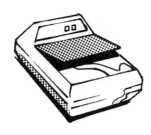

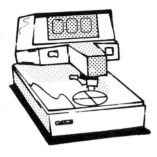

Figure 8-4 Sensitometer and Densitometer
A sensitometer is used to expose a stepwedge of varying photographic densities on unexposed radiographic film (top). A high-quality light source with an accurate timer is a prerequisite for this device. The processed image of the stepwedge exhibits sharply demarcated density variations from clear (white) to black. (See Fig. 11-2.) The stepwedge image is evaluated using a densitometer, which measures the various degrees of density on the processed radiograph (bottom). These variations are transferred to graph paper to form a sensitometric or characteristic curve that illustrates the properties of the film under study. When the densitometer is properly calibrated and there is no film under the sensor, the reading should be 0.00.

Base density is the result of manufacturing parameters and includes the blue tint in the base of the film. The fog density is caused by development of unexposed silver halide crystals during processing. (See Chapter 10.) Although the base of a single sheet of unexposed processed film may appear transparent to the eye, the superimposition of two or more sheets of clear (after processing) film will demonstrate the presence of a base plus fog density.

The minimal density (D-Min) is the least density on the film after exposure and is usually slightly higher than base plus fog density.

The straight line portion of the curve represents the useful imaging portion of the curve. Average gradient reflects both film contrast and latitude. This is measured on the sensitometric curve from 0.25 density above base fog and 2.0 density above base fog and is defined as the slope of the curve. The shoulder of the curve represents the area of greatest radiographic density. Maximal density (D-Max) is read at the shoulder of the curve (Fig. 8–5, right).

Variations in density, demonstrated by the characteristic curve, are a function of exposure (photographic effect). (See Chapter 11.) As exposure rates are changed, the film changes in density.

Contrast and latitude can also be illustrated by the characteristic curve. Film contrast is determined by the manufacturer and influenced by development. (See Chapter 10.) Subject contrast is influenced by the patient (tissue absorption differences). (See Chapter 11.) The combination of subject and film contrast results in radiographic contrast. (See Chapter 11.) Radiographic contrast is the density differences between adjacent areas of the radiographic image. Latitude can be described as the range of exposures in the generally accepted medical density range (0.25–2.0; Fig. 8–5, *right*). As a general rule, an increase in contrast (shorter scale) produces a decrease in latitude, and vice versa.

Types of X-Ray Film

Nonscreen Film

Nonscreen radiographic film responds primarily to the direct effects of x-ray exposure. The emulsion is considerably thicker than the emulsion of screen-type radiographic film. Nonscreen radiographic film requires significantly more exposure than screen film used in combination with intensifying screens. Because of the thicker emulsion, nonscreen film must usually be manually processed (Fig. 8–1B). Increased silver content (thicker emulsion), processing limitations, and high radia-

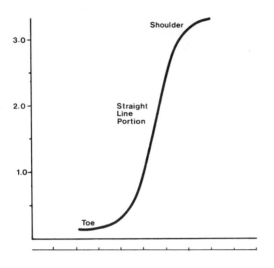

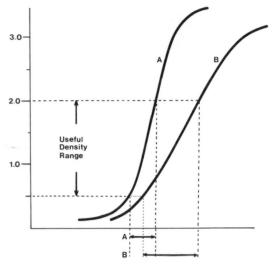

Figure 8-5 Sensitometric Curves *A typical sensitometric curve (left). The vertical axis illustrates increased density; the horizontal axis shows increased exposure. Exposure is expressed logarithmically to confine the graph to a reasonable size. (See Fig. 11-4.)*

The characteristic or sensitometric curve can be described as follows: toe (the inferior portion), ascending or straight line portion (useful density range), shoulder (top of the curve).

Contrast and latitude parameters can be illustrated by the characteristic curve (right).

Film A in the useful density range (0.25–2.0) exhibits poor exposure latitude, whereas film B, also in the useful density range (0.25–2.0), exhibits considerably more latitude.

Abrupt density differences (short scale contrast) will occur with film A. Longer scale contrast (more shades of gray) will occur with film B.

Film speed is determined by the position of the sensitometric curve on the graph. Since the horizontal axis documents increased exposure from left to right, film A would require less exposure than film B to achieve a given density (vertical axis).

tion dosage requirements discourage most radiographers from using this product. For some special purpose examinations, such as evaluation for a metallic foreign body, an increase in x-ray exposure may be justified. A dust artifact on an intensifying screen can mimic or hide a small foreign body.

IMPORTANT: The term *nonscreen technique* is often erroneously substituted for direct exposure technique. Any radiographic exposure using film in a light-proof holder without intensifying screens is a direct exposure. When screen-type film is used in a direct exposure (without screens), it is considerably slower (3–4 times) than nonscreen film in a direct exposure. Screen film requires fluorescent light from intensifying screens for optimal efficiency.

Medical Screen X-Ray Film

Medical screen x-ray film (usually dual emulsion) is designed to be used in combination with intensifying screens. The film differs from nonscreen film in that its emulsion layers are considerably thinner. (Fig. 8–1A).

It is important that a thin film base be used to support the emulsions. The thinner the base, the sharper the superimposed images, with a lessening of the parallax effect (image separation) associated with tube angle techniques. (See Fig. 11–15).

Medical screen x-ray film responds to the fluorescent light given off by activated intensifying screens. Film blackening or density is created primarily by the fluorescent light emitted by the intensifying screens. Radiographic film can be designed to respond primarily to a specific color in the light spectrum. Intensifying screens can likewise be made to emit light (luminesce) in a specific color range (Fig. 8–2).

IMPORTANT: The color sensitivity of radiographic film should be matched to the light emissivity of the screen for optimal results. For example, a primarily blue sensitive film should be used with intensifying screens that are primarily blue emitters.

All radiographic films, whether nonscreen or screen, are sensitive to the direct action of x-rays.

Single Emulsion Radiographic Film

Some radiographic examinations such as mammography or extremity radiography require highly detailed images. A single emulsion film is often used with a single intensifying screen for this purpose. Most single emulsion films have an antihalation backing to absorb "crossover" of light within the cassette, thereby improving image quality (Fig. 8–1D; see Screen: Crossover of Light).

IMPORTANT: The emulsion side of the film must be placed against the intensifying screen. If the antihalation backing is placed against the intensifying screen, there will be a significant decrease in radiographic density.

Film Storage And Handling

When the correct technical factors are used, it can be frustrating to a radiographer if a marginal quality radiograph is produced. Poor storage and handling habits may be responsible for some of these problems.

Heat and moisture hasten the deterioration of radiographic film. High temperatures will produce a foglike density on the processed film. The ideal temperatures for storage of radiographic film vary with unprocessed or processed film. Fresh, unexposed radiographic film should be stored at 50° to 70° F. After processing, radiographs can tolerate higher storage temperatures (60° to 80° F). Both unexposed and processed film should be stored at a 30% to 50% humidity range.

Unexposed radiographic film must be ro-

tated in storage, and older film should be used first. The expiration date of the film is listed on every box of film. Radiographic film fog is often due to out-of-date film. (See Chapter 10.) Film that is out of date can lose both speed and contrast. (See Chapter 11.)

IMPORTANT: High-speed (increased sensitivity) unexposed radiographic films often have a shorter shelf life. Film must be protected from all forms of radiation, including x-ray and light. Radiographic film should be kept in a secure area. These products represent a considerable portion of the department operating budget. The potential for theft parallels the need for security.

Film Artifacts

Poor storage and careless film handling habits can produce radiographic artifacts. Fogging as a result of accidental exposure to light, improper safelight conditions, exposure to ionizing radiation, storage of film at high temperatures, or the use of film beyond its expiration date have been mentioned. Other areas of concern include exposure of radiographic film to chemicals and fumes from gases, formalin, ammonia, and oils.

To avoid physical pressure marks (artifacts), unexposed boxes of film should be stored on their side—not stacked on top of each other. Artifacts such as dark crescent–shaped marks may also be caused by bending or pinching of the film during handling. Static electricity is a common cause of film artifacts. Tree-like static markings occur because of rapid movement of the film in the darkroom. Film pulled quickly from its box often builds up an electric charge sufficient to discharge on the radiographic film as tree-like static. A crown mark is similar to tree-like static. Smudges occur when electrical discharges follow a path formed by either dust, lint, a rough intensifying screen surface, or a roughened work counter (Fig. 8–6).

Other Recording Media

Special recording media is discussed in Chapter 9. Topics that are presented include the

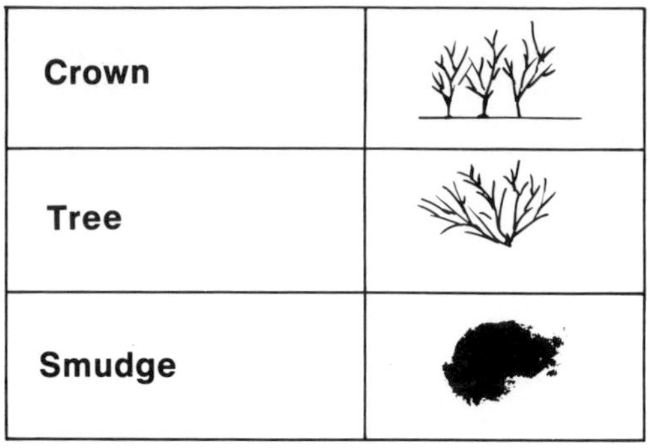

Crown	
Tree	
Smudge	

Figure 8-6   Static Electricity Artifacts
Schematic representation of typical static artifacts are shown, including crown, tree, and smudge markings.
Electrical discharges produce these patterns.

uses of single emulsion of film for both mammography and extremities; single emulsion photographic film for photofluorography, computed tomography, ultrasonography, nuclear medicine, and magnetic resonance imaging; duplicating and subtraction films; radiation therapy portal and verification films; dental products, including periapical, bitewing, occlusal, and pantomography film; and imaging products used with the Polaroid and Xeoradiographic systems.

Intensifying Screens

The emission of light by a material excited by any form of energy is known as *luminescence*. Luminescence, the giving off of light (without heat) is present in both phosphorescence and fluorescence. Incandescence is not a form of luminescence.

One of the properties of x-radiation is that it can cause certain substances to fluoresce or phosphoresce. The terms *fluorescence* and *phosphorescence* are used to describe the luminescence phenomenon that occurs when x-ray energy is converted into light energy by the interaction of x-rays with certain phosphors.

If the light emission ceases almost simultaneously with the termination of the x-ray energy, the process is known as fluorescence. If the phosphor continues to glow after the activating force (x-ray exposure) has been terminated, the process is called phosphorescence.

Properties of Phosphors

Many phosphors are efficient x-ray absorbers and fluoresce with little or no afterglow. Afterglow (screen lag) describes a persistent light after the x-ray energy has ceased. This is not a desirable feature in intensifying screen design.

Photon absorption is affected not only by the type of phosphor used but also by the thickness and packing density of the phosphor layer. For any given phosphor and crystal size, the greater the number of crystals in the path of the x-ray photons, the greater the absorption. Therefore, increasing the screen thickness increases x-ray absorption if packing density remains constant.

Only a portion of the x-ray photons is absorbed by the screens. This absorption can vary from one type of screen to another (Fig. 8–7). The x-ray photons that are absorbed by the intensifying screen are converted into light photons to be used to expose the radiographic film.

Types of Intensifying Screens

The purpose of intensifying screens is to "capture" the remnant radiation that has exited from the patient and to convert this energy into light to expose radiographic film. The amount of radiant energy emitted from the screen is dependent upon the type of phosphor used (Fig. 8–7); the design of the screen (Fig. 8–8); the size and layer thickness of the phosphor (Fig. 8–9); the use of light-restricting dyes (if any) within the screen (Fig. 8–10); the kilovoltage range used for the exposure (see Chapter 11); the amount of total x-ray energy used; and the absorption/conversion ratio of the phosphor (Fig. 8–7). Intensifying screens are used either alone or in pairs.

Screens can be manufactured to emit light that is either primarily blue, green, or ultraviolet. Most screens emit a combination of these colors with one spectrum dominating. For maximal efficiency, the films used with

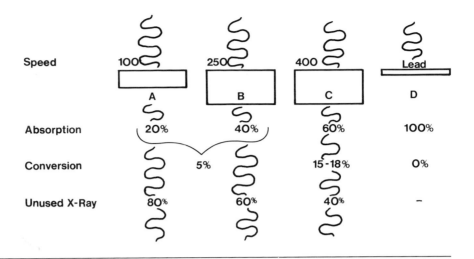

Speed	100	250	400	Lead
	A	B	C	D
Absorption	20%	40%	60%	100%
Conversion		5%	15-18%	0%
Unused X-Ray	80%	60%	40%	–

Figure 8-7 Absorption/Conversion Ratio of Intensifying Screens *Screen film combinations have been arbitrarily labeled as to speed. Most speed comparisons are made against a conventional medium-speed (par) intensifying screen using blue sensitive conventional speed x-ray film, labeled speed 100 (A).*

Before x-radiation can be converted to light, it must be absorbed by the phosphor. An increase in layer thickness will result in an increased absorption of the photons (B). Rare earth phosphors inherently absorb more x-ray than conventional calcium tungstate phosphors of an equal thickness (C).

A thin sheet of lead, the type used to divide cassettes for multiple images, will absorb 100% of the x-ray beam (D). Absorption, therefore, is only a part of the function of an intensifying screen. The x-ray photons that are absorbed must be converted into light that can be used to expose radiographic film. Conventional 100-speed (A) and 250-speed (B) calcium tungstate screens absorb 20% or 40% of the x-ray beam, respectively, converting 5% of what they absorb into useful light. A gadolinium oxysulfide rare-earth intensifying screen (C) of equal thickness to the 250-speed calcium tungstate screen will absorb 60% of the primary beam and convert 15% to 18% of the absorbed x-ray to useful light. A rare-earth screen absorbs more x-ray per equal thickness and converts more of the absorbed energy to light.

the screens must be responsive to the color of light that is primarily emitted (Fig. 8–2).

IMPORTANT: Care must be taken to select the proper safelight filter in the darkroom to match the spectral sensitivity of the radiographic film in use. (See Chapter 10.)

Screens: Construction

Until recently, intensifying screens were made of calcium tungstate or barium lead sulfate. Rare-earth materials such as gadolinium oxysulfide, lanthanum oxysulfide, and lanthanum oxybromide now dominate screen design. Many of the rare-earth elements used in the manufacture of intensifying screens are more available than the term *rare-earth* implies; however, rare-earth phosphors are expensive and difficult to refine from their natural ores. The phosphors must be as pure as possible in order to control spectral light emissivity. After the phosphor is refined, an activator is added to shift the spectral emission to the predominantly desired light output.

Calcium tungstate phosphors emit light at approximately 420 nm (4200 A), primarily in the blue spectrum. Some rare-earth screens, by design, emit light primarily in the green spectrum, approximately 545 nm (5450 A) (Fig. 8–2). In reality, all green emitting screens give off some blue and ultraviolet light as well as green light. Blue intensifying screens (conventional or rare-earth) emit some green and

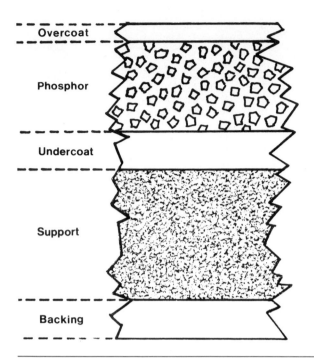

Overcoat

Phosphor

Undercoat

Support

Backing

Figure 8-8 Intensifying Screens
A support (paper or plastic) is used as a base for the intensifying screen. A backing is applied to the support to prevent curling of the screen. An undercoat is used to hold the phosphor layer to the support. The undercoating can be reflective (see Fig. 8-11) or absorptive. The phosphor layer is covered with an overcoat to minimize abrasions resulting from handling.

ultraviolet light. If radiographic films are mismatched to the intensifying screens, the system will function at approximately half speed. A major exception is the Kodak Lanex medium screen impregnated with a yellow dye to minimize screen blur (Fig. 8–10). This dye absorbs most of the blue light emitted by the screens so that the radiographic film is exposed predominantly by green light. If a blue sensitive flim is used inadvertently with a Lanex medium screen, an even further decrease in film blackening occurs. Instead of a half-speed film density, there is a film blackening of approximately one fifth or less of the anticipated density.

For many years, calcium tungstate screens used for detail techniques were deliberate "stained" with a yellow, tan, or pink dye. This produced very slow screens (speed 5 to speed 50; Fig. 8–10). For improved sharpness, some mammographic and extremity screens are manufactured using this principle.

> **IMPORTANT:** When screens are accidentally stained or discolored by age or contaminants such as coffee or carbonated beverages, no sharpness benefit occurs. This discoloration is a localized surface phenomenon rather than a dye impregnation of the entire screen.

Screen Design

ASYMMETRICAL SCREENS

When intensifying screens were made with phosphors that were low x-ray absorbers, symmetrical screens (of equal thickness) were in common use. Rare-earth intensifying

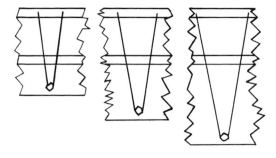

Figure 8-9 Intensifying Screen Design
Intensifying screen crystal size can influence speed. In general, the larger the phosphor crystal, the more light it emits when exposed to x-radiation. Larger crystals produce more unsharpness than smaller crystals. In actual practice, the crystals vary in size, and layer thickness of the crystals is the primary influence on the speed of the intensifying screen. The thicker the layer, the faster the screen.

A single crystal situated posteriorly in each of the phosphor layers illustrates the effect of layer thickness on sharpness. The thicker screen produces more light spreading in the film emulsion than the thinner screen, therefore more image unsharpness.

Note: *Crossover of light to the opposite emulsion with a further increase in the spreading of the light. (See Fig. 8-11.)*

screens absorb considerably more x-ray than do conventional calcium tungstate screens (Fig. 8–7). The anterior intensifying screen in a rare-earth system can absorb a disproportionate amount of x-ray energy compared with a calcium tungstate screen, leaving less x-ray energy available for the posterior screen. In order to equally blacken both emulsions of the radiographic film, rare-earth screens are sometimes designed asymmetrically, with the anterior screen thinner (to absorb less x-ray).

An undercoat is added to the intensifying screens and can be either light reflective or light absorbtive (Fig. 8–8). When the undercoat is reflective, unused light is directed toward the film, with an increase in system speed. Unfortunately, this can also cause some loss of image sharpness (Fig. 8–11).

An overcoat is added to protect the screen from damage (Fig. 8–8).

GRADIENT INTENSIFYING SCREENS

Gradient intensifying screens are often used for full-length vascular studies of the leg or for radiographs of the entire spine (scoliosis evaluation). These screens can be up to 51 in. in length, with speeds varying from one end to the other. For example, a gradient screen may be rated 400 speed at one end and diminish in speed to 100 at the opposite end. The thicker body part is placed over the faster portion of the gradient screen. For a scoliosis study, the faster portion of the intensifying screen is positioned beneath the lumbar region; the slower portions are positioned in the cervicothoracic area. With gradient screens, all regions of the body that are in the x-ray field receive an equal amount of radiation.

IMPORTANT: Compensatory filters should be used instead of gradient screens whenever possible to equalize differences in patient density. (See Figs. 4–10 to 4–12.)

Crossover of Light

It would be helpful if the light emitted by the intensifying screen exposed only the emulsion proximal to the screen. However, light from an intensifying screen passes from emulsion to emulsion through the film base. This effect is called "crossover" of light. As each individual phosphor gives off a cone of light, significant crossover of light with lateral spreading occurs from emulsions to emulsion with a decrease in image sharpness (Fig. 8–11).

When a light-absorbing dye is added to an intensifying screen, the shortest path for light to travel from the fluorescing crystals to the radiographic film is in a perpendicular line. As light spreads laterally, considerably more dye must be penetrated, absorbing some of the "halo" effect of the fluorescing crystals. Assuming that each individual crystal gives off light in the shape of a circle, the thickness of the screen, the presence or absence of light-absorbing dye, and the size of the crystal influence the size of this circle of light. The circle continues to widen as the light spreads from emulsion to emulsion. If a light-absorbing dye is used in the screen binder or on the film base, smaller circles of light are produced (Fig.

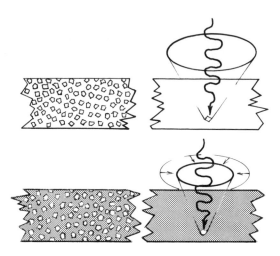

Figure 8-10   The Use of Light-Restricting Dyes in Intensifying Screens   *A typical intensifying screen is shown* (top, right) *with a single phosphor as the light source. The x-ray photon strikes the phosphor, and a halo of light is produced. Light is given off in all directions from the activated phosphor. Some of the light bounces posteriorly and is redirected laterally or frontally from the poste-rior reflective layer. (See Fig. 8-11.) If the intensi-fying screen is impregnated with a dye during manufacturing, the size of the halo of light can be reduced* (bottom, right). *Much of the light that is reflected or spread laterally is absorbed by the dye, restricting the halo of light from each individual crystal. Image sharpness is improved.*

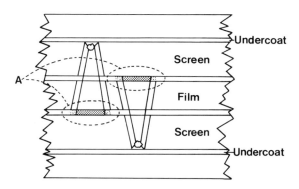

Figure 8-11   Reflection and/or Crossover of Light   *When an x-ray photon penetrates a cas-sette with two intensifying screens, the phosphor gives off light in all directions (spatial). Some of this light can be reflected anteriorly from the pos-terior undercoating to the x-ray emulsion. This light continues to widen (halo effect) and crosses over to the opposite emulsion, producing image unsharpness. (Modified, courtesy of Eastman Ko-dak Company, Rochester, NY)*

8–10). The result is an increase in image sharpness.

Most radiographic film screen combinations permit a 30% or greater crossover of light. New design parameters cut crossover of light approximately in half.

Effective crossover control was first achieved with screens that emitted primarily ultraviolet light, because the silver halide emulsion absorbs a high percentage of the ultraviolet light.

Some manufacturers use special dyes added to the film base prior to the coating of the emulsions to minimize crossover. T-grain (tabular grain) technology uses a dye in the film emulsion to minimize crossover, with an improvement in image sharpness (Fig. 8–3).

In the future, crossover control will become an industry standard, with zero crossover as a goal.

Intensifying Screen Speed

Intensifying screen film combinations are classified according to their speed and resolution. Generally speaking, the slower the intensifying screen, the greater the radiographic detail. (See Chapter 11.)

Most radiographers compare system speed only, for example, speed 250 calcium tungstate to speed 250 gadolinium oxysulfide. Although both of the screens in the given example are the same system speed (250), the rare-earth screen with its higher absorption/conversion ratio (Fig. 8–7) produces a considerably sharper radiographic image. Speed 400 gadolinium oxysulfide intensifying screen produces a radiographic image with approximately the same resolution as speed 250 calcium tungstate intensifying screen. T-grain films, with their improved crossover control, when used with rare-earth screens, further increase sharpness.

Another factor that may affect the speed of intensifying screens is temperature (a theoretical consideration). When room temperature is above 100°F, an intensifying screen will respond slower to x-radiation. When room temperature is below 30°F, the screen will respond faster. It is of interest that the opposite effect occurs with radiographic film. In reality, these effects are probably cancelled out, one by the other. Extreme temperature ranges (30°–100°F) are rarely encountered in radiographic departments.

The speed of an intensifying screen is influenced by the following factors:

1 Type of phosphor.
2 Thickness of the phosphor layer. In general, the faster the speed of the intensifying screen (if all are of the same phosphor type), the less detail on the processed radiograph. This is generally the result of an increase in the phosphor layer thickness (Fig. 8–9).
3 Size of the phosphor crystal (a theoretical concept, not in common use).
4 Absorption/conversion ratio of the screen. For an equal thickness, screens manufactured with rare-earth phosphors not only absorb more radiation but also have a higher light conversion ratio; that is, they convert more of the absorbed x-radiation to image-forming light (Fig. 8–7).
5 Absence or presence of a reflective layer (Figs. 8–8 and 8–11).
6 A light-absorbing layer (as opposed to a reflective layer) between the phosphor and the screen support (Fig. 8–8).
7 Kilovoltage range. Rare-earth intensifying screens are more kVp dependent than other phosphors. Screen speed differences can occur, particularly if the high (150 kVp) and low (30 kVp) extremes of a kilovoltage range are used. Extreme variations in kVp can cause a falloff in light emissivity with some rare-earth film screen combinations. When a technique chart using a rare-earth film screen combination is formulated and low kilovoltages are required (pediatric or extremity radiography), an adjustment must often be made in the mAs factors.

Advantages of the Use of Intensifying Screens

Some benefits that occur when using intensifying screens as opposed to direct exposure techniques include:

1 Shorter exposure times.
2 Reduced patient and operator dosage.
3 Less motion unsharpness.

4 Contrast improvement (shorter scale) when lower kilovoltage values are indicated.

5 X-ray tube life can be extended.

6 Smaller focal spots can often be used.

The increased benefits of using rare-earth film screen technology over conventional phosphors are:

1 An even greater potential for the small focal spots; the use of fractional focal spots (0.3 mm or smaller) for direct roentgen enlargement techniques. (See Chapter 9.)

2 Reduced mAs required for adequate film blackening (less instantaneous load) (see Chapter 4); greater film-blackening effect with lower output generators, such as bedside units (Table 8–1). (See Chapter 2.)

3 Less heat units generated (lower anode thermal loading). (See Chapter 4.)

Reciprocity Law

When using a direct exposure film technique, any combination of mA and time (as long as the product equals the same mAs) produces the same film-blackening effect. This is known as the reciprocity law.

When film blackening is produced by light photons from an intensifying screen, a failure in the reciprocity relationship can occur with very short or very long exposures, such as those used in the posteroanterior (PA) chest exposure (10 msec or less) or with pluridirectional tomographic studies (6 sec – 9 sec).

Radiographic Mottle

Occasionally unwanted fluctuations in optical densities can be seen on a processed radio-graph. This can be described as radiographic mottle (noise). Radiographic mottle can be composed of either film graininess (a rare occurrence), structure mottle (from the screen), or quantum mottle.

Radiographic mottle is rarely due to the random distribution of developed silver halide grains (film graininess).

Structure mottle from variations in intensifying screen crystal sizes is even more rare than film graininess.

Quantum mottle, on the other hand, a variation in optical density resulting from the random distribution of x-ray quanta absorbed by the x-ray receptor, is more common. One can generally categorize the density fluctuations seen on an exposed, processed radiograph as quantum mottle.

Quantum mottle exists to some degree in all screen film radiographs. The faster the system speed or the higher the kilovoltage used, the more likely the visualization of quantum mottle (Fig. 8–12). Increased film blackening, achieved with increased mAs, results in a more homogenous image, and quantum mottle is less likely to be visualized.

Resolution

Visualization of a radiographic detail is influenced by object size and radiographic contrast. Small details require very high contrast for adequate visualization, whereas more gross details can be seen with lesser contrast. Some loss in contrast will occur owing to scatter radiation resulting in decreased radiographic detail. (See Chapter 5.) Additional information on resolution can be found in Chapter 11.

Screen Maintenance

Screens should be cleaned regularly using manufacturers' recommendations. Cleaning eliminates surface marks, which may result in artifacts on the radiograph. This is particularly important if a screen film combination is used to localize small opaque foreign bodies. Dirt or dust particles can mimic or hide small radiopaque foreign bodies. Because artifacts shield the film from the fluorescent light of the intensifying screen, a minus density (white) is produced. Intensifying screen cleaner should never be sprayed directly on an intensifying screen. Excessive spraying or

TABLE 8-1. Film Blackening Effect of Intensifying Screens

mA	Speed			
	100	*400* *4×*	*800* *8×*	*1200* *12×*
50	50	200	400	600
150	150	600	1,200	1,800
300	300	1,200	2,400	3,600
1,000	1,000	4,000	8,000	12,000
1,500	1,500	6,000	12,000	18,000

Figure 8-12   Quantum Mottle
Quantum mottle exists to some degree in all screen film radiographs. It can be a problem in studies in which minute radiographic details might be obscured.

Two representations of quantum mottle are shown. This mottled appearance is not due to film graininess. It is significantly more coarse than film grain and is due to nonuniform light emission from the intensifying screen. On the left is an image made with a relatively fast x-ray system, re-quiring a minimal amount of x-ray for exposure; therefore, the mottled pattern is more pronounced. On the right, a slow intensifying screen was used, which required increased exposure (increased mAs), producing a more homogenous image. Quantum mottle is less pronounced in this image.

Note the improved detail of the plastic bead test object with the slower system. (Courtesy of Eastman Kodak Company, Rochester, New York)

improper drying of the screen can cause screen damage.

Cassette

The cassette, a container for exposed and unexposed radiographic film, is used to protect the film from light. Most cassettes have fronts made of either bakelite or magnesium. Intensifying screens are mounted within the cassette.

A thin sheet of lead foil is often mounted underneath the back intensifying screen to absorb backscatter (Fig. 8–13). (See Chapter 5.)

When conventional cassettes are used for high-detail extremity radiography or mammography, a single intensifying screen is used with an antihalation-backed radiographic film.

Film Screen Contact

Film screen contact must be maintained to minimize blurring of radiographic details ow-ing to lateral spreading of light from the activated phosphors in the screen. Often, poor screen film contact (segmental blurring of the radiographic image) is mistaken for motion blur. Bending or warping of the cassette can cause poor screen contact. Sometimes the weight of a patient placed directly on a cassette can produce a temporary contact problem (Fig. 8–14).

To evaluate screen film contact, a radiograph with a background density of approximately 1.0 should be made of a wire mesh. Wires in an area of poor contact will appear blurred. When viewed, they will seem to be slightly darker than the wires in surrounding areas. When evaluating a radiograph for screen film contact using the wire mesh test, the image should be placed on a viewbox and viewed at a distance of between 10 feet and 12 feet. Diffuse halo-like shadows (poor film screen contact) are more obvious at these distances. If an extended viewing distance is not practical, the images should be viewed at an oblique angle to avoid the excessive amount of light emitted by the viewbox.

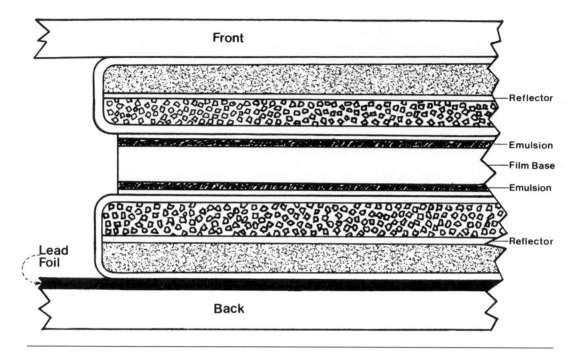

Front

Reflector

Emulsion

Film Base

Emulsion

Reflector

Lead Foil

Back

Figure 8-13 Cross Section of Cassette, Screens, and Radiographic Film *The cassette is a container for both exposed or unexposed film. A pair of intensifying screens in intimate contact with a duplitized x-ray film is shown in a light-proof cassette. The cassette front is usually made of bakelite, magnesium, or some type of low radiation absorbing material. A thin sheet of lead foil is often mounted underneath the posterior intensi-fying screen to absorb backscatter.*

X-ray photons continue to the posterior screen where the reflective or crossover phenomenon is duplicated. The absence of a reflective screen adds to the sharpness of the image. The control of the crossover of light by either dye impregnation of the screen or the presence of a light absorbing dye in the radiographic film (T-grain technology; Fig. 8-3) can improve radiographic sharpness.

Direct exposure film holders are sometimes used for extremity radiography. These non-screen holders protect the film from light and may also contain a lead foil backing to minimize backscatter. (See Chapter 5.)

Low x-ray–absorbing materials that lessen the absorption of the primary x-ray beam are available for cassette fronts and radiographic tabletops. The designers and manufacturers of these products claim a 35% or greater increase in film blackening when compared with conventional cassette front or tabletop materials.

IMPORTANT: While an increase in film blackening owing to the low absorption front material seems impressive, rare-earth film screen combinations produce up to a 1200% increase in film blackening when compared with medium-speed systems (speed 100) (Table 8–1).

Specialty Cassettes

Special cassettes have been designed for mammography, tomography, and unusual positioning techniques.

A reduced exposure mammographic cassette is available, with a polycarbonate and polystyrene front for minimal absorption of the primary beam. The low absorption front is important for screen film mammography because of the low kilovoltage requirements. (See Chapter 7.) Very thin cassette edges permit placement of the cassette in close contact with the chest wall. Vacuum cassettes are also

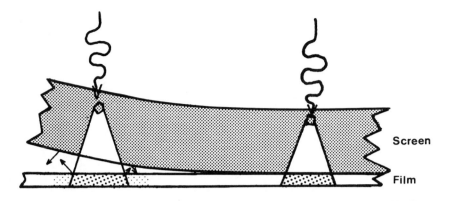

Screen

Film

Figure 8-14   Screen Film Contact
Screen film contact is essential to minimize blurring of the radiographic image. Bending or warping of the cassette can produce poor screen contact. As the screen is pulled away from the film emulsion, the halo of light widens. If the light source (screen) is not in contact with the film, light can reflect in many directions, producing segmental blurring of the image. (Modified, courtesy of Eastman Kodak Company, Rochester, NY)

used with mammographic techniques. There are two types of vacuum cassettes. A flexible reusable vinyl cassette is available, with a built-in vacuum valve and an internal envelope, which can be removed for easy film loading. When reloaded, the end of the vacuum bag can be resealed with a plastic spacer. The air can be evacuated from the bag by means of the vacuum valve, attached to either a hand pump or a motor-driven suction unit.

A second type of thin plastic vinyl bag can be loaded, evacuated, and heat sealed in the darkroom with special equipment designed for this task.

Curved cassettes, available in 8 in. × 10 in. and 10 in. × 12 in. sizes, are used (1) to evaluate the head of the femur in the lateral position when a conventional radiograph cannot be made; (2) to examine the knee in the anteroposterior (AP) position when the knee is flexed and cannot be extended; or (3) to obtain an axillary view of the shoulder.

Multiscreen (book) cassettes can be used for simultaneous multilevel tomographic studies. (See Chapter 7.) These cassettes hold from three to seven pairs of intensifying screens to produce three to seven tomographic sections with only one exposure. A considerable increase (approximately two and one half times the milliampere second value)

over the original exposure value of the single sections is needed to expose the book cassette. Because the beam must penetrate through multilevels of intensifying screens, low kilovoltage levels are not acceptable. Generally, 70 kVp to 75 kVp is the minimal kilovoltage recommended with a book cassette. The images are often of marginal quality, and this technique has not been well accepted. Special intensifying screens arranged in an order of increasing speed from front to back are required. For example, in a five screen pair book, the first screen pair may be 50 speed, the second may be 100 speed; and so on. This progressive increase in screen speed worked fairly well with calcium tungstate screens owing to their low absorption capability. It is difficult to design a book cassette using rare-earth intensifying screens because of the high absorption nature of rare-earth phosphors. The first screen pair absorbs most of the beam, leaving little or no radiation for the remaining pairs of intensifying screens.

A special type of book cassette with closely matched intensifying screens (1.0 mm apart), known as a plesiocassette, holds four pairs of intensifying screens for use in a Bucky tray. The exact 1.0-mm spacing of the pairs of intensifying screens in the plesiocassette produces four equidistant radiographic images

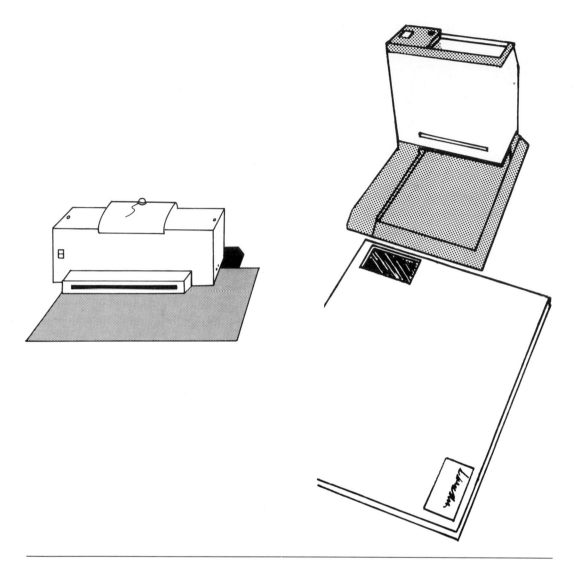

Figure 8-15 Radiographic Film Identification Systems *Most cassettes have lead inserts in a predetermined location to shield a small area of the radiographic film from x-ray. After an exposure is made, this shielded unexposed portion of the film is exposed in the darkroom with an identification printer. The patient information, typed on an identification card, is photographically transferred to the film by means of contact printing prior to processing (left).*

Another type of identification camera, used with specially designed cassettes, records patient information in normal room light (right).

with one exposure. For example when a tomographic fulcrum is set at a specific level such as 10 cm, the first pair of screens in the plesiocassette will image the anatomy at that focal range (10 cm). The second, third, and fourth will image in descending order, 9.9 cm, 9.8 cm, and 9.7 cm of body tissue. With the larger book cassette, corresponding separation (0.5 cm–1 cm) occurs.

Automated Film Handling

Daylight or room-light handling systems use special cassettes that can be loaded and unloaded in an illuminated room. These room-light systems are useful in the emergency ward, neonatal unit, and pediatric and orthopaedic areas.

Radiographic tables that hold boxes of film with a single pair of intensifying screens can also be used to expedite workflow. The automated tables are often linked to a freestanding automatic film processor.

The dedicated chest unit has been available since the mid 1960s and is considered an indispensable part of large radiographic departments. The unit is loaded with a box of radiographic film, and one hundred or more radiographs can be made and processed before additional loading is required. (See Chapter 3.)

Film Identification

Most cassettes have a lead insert in a predetermined corner of the cassette to shield the film from x-ray exposure during the making of the radiograph. In a given product line, this lead blocker is in the same area of every cassette. The shielded (unexposed) portion of the film is used for the photographic transfer of patient information.

Some identification printers can be used only in the darkroom. When the exposed film is removed from the cassette and placed into a given position on a printer, patient information can be photographed (contact printed) from an identification card to the unexposed portion of the film.

Other types of identification cameras permit information to be transferred to the radiographic film under room-light conditions (Fig. 8–15).

Many radiographers use the Kodak X-Omatic cassette in the inverted position (tube side down) as a substitute for a low ratio grid. This technique was described by Sweeney in 1977. (See Chapter 5.) The patient identification area of the Kodak cassette is in a predetermined position when the cassette is properly positioned (tube side up). For example, when the cassette is used in the AP position to radiograph the right femur (lead blocker, superior), the patient identification marker appears on the medical aspect of the right femur. When a similar cassette is used to radiograph the left femur (lead blocker, superior), the pa-

tient identification marker appears on the lateral aspect of the left femur. If the cassette is properly placed (tube side up), even when an identifying lead marker (R or L) is not visualized, the radiologist can determine which femur has been examined by the location of the identification blocker. These relationships reverse when the cassette is inverted (tube side down). The identification blocker appears on the lateral aspect of the right femur

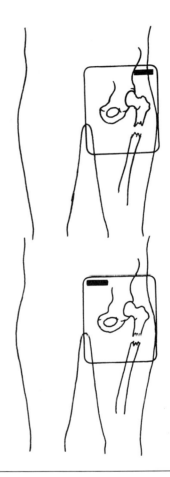

Figure 8-16 Photoidentification of an Inverted Kodak X-Omatic Cassette   *When the Kodak X-Omatic cassette is used in the inverted position (tube-side down) as a substitute for a low ratio grid, proper identifying lead markers (right and or left) are important. When the cassette is inverted, the relationship of the lead blocker to the anatomical area is reversed. If proper lead markers are not used, it is easy to confuse the right and left sides of the patient.*

and on the medial aspect of the left femur (Fig. 8–16).

> **IMPORTANT:** When the cassette is used in the reverse position (as a substitute for a grid), the right-side and left-side identification markers must be seen.

Fluoroscopic Screens

Intensifying screens are used for static imaging. A fluoroscopic screen is required for dynamic evaluation of organs and structures. For fluoroscopic examinations, an x-ray tube is mounted beneath a radiographic table. Radiation passes through the patient to the fluoroscopic screen (see Fig. 3–9) producing a visual image on the screen. The basic phosphor used in the manufacture of fluoroscopic screens is zinc cadmium sulfide. The property of phosphorescence (lag or afterglow) is characteristic of fluoroscopic screen phosphors. The crystals absorb x-ray energy and convert it into visible light, similar to the crystals in intensifying screens. Fluoroscopic crystals are considerably larger in size than are intensifying screen crystals. A fluoroscopic screen can tolerate the unsharpness produced by the larger crystals, because the fluoroscope is primarily used as a positioning device or for organ motion evaluation. Fluoroscopic screens must give off a light (usually yellow-green) that matches, as closely as possible, the color sensitivity range of the eye. This luminescent effect, while in the range that the human eye can see, is not diagnostically useful unless the eyes are adapted to darkness. The brightness of a conventional fluoroscopic screen is a fraction of that of a radiograph as seen on a viewbox. Red adaptation goggles (almost an historical curiosity owing to the advent of the image intensifier [see Chapter 6]) must be used for up to 20 minutes to prepare the eyes for a dimly illuminated conventional fluoroscopic screen. The image-intensified fluoroscope described in Chapter 6 produces brighter images than a conventional fluoroscope and is helpful in reducing patient dosage.

9 Special Recording Media and Techniques

THERE are many types of medical image recording media. In this chapter, we will discuss films used with rapid sequence (serial) changers, direct exposure dental radiographic and pantomographic studies, photofluorography, cineradiography, multiformat cathode ray tube imaging, radiation therapy treatment localization and verification, duplication and subtraction, Polaroid film for radiography and CRT imaging, and electrostatic recording media (xeroradiography).

These recording media often require specialized equipment. A brief description of these products and their application will be presented. The Polaroid and xeroradiograph processes will also be described.

Roll Film or Cut Film for Rapid Sequence Changers

A "serial" film study is made by exposing radiographs at predetermined intervals. If more than one radiograph per second is made, the procedure is known as a "rapid serial" study.

Angiographic studies require the use of serial film or cassette changers to transport the film or cassettes when many radiographs are made in a short period of time. These radiographs are often exposed (alternately or simultaneously) in two planes (anteroposterior, AP, and lateral). A major benefit with the biplane procedure is that only a single dose of contrast material is needed to image the vascular anatomy in both planes. The use of simultaneous biplane exposures compounds the effect of scatter on the radiographic images (Fig. 9–1).

Types of Serial Film or Cassette Changers

Film and cassette changers include the following:

Multiple cassette changer. A two per second (12 cassette maximum) changer was introduced almost 40 years ago. These changers use large sheet x-ray film (11 in. × 14 in.), with cassettes stacked in a "ready" position. There is extra-thick lead foil in the back of each cassette to restrict the "punch-through" of x-ray to succeeding cassettes. When an exposure is made, the cassette is pulled by a moving chain into a "park" position, and a spring mechanism elevates the next cassette to the "expose" position (Fig. 9–2). A four per second capability using a vacuum-type cassette (14 in. × 14 in.) is also available.

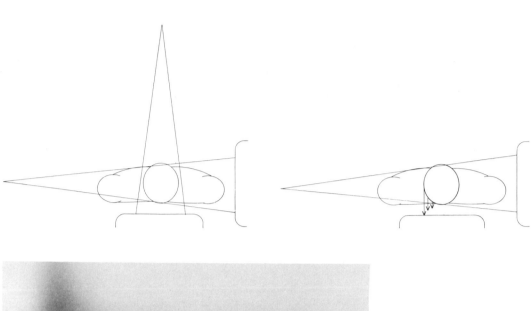

Figure 9-1 Biplane Angiographic Studies
When a simultaneous biplane angiographic study is performed (top), *an increase in density may be noted on the AP radiograph. This increased density decreases in intensity from the entrance beam side of the lateral tube. To determine the amount of scatter generated on the AP image by the lateral beam, a simple test can be performed* (center). *A phantom was positioned for simultaneous AP and lateral projections. While both serial changers were running simultaneously, only a lateral exposure was made* (center). *Note the wedgelike scatter on the AP frame, wider at the entrance point of the lateral beam but diminished in intensity toward the center of the frame* (bottom). *The radiographic density that appeared on the AP film is due to scatter from the lateral exposure.*

When a biplane study (cut film changer) is indicated, an alternate load-alternate exposure biplane technique will avoid cross-fogging of the radiographic films. The frontal magazine should be loaded with film in frames 1,3,5,7, and so on, and the lateral magazine should be programmed with film in frames 2,4,6,8, and so on. When the study is performed, film one is exposed in the AP frame; no film is in the lateral biplane changer at this point. Film two is then exposed in the lateral changer, with no film in the AP frame, and so on. Alternate loading will eliminate biplane scatter problems.

Roll film changer. A roll of x ray film, usually 14 in. wide (about 60 feet in length) is pulled through a pair of intensifying screens in a roll film changer. Prior to exposure, the screens open and the exposed film advances into a receiving magazine. The screens then close to maintain screen film contact, and an exposure is made. The process is repeated as often as is necessary. The exposed films are taken to the darkroom in a take-up magazine (Fig. 9–2).

Cut film changer. A cut film changer (Fig. 9–2) uses a film magazine that is preloaded in the darkroom prior to the angiographic study. Some magazines hold as few as 21 radiographic films; others hold a maximum of 30 films. When activated, a mechanical device advances the film from the preloaded maga-

zine into a pair of intensifying screens. The screens close, and an exposure is made. The exposed film is then advanced to a receiving cassette, which can be removed from the changer and taken to the darkroom for processing.

Full-length cassette changer. Cassette changers holding four cassettes (14 in. × 51 in.) can be used to sequentially image the abdominal aorta as well as lower extremities for serial angiography. Traditionally, different speed intensifying screens have been used in these cassettes to overcome differences in patient thickness. For example, if a high-speed system (400) were used to image the abdomen and a slow system were used to image the distal extremities, the system would vary in speed from top to bottom (400 speed–100 speed). This type of gradient (compensatory) screen has limited application, because as portions of the system speed are slowed down, the patient receives more x-ray than is needed for adequate imaging of a specific part. The distal extremities in the aforementioned example receives approximately four times more radiation than is needed for proper imaging.

The use of a compensatory wedge filter, combined with a single-speed rare-earth screen film combination (up to 1200 speed), is recommended for this procedure in place of compensatory screens (Fig. 9–3). (See Fig. 4–9.) High-speed rare-earth imaging systems provide additional benefits when used for angiography. The increased film blackening (see Table 8–1) produced by these screens permits the use of smaller focal spots. Patient and vessel motion are often stopped by the use of shorter exposure times. More frames per second may be possible.

Occasionally, when an unusually large abdomen is encountered, a high-speed film can be used with the high-speed rare-earth intensifying screens in the abdominal region.

Some Technical Problems That May Be Encountered When Using Serial Film or Cassette Changers

Scatter control is a prerequisite for quality vascular studies. When a body part is so confi-

A
CASSETTE CHANGER

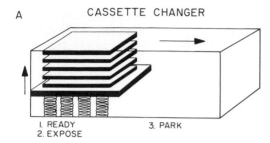

1. READY
2. EXPOSE
3. PARK

B
CUT FILM CHANGER

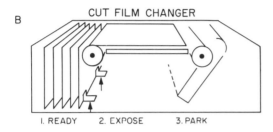

1. READY   2. EXPOSE   3. PARK

C
ROLL FILM CHANGER

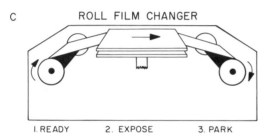

1. READY   2. EXPOSE   3. PARK

Figure 9-2   Serial Film and Cassette Changers
The basic mechanical concepts of serial cassette and film changers are illustrated.

A cassette changer (A) holds 12 (11 in. × 14 in.) cassettes and can be operated as fast as two frames per second or as slow as one frame every two seconds. The cassettes have a thick layer of lead beneath the back intensifying screen to prevent the leakage of radiation to underlying cassettes. The cassettes are positioned, one on top of the other, in a ready position and are elevated to an expose position by a spring-operated tray; then an exposure is made. A chain mechanism pulls the exposed cassette into a park chamber, and the cycle is repeated.

Cut film changers (B) require film magazines holding either 21 or 30 sheets of film (14 in. × 14 in.). Ejection fingers flip the film upward from the sending cassette into a pair of intensifying screens. The screens close and an exposure is made. After the exposure, the screens open, and the film is transported into a receiving magazine.

Most roll film changers (C) have a maximal exposure capability of 6 (11 in. × 14 in.) frames per second. A roll of film, about 60 feet in length, can be advanced into a pair of intensifying screens and an exposure can be made. When the screens open, the film is advanced to a takeup roll.

A 12 per second roll film changer is also available.

gured that the rectangular or square shutter pattern of a collimator is unable to conform to the body structure, an unattenuated primary beam may strike the film screen detector, and undercutting of the radiographic image may occur. An example is the AP Towne projection of the skull used for cerebral angiography (Figs. 9–4 and 9–5). When the unattenuated primary beam strikes the tabletop, scatter is generated. The spatial effect of the scatter causes undercutting of the radiographic image. Lead shielding is often placed on a serial film or cassette changer in an attempt to reduce scatter. Since the scatter arises from the tabletop, the lead shielding (Fig. 9–4) does not significantly improve image quality. The use of a filter material on the tabletop will attenuate the primary beam, minimizing undercutting. Sand, cornmeal, water, rice, or flour bags or lead rubber shielding can be used to attenuate the primary ray. (See Fig. 5–5.)

An undesirable attenuation of the x-ray beam can be caused by an x-ray absorbtive head support or tabletop. Some head supports can absorb as much as 50% of the remnant beam (Fig. 9–6). A simple test to determine beam attenuation by a headboard can be performed using a skull phantom positioned halfway off the headboard. The attenuated portion of the skull phantom image will be underexposed when compared with the unattenuated portion.

Tube angle techniques can increase the unsharpness associated with parallax. (See Fig. 11–15.)

The selection of an appropriate focal spot (to improve radiographic detail) as well as a

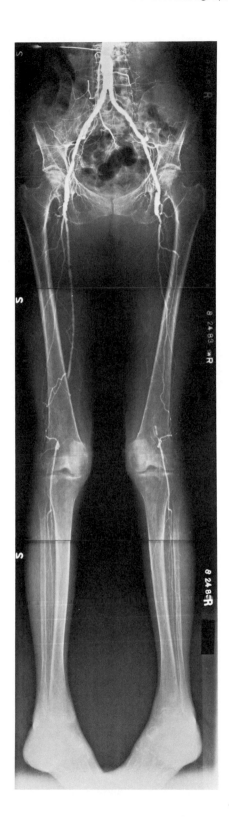

Figure 9-3 Full-Length Arteriography
*Sequential imaging of the abdominal aorta as well
as the lower extremities is possible with a cassette
changer loaded with four cassettes (14 in. × 51
in.). Because of the differences in tissue thickness
from the abdomen to the ankles, a variety of techniques have been developed to balance densities.
(See Fig. 11-6.)*

*Different speed intensifying screens can be
used to overcome differences in patient thickness:
high-speed rare-earth screens for the dense abdominal area and a slower speed screen at the
ankle (e.g., from speed 400 to 100). The distal extremities could receive up to four times more x-
ray than needed for adequate film blackening.*

*The use of a compensatory filter (see Fig. 4-9.)
instead of compensatory (gradient) screens to
help overcome differences in density is suggested.
The vascular study shown in this illustration was
made with a single exposure using a lead acrylic
compensatory filter in the external tracks of a collimator. A technique adequate for abdominal radiography was used. The design of the filter
(wedge) determined the amount of x-radiation
permitted to proportionally expose the lower extremities. With this technique, each segment of
anatomy received the amount of x-ray needed for
proper exposure. (Courtesy of Victoreen Nuclear
Associates, Carle Place, New York)*

short exposure time (to overcome motion)
should be made after tube ratings have been
considered. (See Figs. 4–7 and 4–8.)

Careful attention to radiographic technique
will result in optimal images (Fig. 9–7).

Dental Radiography

Dental radiographic film is used in a direct
exposure technique. The film has emulsion
on both sides (duplitized) and is prepackaged
in a light-tight, usually waterproof, envelope,
containing one or two films. Since it is impossible to label (identify) each dental film
during the procedure, the film manufacturer
impresses a small raised dot on the film and
packet to determine film placement relationships within the mouth.

For specific dental film usage recommen-

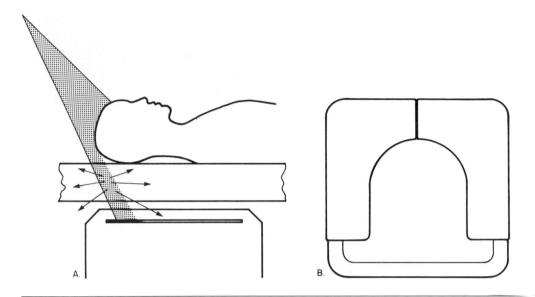

Figure 9-4 Undercutting of the Radiographic Image by a Primary Beam Leak *Since scatter is spatial, an undercutting effect will result if a primary beam leak occurs (A). The shaded area represents a primary beam striking the headboard. Lead shielding is shown placed on the surface of the cassette changer in an attempt to reduce scatter (B). Since a significant amount of scatter radiation originates from the headboard, the lead shielding will have little or no effect on the radiographic image. Although the unexposed borders of the radiographic film shielded from x-ray give the illusion of scatter control, the edges of the radiographic image will be degraded by the undercutting effect of the primary beam leak. The use of primary beam attenuators on the tabletop can lessen the undercutting effect. (See Fig. 5-5.)*

dations, see the Eastman Kodak Company's manual entitled "X-Rays In Dentistry", Cat. 1874759, 1985.

Periapical Film

Periapical film is a direct exposure duplitized dental film used for routine dental radiography to include the roots of the teeth (Fig. 9–8, *top, left*).

Bite-Wing Film

Bite-wing film (direct exposure) is similar in appearance to periapical dental film with a paper "bite-wing" extending at a right angle from the center of the front surface (tube side) of the film packet. The bite-wing is held between the teeth when the occlusal surfaces of the teeth are to be radiographed (Fig. 9–8, *top, right*).

Occlusal Film

Occlusal film (direct exposure), 2¼ in. × 3 in. in size, is used when large segments of the maxilla, mandible, or teeth are to be examined (Fig. 9–8, *bottom*). An occlusal film can also be used to localize calculi in the salivary ducts.

Pantomographic Imaging

A special body section device with the x-ray tube and cassette moving in opposing directions during an exposure can be used to simultaneously image the entire maxilla and mandible (Fig. 9–9). A narrow slit primary beam is used with a long exposure time to produce a linear tomographic image of the upper and lower teeth. The anatomical area visualized with this technique is referred to as a plane or focal trough. The pantomo-

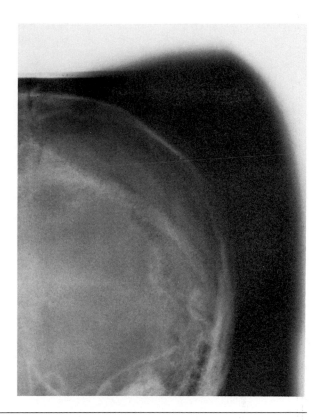

Figure 9-5 The Effect of a Primary Beam Leak on a Skull Radiograph *Since the rectangular shutters of the collimator do not conform to the contours of the skull, an undercutting effect can occur. The left side of the skull is shown with a primary beam leak (about 1 in.) striking the headboard. Note the loss of detail in the skull vault as the scatter from the headboard undercuts the image. The use of a primary beam attenuator on a headboard or tabletop will absorb much of the primary beam, lessening the undercutting effect. (See Fig. 5-5.)*

graphic cassette uses intensifying screens with dual emulsion radiographic film. See Chapter 7 for detailed information regarding tomography.

The Use of Single Emulsion Photographic Film for Radiography

Photofluorographic Imaging

The photofluorographic unit was designed in the early 1940s to detect pulmonary tuberculosis. It is an economical and efficient method for mass survey chest radiography.

A photofluorographic unit contains a single fluoroscopic screen in a light-proof holder. A camera positioned at the back end of the holder is used to photograph the image from a full-size fluoroscopic screen on strip film or cut film. Instead of conventional medical x-ray film with emulsion on both sides, a single emulsion photographic type of film is used to take a miniature photograph of the fluorescing screen (Fig. 9–10). The fluoroscopic image, when recorded on photographic film, results in an image that resembles a radiographic image.

A magnifying lens or a slide projector is required to view the processed miniature rep-

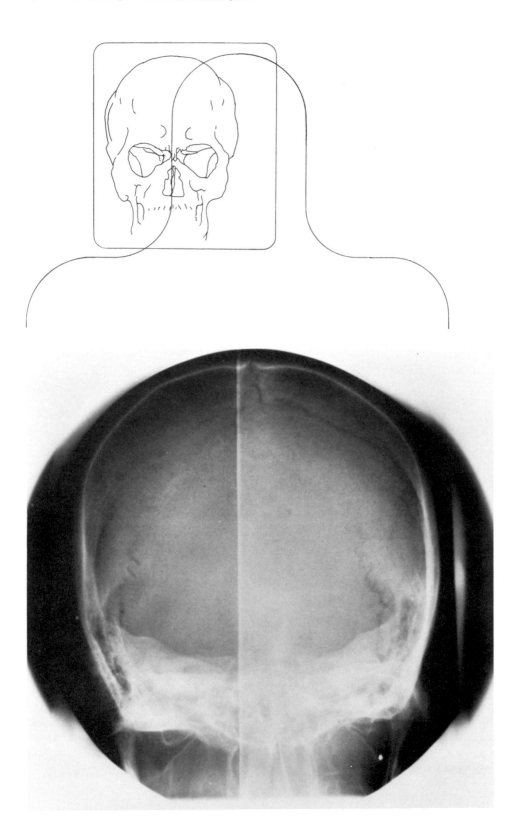

(Fig. 9–12, *bottom, left*). (See Chapter 6.)

Figure 9-6 The Absorption Effect of the Headboard or Tabletop A simple test to determine the absorption effect of a headboard or tabletop is shown (top). A skull phantom is placed on the headboard extension with half the skull positioned off the board. The skull is centered to the film changer, and an exposure is made. The radiograph should show acceptable detail and contrast unless there is significant absorption of the remnant beam by the headboard. The example shown (bottom) suggests that approximately 50% of the remnant beam was absorbed by the headboard. The high absorptive nature of this headboard requires a doubling of exposure factors for adequate radiographic density.

resentation of the chest. Although most modern photofluorographic units use considerably less radiation than older style equipment, screen film chest studies require much less radiation for adequate film blackening.

Cathode Ray Tube Imaging

Single emulsion photographic films with antihalation backings (see Fig. 8–1) are used for television monitor (CRT) imaging. Multiformat cameras can be used to photograph images generated by digital subtraction angiography, ultrasonography, computed tomography, or magnetic resonance. (See Figs. 6–5, 6–11, 6–12, 6–13, 6–14.)

Serial Recording

Images from the output phosphor of an image intensifier (see Figs. 6–1 and 6–2) or a television screen (kinescope) can be obtained using photographic film (Fig. 9–11). Seventy-millimeter, 90-mm, and 105-mm strip film or 100-mm (4 in. × 4 in.) cut film can be exposed at multiple frames per second. When a conventional 9-in. input phosphor is used, these photographic techniques require about 1/20th the exposure needed for a full-size radiograph because of the increased gain of the image intensifier. Lower radiation exposure, less cost per frame, relatively easy film handling, and storage are advantages of strip or cut film imaging. A disadvantage is that the size of

the area to be examined is restricted to the size of the input phosphor of the intensifier

Cineradiographic Film

Often during conventional fluoroscopic viewing, a physiological event occurs so rapidly that it cannot be evaluated. Cineradiography (motion picture imaging) can record the fluoroscopic image in real time or in slow motion. (See Figs. 6–1 and 6–2.)

Cineradiographic units use a grid-pulsed system to control the x-ray tube. (See Chapters 4 and 6.) Exposures as rapid as 1 msec (1/1000th sec) can be synchronized with the open shutter of the motion picture camera.

An automatic exposure control known as an automatic brightness control (ABC) can either increase kilovoltage or milliamperage automatically when considerable differences in body part thickness or density are encountered. (See Chapter 6.)

Cineradiographic films can be exposed at a rate of from 8 frames per second to 60 frames per second or higher. Conventional motion picture sound projectors operate at 24 frames per second. If only 12 frames per second are exposed, a speeded-up impression of the physiologic event occurs when viewed at 24 frames per second. If 60 frames per second are made and projected at 24 frames per second, it takes two and one half times longer to project the study, resulting in slow motion.

Two sizes of cineradiographic film (16 mm and 35 mm) are commercially available. Sixteen-millimeter film will record 40 individual frames per foot, whereas 35 mm film records 16 frames per foot. The 35-mm frame size is approximately four times larger (area) than the 16-mm frame (see Fig. 9–12). The dimensions of each 16-mm frame are 10.5 mm × 7.5 mm, whereas 35-mm film has a frame size of 20 mm × 18 mm. The 35-mm film has a frame size of 20 mm × 18 mm. The 35-mm film has approximately four times more surface area (increased silver halide grains) than the 16-mm film. Since a greater surface area of silver halide grains must be exposed with the 35-mm cineradiographic film, three to four times more radiation is required to achieve the same degree of film blackening.

(*Text continues on p. 158*)

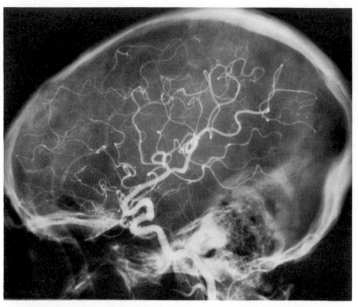

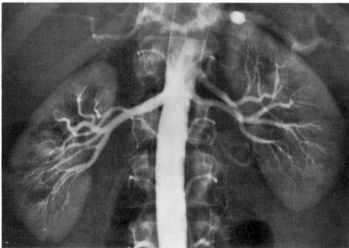

Figure 9-7 Angiographic Images

Careful attention to radiographic technique will result in an optimal study. The illustration shown is a lateral projection of a cerebral angiographic study made using an alternate load biplane direct roentgen enlargement technique (top). A fractional focal spot was combined with an air gap (See Chapter 7.) to produce a 2× linear, 4× area enlargement. A 1200-speed rare-earth screen film combination was used without apparent loss of resolution owing to quantum mottle. (See Figs. 7-16 and 8-12.)

An abdominal aortogram is shown using an 800-speed rare-earth screen film system on a large patient (bottom). The use of a modest kilovoltage value combined with a 12:1 ratio grid produced a relatively high-contrast image. Despite the size and absorptive nature of this patient, careful attention to radiograph technique produced a quality angiographic study. (Courtesy of Eastman Kodak Company, Rochester, New York)

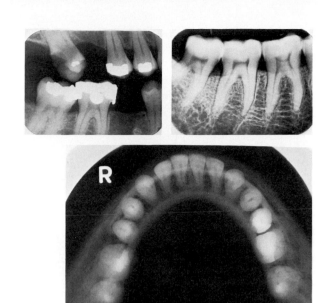

Figure 9-8   Dental Radiographic Images
Typical radiographic images produced by direct exposure dental techniques are shown. A periapical film is used for routine radiography to include the roots of the teeth (top, right). A bite-wing film is used to evaluate the occlusal surfaces of the teeth (top, left). An occlusal film demonstrating almost all the teeth of the mandible is shown (bottom). Large segments of the maxilla, mandible, or teeth can be examined with occlusal films. (Courtesy of Eastman Kodak Company, Rochester, New York)

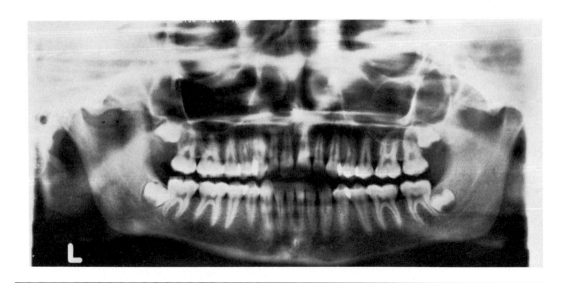

Figure 9-9   Pantomographic Study
Pantomographic units use slit scan tomographic techniques, with the tube and film moving in opposite directions to each other. A radiograph is shown of the maxilla and mandible from one tempromandibular joint to the other. Note the horizontal parasitical streaks (above the inferior orbital ridges) owing to the horizontal linear movement of the tube and film. (See Figs. 7-3 and 7-9.) (Courtesy of Eastman Kodak Company, Rochester, New York)

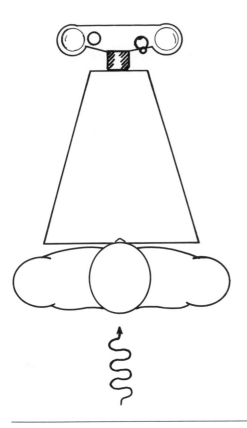
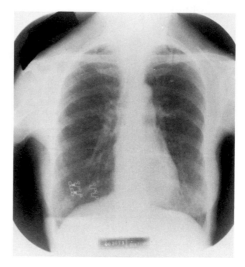

Figure 9-10   Photofluorography
Photofluorographic units consist of a fluoroscopic screen in a lightproof hood (left). A strip or cut film camera mounted at the back end of the hood is used to record the fluoroscopic chest image. A 40-in. FFD is used in conjunction with an automatic exposure device.

An actual-size 70-mm photofluorographic study of an adult female in the PA position made from a full-size fluoroscopic screen is shown (right).
A single emulsion photographic film is used for this study.

The size of the framing mode (framing technique) determines the amount of the area blackened on each individual cineradiographic frame (Fig. 9–13).

Special radiographic accessories, such as projectors, film splicers, and film editing equipment, are required for cineradiography.

Laser Imaging Film

Most new imaging modalities use photographic techniques to transfer an image from a cathode ray tube (television monitor) to single emulsion film. The raster lines of the television screen, electronic noise, and other types of interference are also simultaneously recorded and can diminish resolution. An extremely fine-grain single emulsion laser recording film that is sensitive to laser light has been developed to record data, "written" directly by a laser beam. This eliminates raster lines on the processed image.

Radiation Therapy Imaging

Portal radiographs are often made as part of treatment planning to ascertain the position of the radiation beam and the shielding

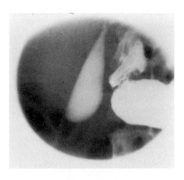

Figure 9-11 Kinescopic Spot Film
An opacified gall bladder imaged from a 1000-line television monitor on 70-mm strip film is shown. Extremely high resolution is possible with fine-line television kinescopic techniques. Kinescopic techniques (photographic imaging from the television monitor) are not in common use. Most cut or strip film images are made directly from the output phosphor of the image intensifier. (See Figs. 6-1 and 6-2.)

blocks. The beam/block relationship to patient anatomy is an important part of treatment. When portal localization radiographs are needed, a single exposure is often made with the radiation shielding blocks in position; a second exposure is then made on the same film with the blocks removed (Fig. 9–14).

Although medical screen film as well as fine-grain industrial-type films are used for radiation therapy imaging, the cassettes used for these techniques are quite different from diagnostic radiographic cassettes. Therapy imaging cassettes do not contain conventional intensifying screens. Early portal imaging systems used lead screens, which ''intensified'' the radiation. A recently introduced portal imaging cassette utilizes a 1.0-mm thick copper front screen in combination with a posterior lead screen. The copper screen intensifies the primary radiation and blocks electrons generated within the patient, keeping them from the film. The lead back screen also serves as an intensifier, providing addi-

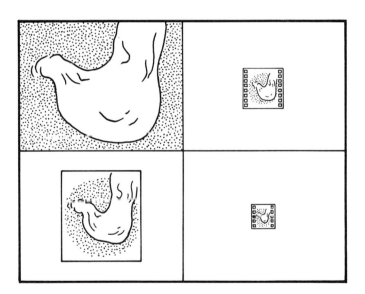

Figure 9-12 Frame Size Comparisons
Four individual frame sizes are represented. The large rectangular drawing illustrates an 8-in. × 10-in. fluoroscopic spot film.

A 4-in. × 5-in. spot segment (four exposures on one 8-in. × 10-in. film) is shown (top, left).

Cut or strip film images are represented by a 70-mm frame comparison (bottom, left). (See Fig. 9-11 for actual frame size.)

The frame size comparison is completed by 35-mm film (top, right) and 16-mm film (bottom, right).

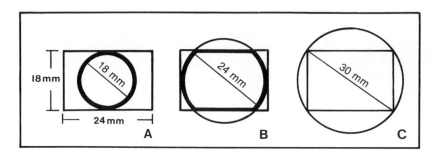

Figure 9-13 Cineradiographic Framing Concepts *Cineradiographic framing can include exact framing* (A), *maximal horizontal framing* (B), *or total overframing* (C).

More than 50% of the film area is used for exact framing (A), *whereas 100% of the film area is used for total overframing* (C).

tional exposure to the film (mostly as a result of backscattering of electrons).

Verification cassettes have anterior and posterior lead screens. A newer version uses a copper front and a posterior plastic screen. The plastic screen does not intensify the radiation but is used as a spacer to ensure contact of the x-ray film with the anterior copper screen. Blur is reduced and resolution is improved, because the image forming electrons are in better contact with the radiographic film.

The techniques and films used for treatment localization and verification differ in the following ways: The radiographic film used for treatment localization is a screen-type film used to minimize radiation to the patient during the treatment localization process (Fig. 9–14). The verification films stay in position beneath the patient throughout the entire treatment. The x-ray film used with the verification system is a direct exposure (fine-grain) slow film. Since the actual radiation treatment exposes the verification film, an extremely slow film is needed (Fig. 9–15). Film in a ready pack envelope is used with the portal localization or verification cassettes. Each sheet of film is prepackaged in a light-proof envelope, and the cassettes can be loaded and unloaded in room light. If an automatic processor is not adjacent to the therapy treatment area or if one prefers to ''batch'' films for processing at a later time, only one of each type of cassette is needed.

Duplication and Subtraction Film and Techniques

Duplication

Duplication images are made for teaching files and legal records and as a courtesy to referring physicians.

This process, photographic in nature, requires a duplicating printer or copier that uses ultraviolet light to make a contact print of a radiographic image (Fig. 9–16, *top*). The image is transferred to a sheet of single emulsion (duplicating) film of exactly the same dimensions.

The printing of any photographic film from a negative results in a positive. Duplication film, however, is sensitometrically designed so that it will reproduce an exact duplication of the image. Since duplication film is single emulsion, the emulsion side must be placed against the radiograph to avoid unsharpness in the printing process. The back of the film is covered with an antihalation coating to stop light from passing through the film (light scattering). (See Fig. 8–1.)

The procedure must be performed under safelight conditions.

Subtraction

Radiographs are summation images, with considerable superimposition of structures. Overlying structures can mask diagnostic information. The subtraction process is used

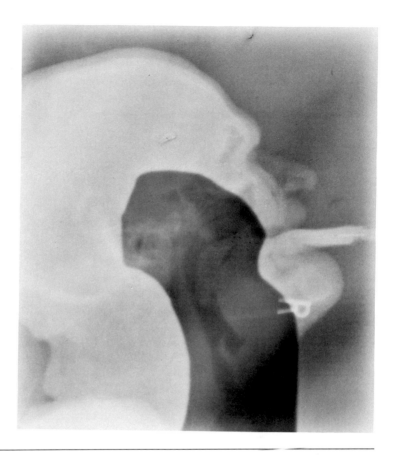

Figure 9-14   Radiation Therapy Portal Locali-zation Image   *A portal localization radiograph of the soft tissue structures of the mouth and neck was obtained prior to radiation therapy. A double-exposure technique was used. The first exposure was made with shielding blocks in place outlining the field size. A second exposure was made with* the blocks removed, and an open field was used to demonstrate anatomy adjacent to the treat-ment area. Note the shape of the actual treatment field designed to minimize exposure to adjacent tissue. *(Courtesy of Eastman Kodak Company, Rochester, New York)*

primarily for vessel evaluation (angiographic techniques).

Subtraction techniques are also photo-graphic in nature and usually use the same equipment (Fig. 9–16, *bottom*) as duplication techniques. Subtraction techniques, however, are considerably more complex to perform. Although these units may have minor differ-ences in design, they all operate in essentially the same manner.

Most duplication/subtraction printers use the following three different types of light:

1 Conventional white light for exposing the subtraction mask and print

2 A bright (white) light for image regis-tration purposes

3 Ultraviolet light to expose the duplicat-ing film

The tasks required for subtraction tech-niques include:

1 The selection of a radiographic image devoid of contrast material that is used

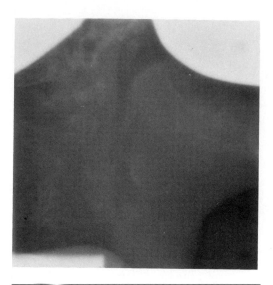

Figure 9-15 Radiation Therapy Verification Image *A portal verification radiograph with treatment shielding blocks in place records the radiation exit dose from the patient for the entire treatment. This radiograph documents the actual radiation treatment and can be used to evaluate localization errors that may occur during treatment. (Courtesy of Eastman Kodak Company, Rochester, New York)*

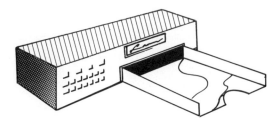

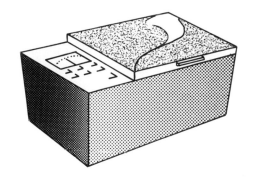

Figure 9-16 Duplication/Subtraction Printers *Duplicating film and a superimposed radiograph are fed into a roller-operated duplicator printer (top) in a darkroom. After exposure of the duplication film by the printer, the film is processed in an automatic processor and an exact duplication of the original radiograph is obtained. Subtraction techniques are also possible with some units of this type.*

A duplication/subtraction printer (bottom) contains three light sources: a bright light for registration of superimposed images, a white light for exposing the subtraction mask and print, and ultraviolet light for exposing duplicating film. This type of printer provides good contact because of equalized pressure over the large surfaces of the film. A timer permits variations in exposure lengths for better control of subtraction densities.

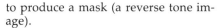

to produce a mask (a reverse tone image).

2 The selection of a radiograph from a serial study after the injection of a contrast medium.

3 The processed mask (step 1) must be superimposed (registered) on the selected angiographic image (step 2).

4 The making of a copy of the superimposed images (mask and angiographic image in register) on subtraction film.

In theory, the mask (reversed image) should cancel out (subtract) the structures common to the mask and the angiographic image. Osseous structures and soft tissues should be subtracted while the contrast ma-

terial remains, since it is unique to the angiogram (Fig. 9–17). It is virtually impossible to produce a "perfect" subtraction image, because slight movement between exposures by the patient can cause registration problems. When subtracting thoracic or abdominal angiographic images, cardiac motion, breathing, vessel pulsations, or changes in position of gas or fecal shadows can cause register difficulties.

Boundary edges on the subtracted image occur if the images (mask, scout, and so on)

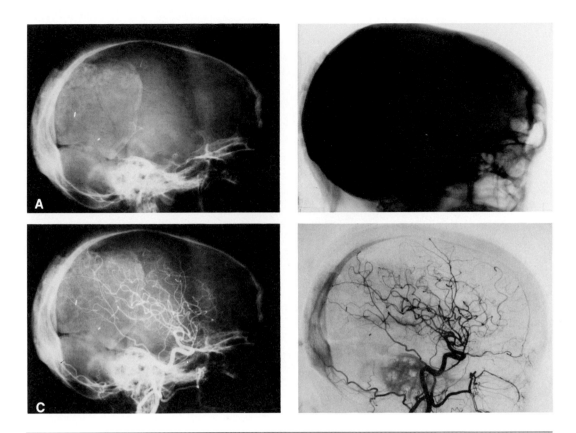

Figure 9-17 Subtraction Technique

Because radiographs are summation Images, there is considerable superimposition of structures. A subtraction printer is used to "cancel out" overlying structures. A radiographic image devoid of contrast material (A) is selected to produce a subtraction mask (a reverse tone image). The mask (D) is then superimposed (registered) on an angiographic image (C). A copy of the superimposed image produces a subtraction film (D). The mask (reversed image) subtracts out structures common to both the mask and angiographic image. Osseous structures are subtracted, but the contrast material remains, since it is unique to the angiographic study. The mask is usually made from a scout film taken just prior to the Injection of the contrast material. (Courtesy of the Genesee Hospital, Department of Diagnostic Radiology, Rochester, NY)

are not properly registered. These edges can interfere with visualization of vascular structures on the final subtracted image. If it is impossible to register all radiographic details because of voluntary or involuntary motion, an effort should be made to register the area of interest.

Some radiographers place the subtracted mask against the angiogram with the emulsion side away from the radiograph. Although this produces a slightly unsharp image, they believe that this slight defocusing effect renders register misalignment less obvious.

If a higher level of subtraction is indicated, a second-order subtraction technique using two masks is suggested. The first-order mask is placed over the scout (base or zero) radiograph, and a second mask is made using subtraction film. The processes second-order mask is carefully superimposed on the first subtraction mask and then taped to the radio-

(Text continues on p. 166.)

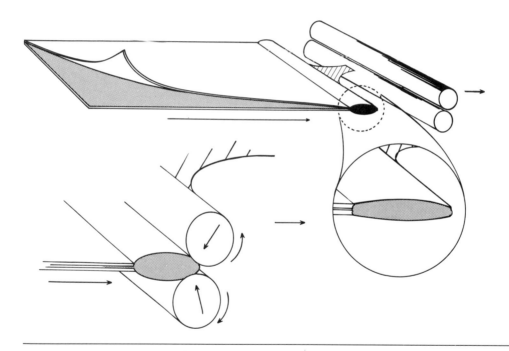

Figure 9-18 Representation of the Polaroid Radiographic Process *The Polaroid radiographic system is a type of instant photography.*

The Polaroid radiographic packet consists of three major segments: a photosensitive emulsion (negative); a metallic foil envelope, which contains a gel-like processing solution; and a receiving sheet, which accepts the image from the exposed negative (top). A Polaroid film is placed (under daylight conditions) in a special cassette, using a single intensifying screen. After an exposure is made, the film requires a special unit for processing. A paper tab is used to pull the exposed photosen-sitive film and the receiving paper through metallic rollers (top) that rupture the pod (insert) and spread the processing agent evenly over the surfaces of the film and paper. The developing gel functions as both developer and fixer. When the process has been completed, the receiving paper is separated from the photosensitive paper and a reverse image results. In the Polaroid image, dense structures, such as bone and barium, appear black.

A reflective Polaroid image requires 10 seconds, and the translucent, plastic-based image approximately 45 seconds to process.

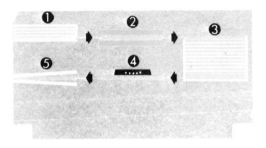

❶ STORAGE BOX STATION (INPUT)

❷ RELAXATION OVEN

❸ INTERNAL STORAGE

❹ CHARGE

❺ CASSETTE

Figure 9-19 Xeroradiographic Conditioner
The xeroradiographic process requires special image receptors, processing, and conditioning equipment. A reusable photoreceptor plate (selenium coated) is the counterpart of x-ray film.

A xeroradiographic plate conditioner functions as follows: The storage box station (1) will hold up to six reusable selenium-coated plates in a standby position. The storage box is taken from the processing unit (Fig. 9-20) and inserted into the conditioner. The plates are transported within the conditioner to the relaxation oven (2) and heated (relaxed) to remove any residual electrical charge remaining from a previous exposure. The plates are then placed in internal storage (3) where they cool to room temperature in a storage magazine that can accommodate up to 16 plates. When an empty cassette is inserted into the conditioner, a plate is moved from the storage magazine to be sensitized (given a uniform electrostatic charge) (4). The plate is now sensitive to x-radiation and light (photosensitive). The charged plate is loaded into a light-tight cassette (5) and released from the conditioner. When the sealed cassette with its charged plate is removed from the conditioner, it can be used for an x-ray exposure. (See Fig. 9-20 for processing functions.) (Courtesy of Xerox Corporation, Xerox Medical Systems, Pasadena, California)

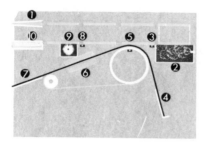

❶ CASSETTE INPUT
❷ DEVELOPMENT CHAMBER
❸ PRE–TRANSFER CHARGE
❹ PAPER FEEDER
❺ TRANSFER CHARGE
❻ FUSING OVEN
❼ PAPER TRAY
❽ PRE–CLEANING CHARGE
❾ BRUSH CLEANING
❿ STORAGE BOX STATION
(OUTPUT)

Figure 9-20 Xeroradiographic Processing Unit A xeroradiographic processing unit functions as follows: The cassette (1) is inserted into the processor using the manufacturer's recommended orientation. Improperly oriented cassettes will not be accepted by the processor. The exposed plate is automatically removed from its cassette, transferred to the development chamber (2), where a charged developing powder (toner) is sprayed on the surface of the selenium-coated plate. More toner is attracted to areas that have a remaining high charge; less toner is attracted to less-charged regions. (See Fig. 9-21.) Pre-transfer charging (3) neutralizes the remaining charge on the plate, and the layer of developing powder is charged negatively to increase the efficiency of the transfer process. A sheet of paper moves from the paper feeder (4) into the transfer position for contact with the plate. At a registration point, the plate and paper meet (5). A transfer charge is passed over the back side of the paper, drawing developer powder to the paper. The paper is then withdrawn from the plate and carried to the fixing station. In the fusing oven (6), the paper surface is heated to permanently fix developer particles to the paper. The finished xeroradiograph exits into the paper tray (7), ready for immediate viewing. Residual powder that may remain on the plate following the transfer is removed by a neutralizing charge (8). This pre-cleaning charge helps to free residual powder from the plate surface. A rotating fine soft brush (9) removes the developer from the plate. The plate is then deposited into the storage box (10), which must accumulate six plates before the storage box can be released to be taken to the conditioner unit. (See Fig. 9-19.) (Courtesy of Xerox Corporation, Xerox Medical Systems, Pasadena, California)

graph to be subtracted. With this multimask technique, accurate registration of the images can be difficult. The use of the bright light in the duplication/subtraction unit helps in the registering of the two masks to the radiograph.

All duplication and subtraction films can be processed in 90-second automatic processors.

ELECTRONIC SUBTRACTION

Digital subtraction techniques use computer technology to produce subtracted angiographic images electronically. The use of a computer to enhance the image permits the injection of smaller amounts of contrast media. (See Fig. 6–5.)

Two television cameras can also be used to simultaneously record both the scout (as an electronically reversed image) and angiographic images. The images can be electronically superimposed for a subtraction effect. Hard-copy images can be recorded from the CRT.

Polaroid (Instant) Photography

Instant photography has been commercially available for more than 30 years. Instant pho-

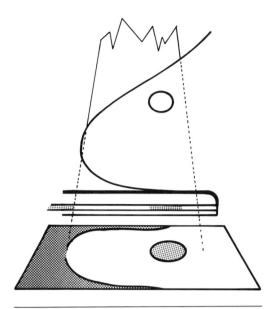

Figure 9-21 *Exposure of a Charged Selenium Plate* A dense circular mass is shown in a breast. The shaded area represents unexposed regions of the xeroradiographic plate. The x-ray beam used for this representation was collimated to the exact shape of the breast. In this illustration, the dense circular lesion absorbs most of the x-rays so that the discharge of the selenium-coated plate surface is minimal. There is little effect on the original surface charge of the selenium plate in the area of the lesion as well as the unexposed portions of the plate outside of the tightly collimated x-ray beam. The x-ray beam passing through the radiolucent breast "erases" much of the charge.

Xeroradiographic systems have a wide exposure latitude due to the development process being particularly responsive to charge differences. In an actual xeroradiograph, density changes would vary throughout the entire image, ranging from soft tissue densities to dense bone structures. (See Figs. 9-22 and 9-23.)

tographic media contain their own development systems. A foil pod containing a special processing gel is ruptured as the exposed film is pulled through a pair of rollers for processing.

Instant black and white photography was used to record medical images from CRT monitors. (See Fig. 6–10.) Transparent photographic sheet films are now in common use for this purpose.

The Polaroid x-ray system works in a manner similar to the Polaroid photographic process. Polaroid radiographic film must be placed in a special radiographic cassette containing a single intensifying screen. After a radiographic exposure, the Polaroid film packet is placed in a special roller processor. The film is pulled through the rollers, and a processing gel is spread over the exposed film (Fig. 9–18). A reverse image (paper print) results. Bone appears black instead of white. This paper print requires reflective light for viewing.

Since the Polaroid x-ray system was available before the introduction of the automatic processor, it was accepted immediately by orthopaedic surgeons for operative x-ray procedures to reduce operating and anesthesia time.

Another type of Polaroid radiographic film on a translucent plastic base can be viewed either by transmitted or reflected light.

Electrostatic Recording Media (Xeroradiography)

The xeroradiographic process and its recording media differs from screen film imaging.

An electrically charged selenium coated plate is used in place of x-ray film in a special light-proof cassette. Whereas ordinary cassettes can tolerate rough handling, the xeroradiographic cassette must be handled carefully to avoid discharging of the plate, which can result in image artifacts. Special conditioning and processing units are required for this procedure (Figs. 9–19 and 9–20).

The selenium plate must be electrically charged in a special conditioning unit. When an exposure is made, the x-ray beam forms a latent image within the electrical charge. X-rays passing through the body electrically discharge the plate in direct proportion to the density (mass) of the overlying tissue (Fig. 9–21). The surface of the exposed plate is dusted with a thermoplastic powder known as *toner* in a processing unit designed for this purpose. The toner adheres to the exposed plate in amounts proportional to the charge remaining on the plate after exposure. The powder image is then transferred and heat sealed in the processing unit to a copy paper (9.5 in. × 13.5 in.). The selenium plate is returned to the conditioning unit to relax the

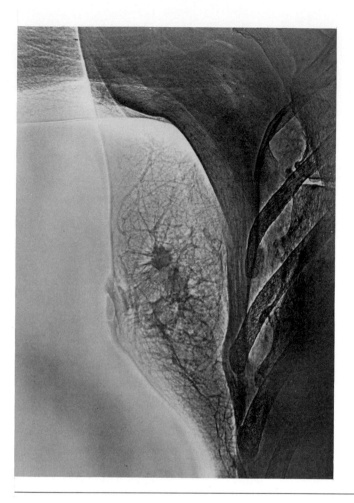

Figure 9-22 Xeroradiographic Representation of the Breast (Positive Mode) *Note the wide exposure latitude exhibited on this image. A stellate carcinoma of the left breast is shown with skin thickening and nipple retraction. The chest wall, including the osseous details of the ribs, can be seen.*

The black densities seen in this image would be blue in an actual xeromammographic study. (See Fig. 9-23 for reversal image.) (Courtesy of Xerox Corporation, Xerox Medical Systems, Pasadena, California)

plate image, after which the cleaned, relaxed plate is recharged for reuse.

Xeroradiography has a wide recording latitude with an edge enhancement effect. In xeroradiography, sharp structural edges are enhanced by the attraction of the toner material on the plate. Immediately adjacent to the sharp-edged structures, little or no powder (toner) is deposited. This effect is known as *deletion*. Sharply delineated edges of ves-

sels, osseous structures, and calcifications benefit from the deletion effect (Fig. 9–22).

Xeroradiographic images are blue and white (positive mode) as opposed to black and white radiographs. In positive mode xeroradiographic studies, blue represents the dense areas, whereas white represents the radiolucent areas. When conditioning the plate, this process can be reversed (negative mode), with white made to represent the more dense areas

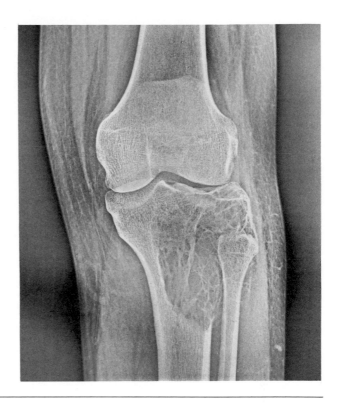

Figure 9-23 Xeroradiographic Image (Negative Mode) *A negative mode xeroradiographic image is obtained by altering conditioning and processing parameters. A negative mode, AP image of the knee, demonstrates a destructive lesion* *encompassing the lateral aspect of the upper tibia. Note the soft tissue visualization throughout the entire image. (Courtesy of Xerox Corporation, Xerox Medical Systems, Pasadena, California)*

and blue the more radiolucent areas (Fig. 9–23).

In the late 1980s, a xeroradiographic process was introduced that produces black and white images similar to conventional radiographs but with the edge enhancement prin-

ciple. A liquid toner is used instead of a powder toner.

Xeroradiographic images, including those produced with the new black and white system, are reflective images (paper prints).

10 Radiographic Processing

THE invisible change in a radiographic film that is caused either by light or x-radiation is called a *latent image*. The latent image is converted into a visible image by the process of development.

Manual Processing

Prior to the design of the automatic processor, all x-ray films were manually developed. Hand processing is still practiced in some low-volume facilities. Under safelight conditions, exposed film is attached to four corners of a metal hanger, placed in the developer, and hand agitated so that uniform development can be obtained. Three to 5 minutes is required for the manual development process.

Developer reduces the exposed silver compounds in the film emulsion to black metallic silver. After a predetermined processing period, development is halted when the film is placed in the fixer. The fixer removes the unexposed silver compounds and hardens the gelatin containing the black metallic silver.

A stop bath (diluted acetic solution) recommended to neutralize the alkaline developer is rarely used. The developed radiograph is briefly agitated in a water bath, then moved to the fixing tank.

The fixing process usually requires approximately 10 minutes, or twice the time of the development process. After proper fixing (clearing and hardening), conventional room lighting can be used. The film is then moved to the wash tank, where 20 or more minutes of washing is required to remove residual fixer.

The radiographs are air dried or placed in cabinets equipped to circulate heated air. Up to 1½ hours are required before a dry radiograph is available for interpretation. The processing cycle is occasionally interrupted for a "wet" reading when an immediate interpretation is required. The radiograph is removed from the fixer (after clearing has occurred), briefly agitated in water, and interpreted while wet. It is difficult to make a proper diagnosis from a wet radiograph, and a final decision is usually withheld until the dry image can be reviewed.

For many years, despite it's limitations, manual processing satisfactorily served the needs of radiology departments. As the workload increased, however, it was recognized that manual processing presented major difficulties. Hand processing techniques took too much time, making it difficult to maintain quality control and to complete the processing tasks in a reasonable period of time.

Automatic Processors

In the 1940s, automated film processors were designed that moved the films on hangers from tank to tank. There was less labor involved but very little saving in time.

In the late 1950s, the first roller transport processor was made commercially available by the Eastman Kodak Company. The 1-hour, or greater, dry-to-dry processing was reduced to 6 minutes (Fig. 10–1).

The purpose of an automatic processor is to transport film through the processing cycles in a controlled manner and to deliver a dry radiograph at the end of the drying cycle. To accomplish this goal, the solutions must constantly be temperature controlled, agitated, and replenished.

Processors can be made to transport films according to the specific needs of the user. Most modern radiography departments use a rapid transport system (approximately 90 seconds) for use with medical x-ray films. Units can be modified to permit a longer processing cycle if needed.

System Design

All manufacturers have specific processor design parameters, which may vary from unit to unit. In this textbook, only the facts common to all processors will be discussed. The details of installation and servicing can be found in the service manuals provided with each model.

Hand processing of radiographs required more than 1 hour. With automatic processors, time of processing is exact because of the constant speed of the motor-drive system. Space to accommodate the drying of large numbers of radiographs presented an additional problem. With hand processing, time, tempera-

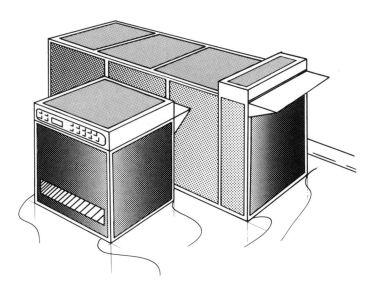

Figure 10-1 The Evolution of the Automatic Roller Transport X-Ray Film Processor The first commercially manufactured roller transport processor (Eastman Kodak Company) had a 6-minute dry-to-dry processing cycle. Today's rapid processing units (90 seconds, dry-to-dry) require con-

siderably less floor space.

The roller racks of this early processor were cumbersome. A ceiling-mounted crane was required to remove the racks from the solution tanks for repair or cleaning.

ture, agitation, and replenishment were difficult to control because of the human factor. Radiographers could, and did, allow films to remain in the developer longer than recommended to overcome underexpose and prematurely removed films from the developer to compensate for overexposed radiographs. This arbitrary approach to development, although not encouraged, was frequently practiced. Safelight viewing of radiographs often resulted in the contamination of the solutions as depleted developer drained back into the developer tank, hastening the exhaustion of the solution. A small amount of fixer, if splashed into the developing solution, can render the developer ineffective.

Two other essentials, agitation and replenishment, were also considered in the design of the automatic processor. The rollers of the transport system and the recirculation pumps continually agitate the solutions. Improper agitation can result in streaks and uneven densities on the radiograph. Replenishment solutions are added as each sheet of film is fed into the processor. The replenishment system is designed so that a precise amount of replenisher (developer and fixer) is fed into the tanks for every centimeter of film that passes over the entrance roller. There are specific recommendations for the proper feeding of sheet or roll films into the processor (Fig. 10–2).

Automatic Processor Sections

The automatic processor consists of three major sections (Fig. 10–3):

1 A film loading area (Fig. 10–3A). The film is fed into the processor in the darkroom. An audible or visual signal is emitted when the

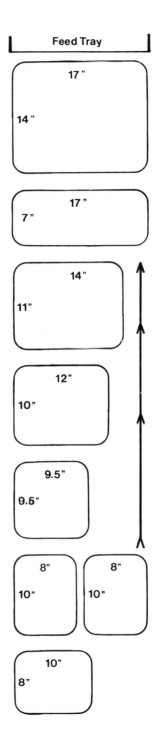

Figure 10-2 *Automatic Processor Film Alignment Feeding Patterns* *Processor manufacturers recommend specific film alignment feeding patterns to maintain proper replenishment rates.*

The feeding patterns shown ensure the recommended amounts of replenishment solutions per square foot of film processed. A change in feeding patterns could result in over- or underreplenishment of the solutions.

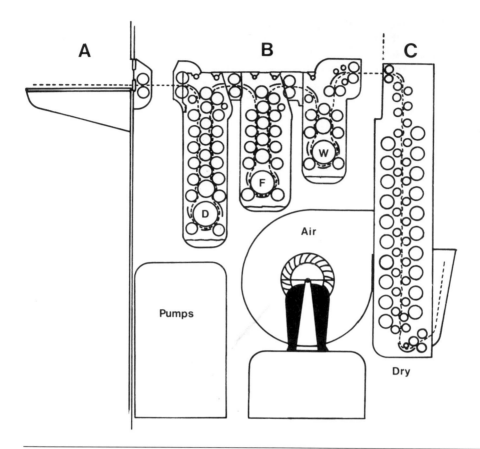

Figure 10-3 Automatic Roller Transport Processing *Three major sections constitute the automatic processor.*

In the darkroom, film is fed into the processor by means of a film feeding tray (A). The remainder of the processor (B and C) is usually installed external to the darkroom. Developer, fixer, and wash tanks with their roller transport components make up a major section of the second portion (B) of the processor. Temperature controls and recirculation and replenishment pumps are vital components of section B. Section C is the dryer portion of the roller transport system. The air blower and heaters along with the dryer roller transport system are the major components of the dryer. A receptacle for processed dry radiographs completes the final segment of the processor.

Most automatic processors are linked to a darkroom. Freestanding processors with special feeding mechanisms can be used with room-light cassettes. These cassettes, which can be automatically loaded under room-light conditions and placed into a special feed mechanism on a free standing processor, eliminate the need for a darkened film feed area.

film completely passes over the entrance roller. This indicates to the darkroom personnel that another film can be fed into the unit. If a second film is prematurely fed into the processor, overlapping of the films could occur. This may result in a jamming of the film somewhere in the roller transport system. Even if a jam does not occur, the overlapped radiographs would be improperly developed or fixed.

2 The film solution processing tanks, roller transport system, temperature controls, and recirculation and replenishment pumps (Fig. 10–3B).

TABLE 10-1. Automatic Processor Systems: Major Purposes

Purposes	Roller	Recirculation Developer	Fixer	Water	Air	Replenishment
Transport film	•					
Control processing time	•					
Control replenishment time	•					
Agitation	•	•	•	•		
Squeegee action	•					
Help prevent film overlap	•					
Develop film		•				
Maintain solution activity and/or concentration		•	•			•
Constant filtration		•				
Temperature control		•		•	•	
Stop development			•			
Clear film			•			
Harden emulsion			•			
Wash film				•		
Control water flow				•		
Control replenishment rate						•
Keep developer overflow clean				•		
Control recirculation		•	•			
Control air recirculation					•	
Dry film					•	
Replenish solutions						•
Prevent and control backflow of replenisher						•
Total Major Purposes	6	6	6	5	3	4

3 Heaters and air blowers to facilitate drying of the radiographs, a roller transport system in the dryer, and a receptacle for the processed, dried radiographs (Fig. 10–3C).

Processor Systems and Cycles

The major purposes and functions of the various components of the automatic processor are outlined in Table 10–1.

THE ROLLER TRANSPORT SYSTEM

The roller transport system consists of a series of gears and chains connected to rollers that are used to transport the films through the processing cycles providing constant, vigorous agitation of the solutions against the film surfaces.

The roller transport system includes:

1 Entrance roller assembly

2 Crossover racks (not used in some processors)

3 Turnaround racks between roller assemblies

4 Squeegee assembly (to remove excess moisture from the film surfaces)

5 Dryer rollers (to transport the film through the dryer section)

THE RECIRCULATION SYSTEMS

The recirculation systems keep solutions evenly mixed and provide chemical agitation to ensure uniform solution coverage of the film while transporting it through the solutions. Overflow solution is carried over the top of the tanks into a well (weir) to a drain.

The system also includes heaters, thermostats, heat exchangers, and filters. In some systems, the temperature of the solutions may be controlled by contact with the common walls of the solution tanks and the temperature of the wash water.

THE WASH SYSTEM

An adequate supply of water is necessary to remove residual fixer from the processed radiograph. Adequate washing helps preserve the radiograph while in storage (improved archival properties). The wash system is not part of the recirculation system. Water is passed through the processor at a constant rate and flows over a weir into the drain.

CHEMICAL REPLENISHMENT SYSTEM

Replenishment keeps the solutions at proper strength and level in the processing tanks while extending solution life. As radiographic films pass through the processor, they change the balance of developer alkalinity and fixer acidity. The automatic replenishment system works accordingly to keep these chemistries in balance. Transport systems can also be affected by improper solution replenishment. If the film emulsion does not swell and harden properly in the solutions, the film can jam in the roller transport system.

Overreplenishment of the developer may result in lower radiographic contrast. (See Chapter 11.) Severe developer underreplenishment may cause film to stick in the dryer.

Overreplenishment of the fixer does not greatly affect image quality but is expensive and wasteful. Underreplenishment of fixer results in poor clearing and insufficient hardening of the emulsion, with possible failure of the film to transport properly. The archival quality of the film can be affected by underreplenishment of the fixer.

Developer and fixer are automatically added to the automatic processor to compensate for the volume of work. As the film passes into the developer, a microswitch in the film detector roller (entrance) closes, activating the replenishment pumps. Replenisher solutions flow into the proper tanks. The rate of replenishment is determined by the film size (Fig. 10–2). After the film passes over the entrance roller, the switch opens and replenishment ceases. The new solutions are blended into the tanks by the recirculating system.

The replenishment system includes a strainer, a device to control backflow, and instrumentation to measure replenishment rates.

AUTOMATIC MIXER AND REPLENISHMENT SYSTEMS

In some large radiology departments that are serviced by an in-house central replenishment facility, bulk chemistry is mixed at a remote location and pumped to the automatic processors.

In departments without a central replenishment facility, developer and fixer replenishment tanks holding up to 50 gallons of each solution are usually located close to the automatic processor.

Automatic mixer and replenishment systems contain concentrated developer and fixer replenishment, which are automatically mixed with water as required, in 5-, 10- or 15-gallon mixing and holding containers. This equipment is simple to operate and can be cleaned and maintained with hot water. Electronic probes sense the chemistry level and mix the precise amount of concentrated solution and water. The dispenser compartments are color- and letter-coded and their openings are shaped to accept correspondingly shaped bottles (Fig. 10–4). One automixer can be used for one or two processors.

THE DRYER

As the film is transported through the dryer section, heated filtered air is directed over both sides of the film by a phlenum (wind box). Humidity and temperature are carefully

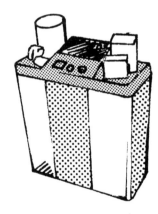

Figure 10-4 Automatic Mixer and Replenishment Units *Processing consistency is ensured with automatically mixed replenishment solutions. Concentrated developer and fixer replenishers can be automatically mixed with water as required. Electronic probes within the automixer sense chemistry levels in the replenishment tanks and add the precise amount of concentrated solution and water.*

The developer and fixer replenishment bottles are of different shapes and colors and are letter coded.

controlled. Proper venting must be provided for dryer heat as well as for chemical fumes.

Automatic standby controls, used to reduce energy costs and water consumption, de-energize the processor when film is not being processed.

Automatic Processing Solutions

The solutions used in the automatic processor have a longer solution life and differ from the solutions used for manual processing techniques.

The Need for Special Solutions

With manual processing techniques, when the film is placed into the developer, its emulsion gets soft and swells. In the stop bath and fixer solutions, the emulsion contracts and begins to harden. As the film is passed from one solution to another, it varies in thickness and stickiness. This is not a problem as long as films do not come in contact with one another.

Film is always in contact with the rollers in the transport systems of an automatic processor; therefore, the degree of swelling and stickiness must be controlled. A film that is too thick slows down the transport system and causes a jam as the next film catches up to it. A film that is too thin could slip in or between the rollers and could also cause a jam. If the film becomes too sticky, it could adhere to or wrap around a roller.

Because of the unique requirements of the automatic processor, special chemicals were formulated containing hardeners in the developer and the fixing solution, which hold the thickness and stickiness of the film within the tolerances needed for automatic processing. These special chemicals along with controlled replenishment and recirculation reduce processing and transport time.

IMPORTANT: Never substitute conventional (manual) processing chemicals for automatic film processor chemicals.

THE DEVELOPER

Developer chemistry (an alkaline solution) used for automatic processing usually contains:

Sulfite (sodium or potassium) — acts as a preservative

Carbonate (sodium or potassium) — acts as a buffer and a source of alkali

Hydroquinone (a developing agent) — helps to provide upper scale density (black)

Metol or phenidone (a developing agent) — helps to provide intermediate or lower scale densities (shades of gray to white)

Hydroxide (sodium or potassium) — the activator in the developer (a source of alkali)

Gluteraldehyde — a hardening agent (not found in manual processing developer solutions)

Potassium bromide — antifoggant and restrainer (used to minimize fog and maintain chemical balance between fresh and seasoned chemicals. It suppresses the activity of the phenidone on unexposed silver crystals, thereby helping to maintain low base fog levels.)

Water — aids in the swelling of the emulsion — is the solvent for the developer chemicals.

THE FIXER

The automatic processor fixer (acidic) solutions are well buffered; therefore, a stop bath is not required. The fixer contains:

Sodium thiosulfate or ammonia thiosulfate (hypo) — used as a silver solvent to remove unexposed silver crystals from the film

Sodium sulfite — used as a preservative for the ammonia thiosulfate

Acetic acid (a source of hydrogen ions) — a buffer

Aluminum sulfate (a hardening agent) — helps to reduce drying time

Water — used as a solvent for the fixer chemicals

Quality Assurance

Often, radiographic equipment seemingly fails to perform properly when, in reality, minor changes in the processor may be responsible for the poor quality radiographs (Fig. 10–5).

In order for the processor to operate efficiently, an established preventive maintenance routine should be faithfully followed.

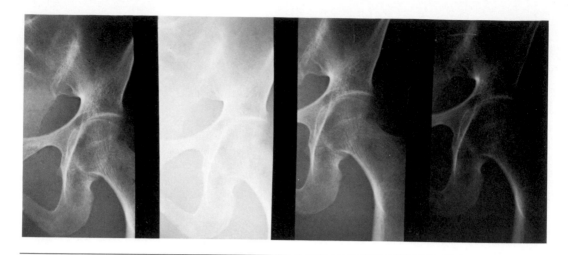

Figure 10-5 Automatic Processor Quality Control *A quality assurance program is of little value if the automatic processor functions are not monitored. Severe differences can occur in radiographic densities as a result of mechanical or chemical problems in an automatic processor. Four radiographs of a pelvic phantom are shown. All were exposed with the same calibrated x-ray unit, cassette, technical factors, and collimator shutter patterns. The four radiographs were im-mediately processed in four different automatic processors and exhibit severe variations in density owing to processor malfunctions.*

When a processor is located at a remote location, for example, the operating room, and severe changes in radiographic density are noted, radiographic techniques are often adjusted. Since we rarely have the opportunity to compare images from processor to processor, daily quality assurance testing of the processor is essential.

Daily and weekly cleanup procedures will result in a well-maintained processor, which will require minimal servicing.

Developer and fixer replenishment tanks must be covered with evaporation lids to reduce chemical evaporation. If a processor is used in a low-volume area, evaporation covers are critical. Evaporation can cause oxidation of the developer, diminishing its chemical activity.

Dried precipitation from evaporated chemicals on the rollers can cause transport problems. A single dirty roller can cause a breakdown in the automatic processor.

It is advisable to change processing solutions at least every 6 months. More frequent changes may be required, depending upon the workload of the department. When the solutions are being changed, a more thorough cleaning and inspection should be made using a maintenance checklist.

Some quality control tasks that require careful attention include the monitoring of the developer activity, the length of development, and factors that affect chemical activity, such as replenishment rates and solution contamination.

The processor activity should be evaluated by a sensitometric film strip exposed from a sensitometer. (See Fig. 8–4.) An x-ray machine is sometimes used to expose a stepwedge image to monitor the processor. The sensitometer is recommended for this task, because the x-ray machine would also require evaluation for output accuracy.

A densitometer (see Fig. 8–4) is used to evaluate the sensitometric readings from the processed image. Speed, contrast, and fog should be evaluated daily, and a log should be maintained.

Replenishment rates can be easily measured by disconnecting the replenishment lines and catching, in graduated beakers, the replenisher that is fed into the processor as a film is passed over the entrance roller.

A processor quality assurance program can

help to minimize the repeat rate, patient exposure, and departmental operating costs. The combination of film quality (controlled by the manufacturer), chemistry, and mechanical monitoring coupled with a technical quality assurance program should result in radiographs of uniformly high quality.

Safelight Filter Selection

Care must be made in the selection of safelight filters. Special filters are required to match the spectral sensitivity of the film in use.

For years, the Eastman Kodak Wratten Series 6B Safelight Filter was in common use. This filter was designed to be used with blue sensitive medical x-ray films. With the introduction of orthochromatic sensitive medical x-ray film, a filter had to be designed that could be used with blue and green sensitive products. This filter is the Kodak safelight filter type GBX-2.

A dark green filter is available for photofluorographic and cinefluorographic panchromatic films. These films should be handled in total darkness until at least one half the development time has expired.

IMPORTANT: The use of a safelight designed for blue sensitive film with orthochromatic x-ray film (primarily green sensitive) results in fogging of the film. Light bulb wattage level information and a simple safelight test kit are available from most film sales representatives.

Silver Recovery

Silver recovery is a simple process, and the recovered silver can be sold to provide an additional source of revenue for the radiology department.

The residual silver halide in the fixing solution of the processor can be collected by either a metallic replacement cartridge or an electrolytic plating cell. These reclamation procedures can be carried out "in house." Chemical precipitation of used fixer is generally performed in commercial facilities or in departments with centralized collecting systems.

To collect the silver from the fixing solution, a drain is connected to the fixing tank. Instead of emptying the exhausted fixer solution into the main drain, it is allowed to flow into a collecting receptacle or directly into a silver recovery unit.

If solution is being passed into an electrolytic silver recovery unit, it is necessary to provide a broken connection (an air space) in the tube so that no electrolytic action can follow the solution back to the processor and cause corrosion or plating of silver in the processor.

Another form of silver recovery is the removal of the black metallic silver on processed radiographs or the unprocessed emulsion of unexposed film. The film is usually purchased by reclaimers who are equipped to remove the silver in an efficient, cost-effective manner, either by burning or by chemical methods.

Cine or Strip Film Processing

Professional cine processors are available that can accommodate films from 8 mm to 70 mm. They are similar to medical x-ray film processors in that they control time, temperature, agitation, replenishment, and wash water flow rates. Special drive transport systems ensure proper film tension and help to eliminate film breakage during transport.

Seventy-millimeter or 105-mm fluoro spot films and 14 in. wide roll film used for serial angiography can be taped to a lead sheet of x-ray film and processed in a conventional automatic processor. The leader should be 7 in. or longer and as wide or wider than the roll film to ensure proper transport through the automatic processor. Scotch Brand Electrical Tape No. 850 (1 in. wide) can be used to butt-splice the roll film to the leader film.

IMPORTANT: The adhesive side of the tape must not come in contact with the roller transport system.

11 Radiographic Quality

IMAGE quality is the term used to describe the radiographic image and refers to those qualities that are present (in varying degrees) in all images. The quality of the radiograph helps to determine the diagnostic information available for interpretation.

All radiographic images exhibit photographic and optical density (overall blackness), radiographic contrast (differences between two or more densities), definition (sharpness of the structure being radiographed), and distortion (size or shape of the image relative to the true size and shape of the object being examined). If these imaging qualities are optimum, they will be easy to discern on the processed radiograph. The physical parameters that control or affect image quality can be adjusted by the radiographer to accommodate the preferences of the interpreter.

Radiographic images are transparencies; therefore, their light-absorbing properties are measured as transmission densities. When a reflective support is used to record the image, such as in Polaroid or electrostatic imaging (Xerox) techniques (see Chapter 9), reflection densities are measured.

A proper blend of technical factors affect the appearance of the radiographic image.

Some of the factors used in the production of a radiograph are standard, while others must be changed depending upon patient condition, size, ability to cooperate, and equipment limitations. The characteristics of density, contrast, definition (detail), and distortion can be controlled and affected by many technical factors and radiographic accessories.

The application of the principles of exposure is a measure of the art and skill of the radiographer. Image quality will be discussed in terms of how radiographic principles affect the radiographic image and the relationships of controlling factors to each other.

There are four primary exposure factors that are used to change the photographic effect of the image. They are kilovoltage (kVp), milliamperage (mA), time (seconds), and distance.

Kilovoltage affects the quality of the x-ray beam. As the kilovoltage levels are increased, changes occur in the energy spectrum (shorter wavelength radiation). (See Chapter 1.) The overall number of photons of all energies increases, with a significant increase in the number of higher energy photons. More higher energy photons will penetrate the part under study; therefore, a greater effect is produced on the radiographic image. When a longer wavelength (lower kVp) technique is used, more of the low energy photons are absorbed by the body.

The energy spectrum is not changed by a change in the milliampere value. As milliamperage is raised, the quantity of x-ray production is increased, but the energy of the photons is not affected. The combination of mA and time (exposure length) determines the total number of x-rays produced (quantity). Milliamperage and time (seconds) can be varied to maintain a preselected mAs with no change in radiographic density. (See Chapter 13.) Occasionally, a high milliampere value combined with a short exposure time is needed to stop motion. Several problems can occur with extremely short exposure times and high ma values. These include ''blooming'' of the focal spot (see Chapter 4) or ''capture'' of the grid in motion. (See Figs. 5–15 and 5–17.) Minimal response time difficulties can also occur with automatic exposure devices (AED). (See Chapter 2.) As with all technical factor selection, the radiographer must do more than simply select kVp, mA, and time. A compromise is often necessary.

Image quality and diagnostic quality are not necessarily synonymous. Although a radiograph may seem to possess excellent image quality, it may not be a diagnostic image. For example, a short-scale contrast (abrupt black and white) image of the lung fields may mask subtle pulmonary vascular details. A short-scale contrast image of an extremity may fail to demonstrate a subtle soft tissue change. On the other hand, a radiograph that is not of optimal radiographic quality may be adequate for diagnostic purposes. If an infant were examined for a metallic foreign body such as a straight pin, a short exposure time might be used to overcome motion of the pin (owing to peristaltic activity or patient motion). If a high kilovoltage study (85 kVp or greater) were used without a grid for this study, the overall appearance of the radiograph would be photographically unattractive but diagnostically adequate.

If a child were suspected of ingesting a coin, it is important that the entire alimentary tract be evaluated. When the first image is made of the abdomen and the coin is not found, cervical and chest radiographs are taken. The coin, if lodged in the esophagus, could migrate to the abdomen while the abdominal radiograph was being processed. When chest and cervical area studies are made, a negative study could also result. A large format (14 in. × 17 in.) study using high kVp and low mAs helps to avoid this problem while minimizing exposure to the child. An infant can often be placed diagonally on the cassette, to image the entire alimentary tract from the nasal cavity to the rectum. Although the technique used for this single exposure is not one that would be recommended for any one specific area, the anatomical details would still be visible in relationship to the high contrast metallic foreign body.

Variations in focal film distances are rarely deliberately used to affect image quality. A minor increase in focal film distance may require a major change in technical factors (see Table 11–1). If distance is changed with a grid technique, the radiographer must remember that grid focal ranges are determined by grid ratio. (See Table 5–1.)

Formulas needed to accomplish technical changes are presented in Chapter 13. The purpose of grouping all formulas together is to provide easy access when they are needed as a reference for conversion of technical factors. Chapter 14 will be devoted to the application and evaluation of the imaging principles presented in this textbook.

Radiographic Density

Density as applied to mass per unit volume (see Chapter 1) should not be confused with photographic or optical density.

Photographic density is defined as the log of the intensity of the incident light falling upon the image to the intensity of the light transmitted through the image. (See Chapter 13.) Radiographic density is usually described in terms of the overall blackening of a processed film.

The radiologist refers to density as anatomical or pathological changes that absorb x-ray (Fig. 11–1), for example, a solid mass within the lung that stops x-ray from reaching the detector, decreasing film blackening.

X-ray absorption is dependent upon the atomic number as well as part thickness of this absorber, whether it be a solid tumor, an

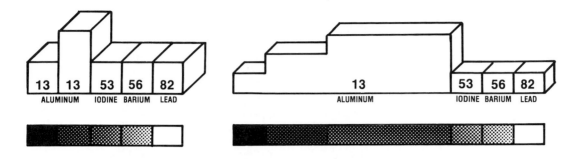

Figure 11-1   The Effect of Absorption on Radiographic Density *Physical density (mass per unit volume) should not be confused with photographic or optical density. Five different materials (four different densities) are shown (left). The atomic number of each material is shown. The four materials, aluminum, iodine, barium, and lead are displayed as equal size objects. A rectangular-shaped structure of aluminum shown in position two represents 2× increase in thickness compared to the other objects. Note the difference in the densities produced in the simulated stepwedge. The x-ray beam produces a blackened step for the first thickness of aluminum, since most of the radiation would pass through this substance. The double thickness of aluminum absorbs more x-ray and therefore attenuates the x-ray beam to a greater degree. Note iodine, (atomic number 53) and barium (atomic number 56) absorb a similar amount of radiation. Lead, on the other hand, absorbs almost all the x-radiation in this example. An object having increased mass determined by the atomic number and or tissue thickness will absorb more x-radiation, with decreased film blackening (radiographic density).*

Equal thickness of dissimilar materials are used to demonstrate subject contrast. A representation of an aluminum stepwedge adjacent to the iodine, barium, and lead objects is shown. The aluminum stepwedge varies in multiples of two. Step two is 2× thicker than step one; step three is 4× thicker than step one. The first step appears black; step two, less black; step three appears gray owing to the increase in absorption resulting from the 4× thickness of the aluminum. The third step almost matches the radiographic density of the iodine and barium steps adjacent to it. The iodine, barium, and lead are of the same thickness (equal in thickness to step one of the aluminum wedge), yet they absorb different amounts of x-ray. The differences in adjacent densities shown represent contrast. When multiple density changes are seen, long-scale contrast is present. Abrupt density differences indicate short-scale contrast.

osseous change, or fluid. The radiographer thinks of the term *density* as referring to overall film blackening (an optical or photographic property). A radiolucent area (decreased absorption) would produce an increase in film blackening.

The image as viewed by transmitted light, usually on a viewbox, consists of variations in the amount of black metallic silver remaining on the film after chemical processing (Fig. 11–2). The exposed silver emulsion is converted into black metallic silver by the process of development. The degree of blackness on a radiograph is determined by the amount of exposure reaching the emulsion of the film. (See Chapter 10.)

The overall blackness and relationship of the intensity of the incident light from the viewbox to the light transmitted through the film can be measured. (See Chapter 13.)

Differences in density represent the contrast within the image. Images with only a few density variations are said to exhibit short-scale contrast. Greater density variations result in longer-scale contrast. (See the section entitled Contrast.)

To graphically portray the response of x-ray film to known amounts of exposure, density may be measured by a densitometer (see Fig. 8–4) and plotted on a graph. The resultant curve drawn from the graph is called an H & D curve, sensitometric curve, or characteristic curve. (See Fig. 8–5.)

Radiographic film has a blue tint in its base, which adds to overall density. (See Chapter 8.) An increase in density can also be

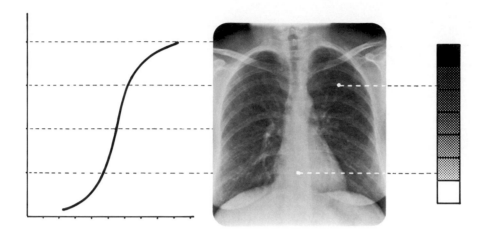

Figure 11-2   Optical Density

A densitometer is used to measure the response of x-ray film to known amounts of exposure. Overall blackness (optical density) and the relationship of the intensity of the light transmitted through the radiographic film to the amount of light incident to the image from the viewbox can be measured. These measurements can be plotted on a graph known as a characteristic curve (left). Radiographic density increases as exposure is increased.

Exposure factors are represented logrithmically at the bottom of the illustration. (See Fig. 11-4.) A chest radiograph as viewed by transmitted light is shown (center) with a representation of a stepwedge of the differences between densities (contrast) (right). Dotted lines from the sensitometric curve pass through representative areas of density on the chest radiograph and are aligned to representative densities on the stepwedge.

caused by the development of unexposed silver halide crystals (chemical fog). (See Chapter 10.)

Density and mAs

Radiographic density, as a result of x-ray exposure, is primarily controlled by mAs. Milliamperage is used to control the number of electrons made available for interaction with the target and time is used to control the length of exposure. Milliamperage and time are inversely proportional to each other; therefore, it is easy to maintain a given density when either variable must be changed. Increasing mA or time will cause a corresponding increase in radiographic density. (See Chapter 13.)

> **IMPORTANT:** A 30% to 40% increase in mAs is required to detect a visible density change on a radiograph.

Radiographic density can also be affected by other exposure factors, such as distance kilovoltage, the use of radiographic accessories, and processing.

Density and Distance

Distance is rarely selected as a factor to control or influence density. In practice, it may be necessary to adjust mAs because of distance restrictions imposed by the patient's condition or the use of a grid or by other equipment limitations. (See Fig. 3–7.) Changes in the focal film distance can greatly affect density. Because less radiation reaches the film as the FFD is increased, mAs must be changed to compensate for changes in distance (Fig. 11–3). The intensity of the x-ray beam varies inversely with the square of the distance. (See Chapter 13.)

> **IMPORTANT:** Doubling of the distance would result in a reduction of radiographic density by a factor of 4 (four times the mAs would be required to maintain the given density; Table 11–1).

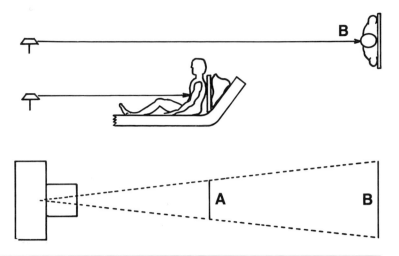

Figure 11-3 **The Effect of Focal Film Distance on Density** *The intensity of the x-ray beam varies inversely with the square of the distance. (See Chapter 13.) If the exposure factors used for a bedside chest* (A) *at 36 in. resulted in a proper radiographic density, a 4× increase in exposure* factors would be required to duplicate this image at a 72-in. FFD (B). See Table 11-1 for representative distance relationships. A shortened focal film distance (A) can produce geometric imaging problems. (See Chapter 13.)*

TABLE 11-1. Distance (D) Relationships

	Field Size: Directly Proportional to D	Area Coverage: Directly Proportional to D^2	Density: Inversely Proportional to D^2	Beam Intensity: Inversely Proportional to D^2	Exposure Value: Directly Proportional to D^2
1/2 (D)	2 in. × 2.5 in.	5 sq. in.	4.0	4 (R)	1/4 (mAs)
(D) Value	4 in. × 5 in.	20 sq. in.	unit of density	R	mAS
2 (D)	8 in. × 10 in.	80 sq. in.	1/4	1/4 (R)	4 (mAs)

DISTANCE RELATIONSHIPS

Representative distance changes are shown in Table 11–1, with D indicating the distance for a normal study. Field sizes change in a linear fashion, whereas area coverage is directly proportional to the distance squared. For example, the doubling of the distance produces a 2× linear, 4× area field coverage. Density and beam intensity (film blackening and dosage) vary inversely to the distance squared. (See Chapter 13 for related formulas.)

The density and beam intensity changes in this table are accomplished with adjustments in distance only. In practice, when distance is changed, technical factors are adjusted to maintain the desired radiographic density.

Under the heading labeled Exposure Value in Table 11–1, adjustments needed in the mAs values to overcome changes in distance are shown. The exposure changes are directly proportional to distance squared.

Variation in kilovoltage is not shown as part of this table, because kilovoltage is not linear. It is difficult to recommend changes in kilovoltage over the wide range of focal film distances shown. (See Fig. 11–4.)

Kilovoltage and Density

The kVp relationship to radiographic density is not linear. At lower kilovoltage levels, an increase of less than 10 kVp is sufficient to double the density on a radiograph. At higher kVp levels, much more kilovoltage is needed for a doubling effect if all other factors remain constant. A 15% change in kVp is required to double or half density. (See Chapter 13.) Compare this change with the linear relationship associated with the adjustment of mAs to control density (Fig. 11–4).

Minor changes in technique should be made with caution when using a high-speed rare-earth screen film combination. Technical changes with a 1200-speed system will have 12 times the effect of a change made with a 100-speed system (see Table 8–1), with a corresponding reduction in exposure latitude (Fig. 11–4).

The kVp range determines the penetrating

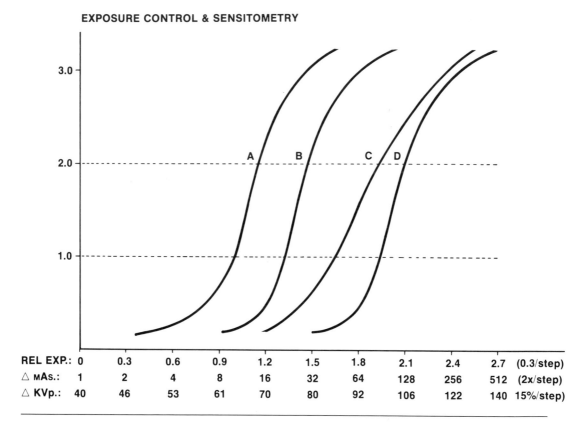

EXPOSURE CONTROL & SENSITOMETRY

REL EXP.:	0	0.3	0.6	0.9	1.2	1.5	1.8	2.1	2.4	2.7	(0.3/step)
△ MAs.:	1	2	4	8	16	32	64	128	256	512	(2x/step)
△ KVp.:	40	46	53	61	70	80	92	106	122	140	15%/step)

Figure 11-4 The Relationship of Exposure Factors to Radiographic Density *Typical sensitometric curves are labeled A, B, C, and D. Relative exposure values are used to logrithmically indicate the doubling of radiographic exposure values (2× increase in exposure per 0.3 step). Logrithms are necessary to confine the scale to a reasonable size. The doubling of density by a change in mAs is conceptually easier to visualize than a* logrithmic change, since mAs changes are linear. Kilovoltage is not linear and requires an approximate 15% change to double radiographic density. The doubling or halving of mAs or a 15% incremental change in kilovoltage produces approximately the same effect on radiographic density. These changes are related to logrithmic increments in this illustration.*

ability of the x-ray beam (Fig. 11-5). Increased kVp results in the production of radiation with a shorter wavelength, increased penetration, and greater Compton effect (scatter). (See Fig. 1–8.) The scatter generated by an increase in kVp is also reflected in the density on the radiograph, since scatter radiation produces a supplemental density. It is difficult to measure the effect of scatter in each given situation.

IMPORTANT: The kVp must be sufficient to penetrate the object. No reasonable amount of mAs can compensate for inadequate kVp.

Density and Processing

Changes in development time, developer temperature, transport time (in automatic processing), and the degree of concentration or exhaustion of developer can affect radiographic density. Chemical fog owing to overdevelopment or chemical imbalance may produce a supplemental density on the radiograph. Cold or weak solutions can result in films that are underdeveloped and lack adequate density. Film storage conditions can also affect radiographic density. (See Chapter 8.)

Density and Filtration

Any material that attenuates the x-ray beam will reduce density on the radiograph. Depending upon the type of filtration, its method of use, and its purpose, this effect may or may not be obvious. Low-energy wavelengths that are filtered out by inherent and added tube filtration do not appreciably affect density. Wedge, trough, and other compensating filters, however, are often used to affect density changes on a given portion of the radiograph. (See Fig. 4–9.) Absorptive tabletops or cassette fronts have a filtration effect on the x-ray beam and can decrease radiographic density. (See Fig. 9–6.)

Density and Intensifying Screens

Intensifying screens are designed to increase the efficiency of the x-ray beam and are frequently used to influence radiographic density. High-speed rare-earth screen film combinations are frequently used to compensate for low output equipment. (See Chapter 8.) An added benefit is the reduction of dosage to patient and operator.

Density and Scatter Radiation

Scatter radiation, although detrimental to image detail by masking useful information, also adds to radiographic density. Controlling scatter radiation (all other factors unchanged) reduces radiographic density. (See Chapter 5.)

Grids reduce the overall density on a radiograph by preventing scatter from reaching the film and by absorbing some primary as well as most secondary radiation. (See Chapter 5.) To maintain a given density, the use of a grid requires an appropriate increase in exposure factors (usually kVp). (See Table 5–1.)

Beam restriction by the use of cones, collimators, or diaphragms limits the production of scatter radiation, improving radiographic contrast (shorter scale). (See Fig. 5–6.) By reducing the supplemental density created by

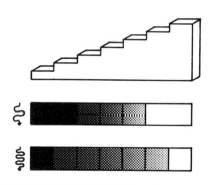

Figure 11-5 Penetrating Ability of Kilovoltage A representation of an aluminum stepwedge is shown. Two simulated x-ray beams show the effect x-ray wavelengths have on penetration. The longer wavelength (low kVp) results in shortscale contrast, which produces sharp demarkations between structures. Kilovoltage must be adequate to penetrate the part under study to visualize radiographic details within the structural borders. The shorter wavelength (high kVp), which is more penetrating, produces multiple density changes from black to white with intermediate shades of gray, demonstrating a wider range of structures (latitude).

scatter, density is also reduced. A compensation in technical factors is required to maintain a given density. (See Fig. 12–1 and Table 14–2.)

When an AED is used, the effect of collimation on radiographic density is obvious. (See Chapter 2.) When the added density created by scatter is reduced by tight beam collimation, the AED will adjust for the change in density by lengthening the exposure time until the predetermined density has been reached. It follows that the degree of collimation affects radiographic density.

Undercutting of the image by scatter can cause the AED to prematurely shorten the length of the exposure, resulting in an underexposed radiograph. (See Fig. 2–12.)

Density and the Patient

The density (mass per unit volume) of the patient or of the part under study can affect radiographic density. Thicker body parts absorb more radiation. (See Fig. 12–4.) This factor is generally thought of in terms of differential absorption, which is related to radiographic contrast, since kVp is often used to compensate for thicker body parts (Fig. 11–6). Information on the effect of pathology on radiographic techniques can be found in Chapter 12.

Density and Heel Effect

The position of the x-ray tube can have an effect on radiographic density. This variation in intensity is known as the *heel effect*. The heel effect is less noticeable when increased focal film distances or small field sizes are used because the beam is more uniform nearest central ray. (See Figs. 4–3 and 4–4.)

Contrast

Radiographic contrast is an important image quality that takes into consideration subject contrast and film contrast and is defined as the differences between two or more adjacent densities on a radiograph (Fig. 11–7).

Subject Contrast

The ratio of the x-ray intensity transmitted through one segment of the part in a study

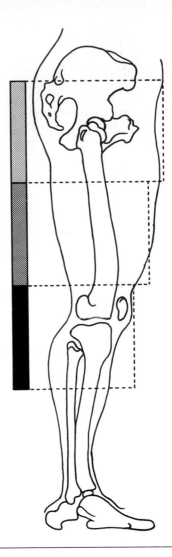

Figure 11-6 The Effect of Differential Absorption on Density *Thicker body parts absorb more x-radiation. A body part can vary in thickness as well as mass density. A representative illustration from the acetabulum to the thinner portion of the lower leg is shown. The thicker hip area requires more x-radiation than the knee. (See Fig. 12-4.) If an adequate exposure were used to image the hip, the femoral area would be approximately 2× overexposed and the knee approximately 4× overexposed. Conversely, proper exposure for the knee would result in an underexposed hip radiograph. Individual exposures of each region should be made for adequate density and contrast. If the entire leg must be visualized for orthopedic measurement (see Fig. 4-12), the use of a compensatory filter near source (see Fig. 4-9) can be used to overcome the gradation (stepwedge-like) differences in tissue density from hip to the mid portion of the lower leg.*

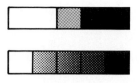

Figure 11-7   Radiographic Contrast
The difference between two or more adjacent densities on a radiograph is defined as radiographic contrast. The term contrast *is used to describe short-scale contrast* (top) *usually associated with low kVp, high mAs values. Long-scale contrast* (bottom) *is associated with high kilovoltage, low mAs techniques. A higher kilovoltage range that produces long-scale contrast can be of advantage when the subject contrast contains many subtle densities. In the chest, long-scale contrast is preferred; the heart must be penetrated for mediastinal details and the lungs not overexposed. When a low kilovoltage technique s used for chest radiography, the ribs will appear chalk-like, the lungs blackened, and the mediastinal structures underpenetrated.*

to that transmitted through a more absorbing adjacent segment is known as subject contrast. The density and atomic number of the part affects subject contrast. Radiation quality also affects subject contrast. Kilovoltage settings, total filtration, and the tube target material all influence beam quality. (See Chapter 7 for tungsten and molybdenum tube target material comparisons.)

A major influence on subject contrast is the effect of scatter radiation, which can be controlled by collimation, grid, or compression techniques. The use of contrast media to outline organs or vessels also influences subject contrast. (See Chapter 12 for specific information about the selection of technical factors for use with radiopaque or radiolucent contrast media.)

If a single radiograph were taken of two identical objects of equal thickness and material content, no density difference should be evident. If the two objects do not exhibit density differences, contrast is not present. One could choose objects of dissimilar materials or unequal thickness to demonstrate the absence of radiographic contrast. Equal thickness of dissimilar materials (different atomic num-

bers) will radiographically demonstrate subject contrast (Fig. 11–1).

Contrast can be better understood if we first consider only the density difference between black and white ("short-scale" contrast).

If one were to sensitometrically evaluate a clear processed film, a sensitometric reading would begin at D-Min. A totally blackened radiograph would be read at D-Max. (See Chapter 8.) If the conditions that produced the first two radiographs could be reproduced resulting in the two densities being adjacent to each other on the same radiograph, short-scale contrast (difference in densities) would be evident (Fig. 11–7).

As a greater number of density changes are produced, the contrast scale increases. The longer the scale of contrast, the wider the range of structures that can be imaged (latitude; Figs. 11–5 and 11–7).

Film Contrast

Film contrast refers to the contrast inherent in the radiographic film. Processing conditions, fog level, as well as other sources of radiation can affect film contrast. (See Chapter 10.)

A radiographer cannot control film contrast, since it is a design parameter. Radiographic film can be manufactured to exhibit high (short-scale) or low (long-scale) contrast (Fig. 11–8). (See Fig. 8–5.)

Kilovoltage and Contrast

Kilovoltage is used to control both radiographic contrast and penetration. Kilovoltage determines whether the radiation will be of sufficient strength to penetrate the object (short wavelength) or whether the radiation consists of long wavelengths, some of which would be absorbed by the object. In the diagnostic kilovoltage range, two x-ray interactions with matter are significant: photoelectric effect (absorption), and Compton effect (scatter). (See Figs. 1–7 and 1–8 and Table 1–2.)

As kilovoltage is increased, the number of photons of all energies up to the peak kilovoltage is increased, adding additional high-energy photons to the beam. Above 80 kVp, the primary interaction is Compton effect, which reduces short-scale contrast.

Scatter radiation is detrimental to radio-

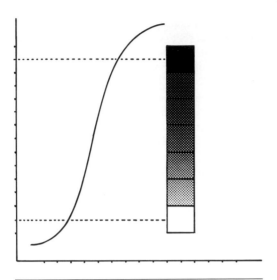

Figure 11-8 Sensitometric Representation of Radiographic Contrast *A typical sensitometric curve is shown, with dotted lines representing the useful density range for medical radiography. The first dotted line, just above the toe of the sensitometric curve, is represented by the whitest portion of the stepwedge. The upper dotted line, crossing through the highest density portion of the stepwedge, is represented as black. As the curve ascends from the toe to the shoulder, there is an increase in density. Fine dotted lines link segments of the curve to related densities on the stepwedge. The differences between the seven density steps in this illustration denote radiographic contrast. For additional sensitometric information see Chapter 8.*

graphic contrast, since it affects the whiter areas on the radiograph to a greater degree than the blacker areas. Segments of the image that have reached D-Max cannot get blacker.

Beam Filtration and Radiographic Contrast

Filtration attenuates the low-energy photons in the beam by the photoelectric process. (See Chapter 1.) Small increases in aluminum filtration do not appreciably affect contrast, because low-energy photons would not have contributed to the image but would have been absorbed by the patient. If the amount of added filtration is sufficient to reduce density

on the radiograph, shorter-scale contrast results.

Intensifying Screens and Contrast

Radiographic contrast is affected by the use of intensifying screens. The fluorescent effect of the screens on the film results in the production of a shorter scale of contrast compared with images made by the direct action of x-radiation alone. When sensitometric test radiographs are made and evaluated, the slope of the characteristic curve will change more abruptly on screen film images, indicating a shorter scale of contrast.

Contrast and Scatter Control

The elimination of scatter helps to produce a radiograph with shorter scale contrast. Scatter radiation does not affect the entire image in a uniform manner. The lower density areas on the film, however, lose contrast because of the supplemental density caused by the scatter.

Beam restriction limits the area of tissue interaction with the primary beam. The smaller the field size, the less scatter radiation generated, resulting in shorter-scale contrast. (Fig. 11–9). (See Chapter 5.)

The purpose of a grid or Bucky is to prevent most scatter radiation from reaching the x-ray film.

Processing and Contrast

Processing solutions can affect radiographic contrast. Solutions that are too hot can produce chemical fog. If the time of development is too great, owing to emersion in the solutions for a longer period of time than is required (transport time in an automatic processor or increased development time in manual processing), the lower density regions of the radiograph will continue to be affected by the developer chemicals, and short-scale contrast will decrease. Proper processing (time/temperature) is required to maintain contrast as well as density. (See Chapter 10.)

Controllable Factors

The radiographer is able to control several factors that affect radiographic contrast (Table 11–2).

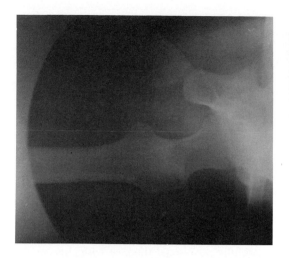 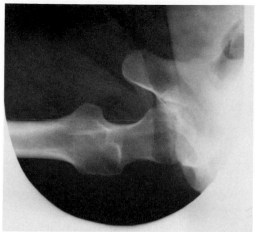

Figure 11-9 Contrast Improvement With Scatter Control *Scatter diminishes radiographic contrast. A reduction in field size will limit the amount of tissue that can interact with the x-ray beam to produce scatter.*

An attempt was made to demonstrate the relationship of the head of the femur to the acetab- *ulum. The tightly coned grid view exhibits excellent radiographic contrast and recorded detail (right). The non-grid, larger field image demonstrates the effect of scatter on contrast as well as detail. The relationship of the head of the femur to the acetabulum is not well seen on this poorly collimated image.*

TABLE 11-2. Radiographic Contrast (Short-Scale)[*]

Controllable Factors	Recommendations
Kilovoltage	Sufficient to penetrate the part under study
Scatter control (A) Collimation (B) Grid or Bucky	Restrict field size to cassette size or smaller Match grid ratio to highest kVp to be used Use recommended focal range
Extra focal radiation	Restrict the x-ray beam as close to source as possible (see Fig. 5–9)
Compression	Use to flatten tissue to reduce scatter; helpful in mammography (see Chapter 7) May be contraindicated in some examinations

[*]Some factors that are controlled by departmental preferences or quality assurance practices include selection of filtration material, film screen products, processor temperatures, and the use of contrast media.

Recorded Detail

Recorded detail is a visual quality. The sharpness of the structural edges of the radiographic image (definition) is usually referred to as *detail*.

Detail in a radiograph can be affected by geometric limitations and by those controllable factors (Table 11–3) that make the details visible to the observer.

In some instances, the structures in an object are recorded with all details transferred to the film (good geometric detail), but because of technical limitations, the information may not be visible (visibility of detail).

Radiographic sharpness (detail) is used to

TABLE 11-3. Radiographic Detail (Geometric)*

Controllable Factors	Recommendations
Focal spot size	As small as possible
Position of object	Perpendicualr to central ray to minimize distortion (see Fig. 14–7)
Focal object distance	As great as possible within grid focal range
Object film distance	As short as possible to minimize enlargement
Plane of the object	Parallel to receptor

*Since the x-ray beam widens as it travels from the actual focal spot to the image receptor, there is often unequal distortion of portions of the anatomy. Some degree of magnification occurs with all studies.

describe the impression of the boundaries or edges of structures on a radiograph. The boundary of a structural edge of an image can appear blurred owing to lateral spreading of the image, whether by motion, geometry, or inherent receptor blur. Geometric blurring is influenced by focal film distance (Fig. 11–3) focal spot size (Fig. 11–10), object film distance (Fig. 11–11) and so on.

Measurement of resolution and perception of sharpness are subjective. Photographic scientists have developed complex objective testing procedures, which, by their nature, are film design parameters.

A technique known as *modulation transfer function (MTF)* can be used to measure image detail (resolution) from a radiograph made of a metallic test pattern. With this evaluation method, an attempt is made to reproduce the sharp edges of the test pattern with no loss in contrast. Visibility of detail is greatly influenced by contrast. This measurement technique helps physicists to determine the limitations of an imaging system. Performance and evaluation of tests such as line spread function (LSF) and MTF should not be attempted without appropriate training. These tests require specific test tools and must be carried out according to manufacturers' recommendations. A detailed explanation of MTF and LSF is not the intent of this textbook.

A more useful approach would be concern for individual components of the imaging chain to avoid compromising image quality. If a radiographer carefully selected the proper technical factors to obtain an optically sharp image; used the sharpest screen film system; carefully positioned the part with concern for object film distance, focal film distance, and central ray alignment; collimated appropriately and used the proper grid in an attempt to improve radiographic contrast; but did not use a small focal spot, the result could be a poor-quality radiograph. The weak link in this example is the focal spot size, which diminished the total MTF of the system.

Any unwanted fluctuation in optical density (mottle) on a screen film study can be categorized as radiographic noise and consists of receptor graininess, quantum mottle, or structure mottle. (See Chapter 8.) Although screen or film graininess is rarely seen, quantum mottle can severely damage image resolution. (See Fig. 8–12.)

Four basic categories of unsharpness may be present on a radiograph and may contribute to a loss of detail. Unsharpness can be caused by image geometry, the effect of the shape of the structure on beam absorption, characteristics of the intensifying screen, and motion artifacts.

Geometric Unsharpness

Geometric sharpness is defined in terms of the umbra (distinct shadow) evident on an image. Ideally, radiation should originate from a point source; however, x-radiation usually arises from a focal "area" on the target called the *actual focal spot* (Fig. 11–10) (see Fig. 4–3) and travels in straight lines, in a divergent beam. (See Chapters 1 and 4.) An object in the path of the beam may not be imaged as a distinct shadow because of the widened

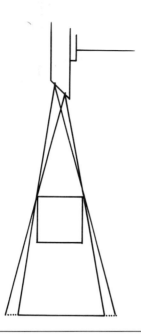

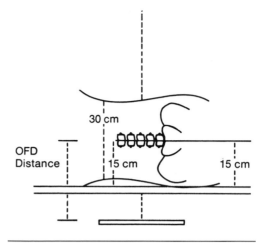

Figure 11-11 Tabletop/Bucky Tray (TT/BT) Relationship Every effort should be made to position the object under study as close to the image receptor as possible for optimal recorded detail. In this illustration, a patient is seen in the lateral position for an examination of the lumbar vertebrae. The patient measures 30 cm through the thickest portion of the abdomen. The lumbar vertebrae are mid way between both lateral aspects of the abdomen, resulting in a 15-cm object-to-tabletop distance. An additional increase in OFD is caused by the TT/BT distance, which can vary from 6 cm to 13 cm. The vertebrae in this illustration are 15 cm from the tabletop, with an additional 13 cm to the Bucky tray for a 28-cm OFD. A small focal spot (0.6 mm or smaller) is essential to maintain image sharpness with an increased object film distance. (Courtesy of Eastman Kodak Company, Rochester, New York)

Figure 11-10 The Effect of Focal Spot Size on Image Sharpness Ideally, radiation should originate from a point source for optimal sharpness (recorded detail). Since x-radiation arises from a focal area on the target, greater than a point source, structural edges may appear unsharp. The widened divergent beam passing over the edges of the structure produces a penumbral effect immediately adjacent to the sharp umbral shadow. The degree of unsharpness is dependent upon the size of the focal spot and the distance that the object is placed from the recording media. As the object is brought closer to the detector, or, if the focal film distance is increased, recorded detail improves. The optimal image would be generated by increased focal film distance, minimal object film distance, and the smallest possible focal spot size. (See Chapter 13.)

In this illustration, the object is positioned approximately two thirds of the distance from the focal spot and one third of the distance from the image detector. This results in approximately a 50% enlargement of the part. In practice, this relationship would not be acceptable unless a fractional focal spot (0.3 mm or less) were used for direct roentgen enlargement techniques. (See Chapter 7.)

divergent beam passing over the edges of the structure. The recorded image may possess a region of unsharpness (penumbra) immediately adjacent to the umbral shadow. The degree of unsharpness is dependent upon the size of the focal spot, the distance the divergent beam travels from the source to the object, and the location of the object in relation to the detector (Figs. 11–11 and 11–12).

Even when the OFD is minimal, nothing can be done to overcome the tabletop/Bucky tray (TT/BT) distance. Many radiographic tables have from a 6-cm to a 13-cm TT/BT relationship. The part under study, although in

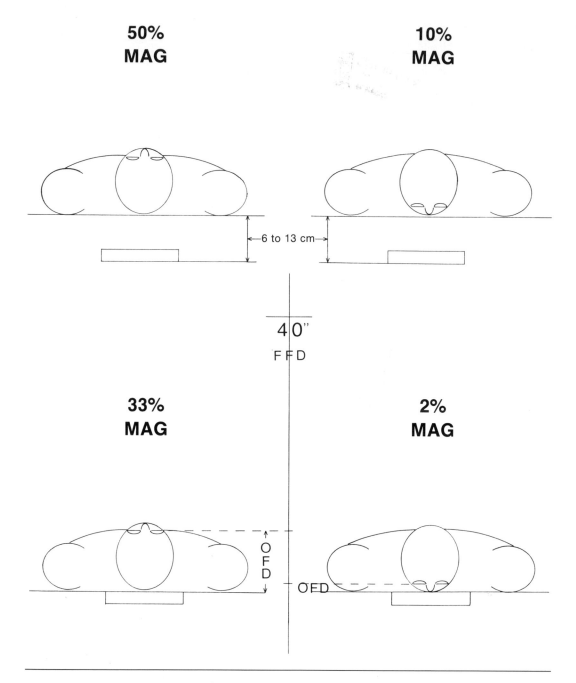

Figure 11-12 Table Bucky vs. Grid Cassette Placement A patient is positioned supine (top, left) and prone (top, right) for orbital evaluation. In the supine position, the orbits are approximately 20 cm from the tabletop. In the prone position, the orbits are almost in contact with the tabletop. The tabletop/Bucky tray distance increases the OFD. At a 40-in. FFD in the supine position, an approximate 50% enlargement of the orbits will occur, and an approximate 10% enlargement will occur in the prone position owing to the increased TT/BT distance.

If the patient were then examined in the supine and prone positions using a grid cassette (bottom), the increased OFD generated by the TT/BT spacing would no longer exist. In the supine position (bottom, left), a 33% magnification occurs. In the prone position (bottom, right), the part is positioned directly on the grid cassette, minimizing the OFD, with only a 2% increase in enlargement.

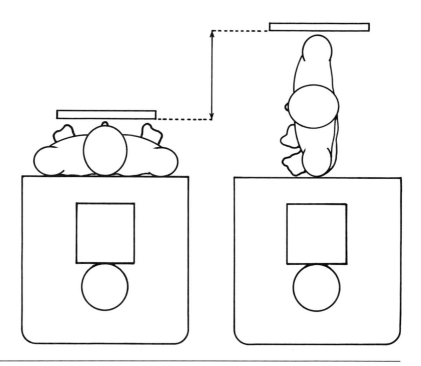

Figure 11-13 Fluoroscopic Spot Film Tunnel Geometry *The size or position of the patient or both determines the FFD used for fluoroscopic spot films. The relationship of the part to the detector influences image sharpness. In the left lateral position (right), anatomical structures on the left side of the patient will be greatly magnified. The structures on the right side of the patient should be somewhat sharper because of the reduced OFD and increased FFD.*

When a small focal spot (0.6 mm or less) is used with a fluoroscopic spot film tunnel, image sharpness is improved. The unsharpness associated with the shortened FOD (approximately 20 in.) is minimized (left). (See Figs. 5-14 and 12-7 right.)

intimate contact with the radiographic table, can be as great as 13 cm from the image detector. When a patient measuring 30 cm is placed in the lateral position for a lumbar spine, the center of the vertebral column is 15 cm from the tabletop, with a 28-cm object film distance. Unless a small focal spot (0.6 mm or smaller) is used, significant unsharpness will result (Fig. 11–11). When the patient is radiographed in the anteroposterior (AP) supine position for the orbits (20 or more cm from the tabletop), there is at least a 30-cm or greater object film distance. The part under study can be magnified as much as 50% (Fig. 11–12). Although a radiographer would not consider the making of a radiograph of a hand situated 30 cm from the cassette with a large focal spot, this is what occurs when the orbits and lumbar spine are evaluated using a 13-cm TT/BT distance.

When using a fluoroscopic spot tunnel (see Fig. 3–9), the size or position of a patient determines the FFD. Because of the shortened TOD (approximately 20 in.), image unsharpness can occur. The use of a small focal spot helps to minimize image unsharpness.

GEOMETRIC UNSHARPNESS AND HEEL EFFECT

In addition to the penumbral unsharpness caused by the size of the focal spot and the position of the part, one must also consider the variation in sharpness along the projected x-ray field. (See Figs. 4–3 and 4–4.) The projected focal spot increases in size (along the axis of the x-ray tube) from anode to cathode.

GEOMETRIC UNSHARPNESS AND EXTRA FOCAL RADIATION

Off-focus radiation adds to image unsharpness. Structures outside the collimated shutter pattern are often seen as indistinct shadows. The extraneous details, while asthetically unattractive, do not influence diagnosis. Unfortunately, a portion of the primary x-ray beam consists of off-focus (extrafocal) radiation and adds to the unsharpness of the image. Off-focus radiation can be controlled by positioning the primary shutters of the collimator or by placing an aperture diaphragm as close to source as possible. (See Figs. 5–9 and 5–10.)

Absorption Unsharpness

Absorption unsharpness is the term used to describe the effect produced when a three-dimensional object is radiographed and recorded in a two-dimensional plane (Fig. 11–14). The unsharpness of the recorded image is caused by variation in the absorption of the beam throughout the structural edges and the location of the object in the path of the beam.

The combination of the penumbral effect and the absorption effect results in the radiographic demonstration of indistinct borders in many internal body structures (Fig. 11–14).

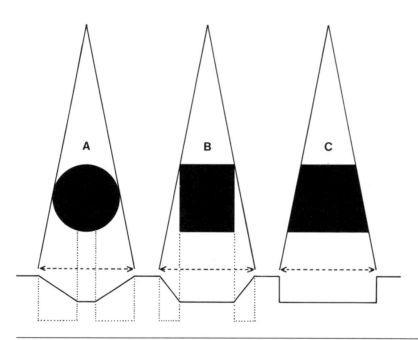

Figure 11-14 Variations in Absorption of Structural Edges *Three different shaped objects are shown: a sphere (A), a rectangular object (B), and a wedge-shaped structure, approximating the pattern or shape of the divergent x-ray beam (C). All three objects are positioned with an increased OFD. Note that the three objects produce approximately the same size x-ray shadow.*

The circular structure (A) absorbs more x-ray in the center and less x-ray bilaterally, producing unsharp overexposed edges of the image. The rec- *tangular object (B) is enlarged, and again the lateral aspects of the beam image the upper edges of the object, resulting in a penumbral effect. The object that conforms to the beam shape (C) appears as the sharpest image in the series, because absorption is equal throughout the entire structure and artificial boundaries or edges are not created by structures proximal to the x-ray source. If the object in C were inverted, the borders associated with B would occur.*

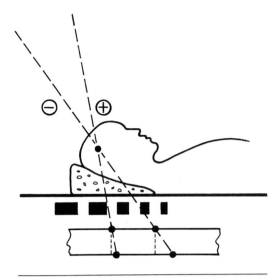

Figure 11-15 Tube Angle Technique Concerns
A concern with tube angulation techniques is the potential for image unsharpness owing to the parallex effect. A black dot in the skull in this illustration represents an area of pathological interest. A shallow tube angle (10 degree) is shown with the dot projected on to a dual emulsion film. Note the separation of the image from the anterior to the posterior emulsions. When a tube is angled from zero to 10 degrees, the unsharpness attributed to the parallex effect is less than the intrinsic unsharpness of the film screen combination. When the tube angle is increased beyond 10 degrees, the detection of unsharpness associated with the parallex effect increases. Whenever possible, a perpendicular beam should be used to minimize the parallex effect. When the tube angle is increased to 25 degrees, there is a greater separation on the image represented by the black dots. If a small focal spot (0.6 mm or smaller) is available, the skull can be elevated (increased OFD) on a 15-degree sponge as shown in this illustration. The 25-degree tube angle can then be lessened to 10 degrees, minimizing the parallex effect.

In this illustration, differences in sharpness are shown across the field (cathode to anode). These differences in sharpness are related to the heel effect. At the anode end of the x-ray tube, the focal spot is smaller than the effective focal spot as measured at central ray; at the cathode side, the focal spot is larger. Image sharpness varies in this illustration from the top (less sharp) to the bottom (more sharp) of the skull. (See Fig. 4-4.)

There is also a variation in intensity across the long axis of the x-ray tube; therefore, film blackening is not uniform. (See Fig. 4-3A.)

Intensifying Screen Unsharpness

The degree of unsharpness resulting from the use of intensifying screens is dependent upon the type of phosphor used in the manufacturer of the screen, the size and layer thickness of the phosphor, the use of light restricting dye (if any), and the degree of film screen contact present in the system. (See Fig. 8–14.) Tube angulation techniques can result in an increase in unsharpness owing to the parallex effect (Fig. 11–15).

Motion Unsharpness

Motion of any type will diminish recorded detail. Motion (voluntary or involuntary) can originate in the patient. Immobilization of the part and short exposure times can help to minimize this problem.

Motion unsharpness can also occur at the source of the radiation as a result of vibration in the imaging equipment. Improper use of locks on equipment can cause vibration of the x-ray tube or crane. Defective Bucky lock assemblies can permit motion of the cassette in the Bucky tray, resulting in unsharpness. Rotating anode tubes with damaged bearing assemblies can result in vibration of the anode and produce unsharpness on the recorded image. (See Chapter 4.)

Motion can be deliberately used to advantage to blur out structures, as described in the section on tomography. (See Chapter 7.)

Shallow breathing techniques using low milliamperage and long exposure times can be used to blur out the pulmonary markings and ribs for studies of the thoracic spine and sternum. (See Figs. 14–4 and 14–5.)

Visibility of Detail

Recorded detail and contrast are greatly dependent upon each other. A quality radiograph must possess sufficient contrast to render the structural details visible. Reduction in contrast can result from scatter radiation (see Chapter 5) or underpenetration of the object.

Chemical fog generated by processing difficulties (see Chapter 10) and other types of fogging of the image can also reduce the visibility of recorded detail.

(Text continues on p. 201.)

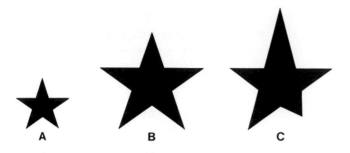

Figure 11-16 Magnification-Distortion Relationships Distortion is the radiographic differences (misrepresentation in size or shape) in a radiographic image when compared to the object under study.

A star is shown (A) as a normal-sized radiographic image. If the object under study is magnified (B), equal (overall) enlargement occurs—an increase in the size of the object without a change in the shape of any of its parts. When portions of or all of the structure under study are distorted (elongated or foreshortened), shape distortion occurs (C). This effect can be due to the angulation of the part, detector, or x-ray tube. The star shown in C exhibits an elongated distorted point as well as a foreshortened point.

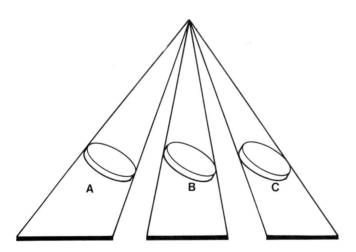

Figure 11-17 Tube Angulation/Part Relationship A flat disc with an increased object film distance is tilted at an angle and radiographed with an angulated beam (A), a beam that is perpendicular to the detector (B), and a reverse angle beam (C). Note the changing shape of the disc, from elongation (A) to foreshortening (C), depending upon the position of the x-ray tube. See Fig. 11-20 and Fig. 14-6 for clinical applications of this principle.

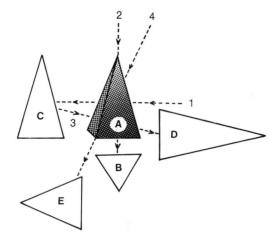

Figure 11-18 Shape Distortion
A three-dimensional pyramid is shown (A). Central ray (1) is positioned perpendicular to the apex of the pyramid for the projection represented by a two-dimensional triangle (C). The exact size of the base of the pyramid is represented (B). When an image is made from position (2), a representation of the side of the pyramid is shown without shape distortion (B). When an angled projection (3) is used, an elongated image results (D). An image obtained with central ray at position 4 will be fore-shortened (E). A clinical example of this shape distortion can be seen in Figure 11-20.

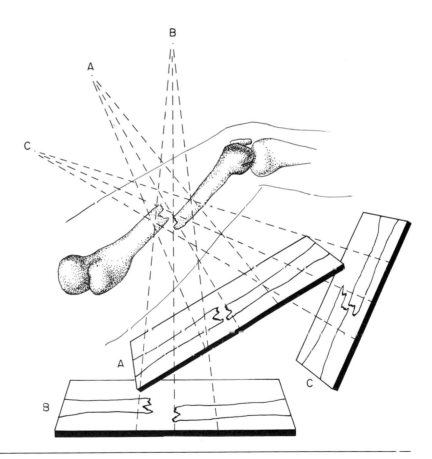

Figure 11-19 Distortion Associated With Tube, Receptor, and Object Alignment *Attention must be given to the relationship of the alignment of the tube, receptor, and object. The x-ray tube and receptor in A are in proper alignment with central ray perpendicular to the film. The* slight separation of the fragments of the femur is demonstrated. The tube-receptor relationship of B gives the illusion that the fragments are further separated. The tube-receptor angulation technique in C gives the impression of overlapping of the fragments.

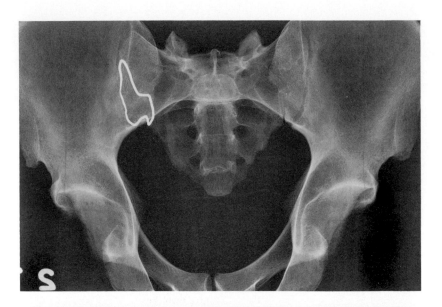

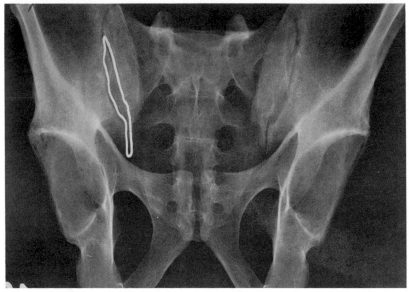

Figure 11-20 A Clinical Application of Distortion On occasion, distortion can be used to clinical advantage. A soft wire was shaped to conform to the actual sacroiliac joint on the right side of a dried pelvic specimen.

A conventional AP projection of the pelvis was made (top). The relationship of the sacroiliac joints to the pelvis is not well visualized.

The x-ray tube was then angled 35 degrees cephalad elongating the pelvis (bottom). Note the elongation of the metallic wire and the sacroiliac joints, which are now well visualized.

Another clinical example of the value of distortion can be seen in Figure 14-6.

(Courtesy Eastman Kodak Company, Rochester, NY)

Distortion

Distortion is the radiographic difference (misrepresentation) in size or shape compared with the actual object. Image distortion must be considered when evaluating image detail (Figs. 11–16 to 11–19).

Distortion can sometimes be used to advantage (Fig. 11–20).

Distortion may be categorized into two major types: size and shape.

Size Distortion

Equal (overall) enlargement of the image (magnification) is one form of distortion (size). With magnification, the shape of the object is accurately reproduced; however, the recorded details of the image are enlarged (Fig. 11–16).

SIZE DISTORTION AND DISTANCE

The relationship of the distance of the object to the film plane affects the size of the object. The closer the object is placed to the film, the less magnification evident on the image. (See Chapter 13.) If the object is moved further away from the recording plane, magnification increases (Fig. 11–16). Focal film distance (FFD) and object film distance (OFD) relationship can determine image size (Figs. 11–11 and 11–12). If an object cannot be placed in close proximity to the recording plane, size distortion (magnification) can be reduced by increasing the FFD. (See Chapter 13.)

Image distortion can be particularly troublesome when attempting to localize a foreign body. (See Fig. 14–7.)

SIZE DISTORTION AND FOCAL SPOT SIZE

The closer the focal spot size approaches a point source, the less penumbral effect and the greater the detail on the magnified image. The degree of magnification of the image or the size of the object being radiographed can be determined mathematically. (See Chapters 7 and 13.)

Shape Distortion

Any angulation of the x-ray beam, the recording plane, or the object in the path of the beam will result in distortion (true distortion) on the recorded image (Figs. 11–16 – 11–20).

Distortion can also be used to project superimposed anatomy away from the area of interest. (See Figs. 12–3 and 14–6.)

Depending upon the position of the x-ray tube and the patient, the image will demonstrate either elongation or foreshortening (Figs. 11–18 and 11–19).

It is sometimes necessary to deliberately distort anatomy when an air–fluid level interface must be seen. (See Fig. 3–8.)

Total Unsharpness

All forms of unsharpness detract from the resolution of the image.

The recording media should be able to produce well-defined structural outlines (resolution). To evaluate total resolution (MTF), the product of the components that enter into the resolution of the imaging system must be considered. Some factors that many affect resolution include focal spot size, geometric enlargement and distortion, motion, and screen film unsharpness.

12 Technical Factor Selection

THE selection of a combination of technical factors to produce an optimal radiograph is a complex art. In an article entitled "Evolution of The Technique Chart," Harold G. Petsing made the following statement, "One of the problems coincident with the art of radiography has been the search for satisfactory and practical methods of selecting and recording desirable techniques for different anatomic regions." This statement, published in The X-Ray Technician, in January of 1940, is still appropriate almost a half century later.

An experienced radiographer can project an expected outcome in a clinical situation, and, based on solid knowledge of the principles of exposure, can modify technical factors to arrive at acceptable compromises. Technique charts offer baseline values for specific examinations.

The technical suggestions made in this chapter are based on the presumption that x-ray units are calibrated regularly and that automatic processors are maintained according to manufacturers' recommendations. (See Chapters 3 and 10.) Hotte et al, in "A Sensitometric Evaluation Of Film/Chemistry/Processor Systems In The State Of New Jersey," HHS Publication (FDA) 82–8189 (April 1982), state that a fourfold variation in exposure

range can be due to processor conditions. Improper processing conditions of this magnitude can negate the film blackening effect of high-speed rare-earth imaging. (See Fig. 10–5.)

Only after adequate calibration of the equipment has been ensured, should technical factor selection be considered. The selection of technical factors and the screen film combinations used can influence the amount of radiation received by patient and operator. One must be aware of how to lower dosage and still produce a quality radiographic image.

A technique chart is not intended to be used interchangably from x-ray room to x-ray room. Even with identical equipment, a variation in calibration may affect techniques.

IMPORTANT: Every radiographic unit must have its own technique chart. If an upright Bucky is used in the same room with a table Bucky having a different ratio grid (see Chapter 5), separate technique charts will be required.

Although the type of technique chart to be used is often based upon the preference of the interpreter, the quality of the image can

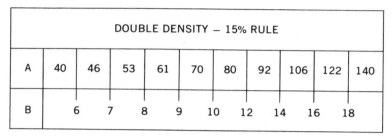

A	40	46	53	61	70	80	92	106	122	140
B		6	7	8	9	10	12	14	16	18

DOUBLE DENSITY — 15% RULE

A. Original Kilovoltage Value
B. Increase in kVp Needed to Double Density

Figure 12-1   The 15% Rule Versus "A Rule of Thumb" for Density Changes   *Kilovoltage values ranging from 40 kVp to 140 kVp are shown* (A) *with a 15% increase in kilovoltage* (B) *to double radiographic density. "A rule of thumb" adjustment of kVp is sometimes substituted for the 15% kilovoltage change. (See Chapter 13.) This rule states that radiographic density can be maintained if an adjustment of one half mAs is accompanied by an increase of 10 kVp. The reduction of 10 kVp and the doubling of mAs has the same effect on density. In the typical kilovoltage range (60 kVp to 80 kVp) used for most medical radiographs, this "rule of thumb" approximates the 15% calculation. As kilovoltage is lowered to the 40 kVp range or elevated to 125 kVp or greater, the 10 kVp adjustment no longer approximates the 15% change.*

be influenced by technical factors under the control of a radiographer. (See Chapter 11.)

Technical factor adjustments should be made after consideration of the following rules or principles of radiographic exposure:

1 To maintain a given density, (a) increase kilovoltage by 15% and reduce mAs by one half, or (b) decrease kilovoltage by 15% and double mAs (Fig. 12–1 and Table 12–1).

2 When kVp is increased, short-scale contrast decreases (see Fig. 11–7); a wider latitude technique results.

3 The use of a grid or Bucky improves contrast; a grid will also absorb some primary radiation, producing a decrease in radiographic density.

4 As film screen combination speed increases, there is an increase in radiographic density (see Table 8–1), with a possible decrease in radiographic detail. This statement does not take into consideration the high absorption/conversion ratio of rare-earth phosphors. (See Fig. 8–7.)

5 A smaller focal spot results in increased detail but may require a lower

TABLE 12-1.   Technical Factor Manipulation to Maintain Density*

mA	Second	kVp	S/F Speed
100	1/2	70	200
200	1/4	70	200
400	1/8	70	200
400	1/16	82	200 (may require large focal spot)
200	1/16	82	400
100	1/8	82	400
100	1/4	70	400

*Any of these technical factors will produce a similar radiographic density. The higher kVp images would exhibit longer-scale contrast; the shorter exposure times would help to stop motion.

mA value and an increase in exposure time. (See Chapter 4.)

6 An increase in FFD improves recorded detail but decreases radiographic density (Table 12–2).

7 An increase in OFD or a decrease in FFD results in image enlargement, with an increase in unsharpness. (See Figs. 11–11 and 11–12.)

8 Any increase in scatter diminishes radiographic contrast and visibility of detail. (See Chapter 5.)

Table 12-2. FFD Conversion Table*	40 in.	48 in.	72 in.
40 in.	—	1.44	3.24
48 in.	0.69	—	2.25
72 in.	0.24	0.44	—

*Minor variations in FFD can produce significant changes in radiographic density. Most FFD conversion tables list many distances, most of which are not in common practice. Distance changes of 40 in., 48 in., and 72 in. are shown. If a 72 in. chest study needed to be repeated at 40 in. or 48 in., the conversion factor multiplied by the original mAs would indicate the technique conversion needed to maintain the original density. If, for some reason, the original 40 in. study had to be repeated at 72 in., more than a 300% increase in mAs would be required if kilovoltage remained constant. If a 72 in. study were repeated at 40 in. and kilovoltage remained constant, approximately one fourth the mAs would be required. It is not necessary to memorize this table. The calculations can be made using the formula for mAs/distance/intensity. (See Chapter 13.)

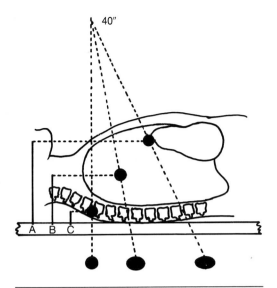

Figure 12-2 **The Divergent Effect of the X-ray Beam** *In this representation of the lateral chest, three dark circles represent pathological lesions, with central ray passing through the most posterior circle. Since these representative lesions are at different positions from the tabletop, they will be enlarged to different degrees. Due to the divergent effect of the x-ray beam, the circles will also appear distorted (elongated) on the radiograph. The posterior circle (5 cm from tabletop) is the most accurate representation. The central circle (10 cm from tabletop) is enlarged and slightly elongated. The anterior circle (15 cm from tabletop) is also enlarged and more elongated owing to its position relative to central ray. When a patient is being examined for multiple lesions, a positioning compromise must sometimes be made. In the above illustration, central ray should pass through the central circle to minimize distortion and elongation of the remaining circles.*

9 Any type of extraneous fog (e.g., chemical, visible light, safelights) increases overall density, diminishing radiographic contrast and visibility of detail.

10 Angulation of a part, image receptor, x-ray tube, (Figs. 12–2 and 12–3) or the divergent effect of the x-ray beam can produce anatomical distortion. (See Figs. 11–17 and 14–7.) Angulation of the x-ray tube results in an increased FFD.

Errors in technical judgment or in equipment calibration can negate the effect of a technique chart. Radiographers are sometimes disappointed when application of radiographic principles of exposure results in less than an optimal quality image.

Although a major technical error is usually easily recognized, several small technical errors can collectively result in an unacceptable image (Table 12–3).

Technique Charts

Technique charts are guides for providing the exposure factors needed to produce an image that meets the given standards of a radiology department. They are formulated so that predetermined contrast and density ranges can be consistently produced by all radiographers on all radiographic equipment within the department. In a large facility, where many radiographers rotate from room to room, technique charts not only are helpful but also are essential to consistently maintain image quality. Radiographers should not rely on a "favorite" technique for a given body part. A technique that may produce an acceptable image with one x-ray unit many not be acceptable with another.

A technique chart should indicate the following:

1 Tube warm-up procedures as recommended by the manufacturer, and the

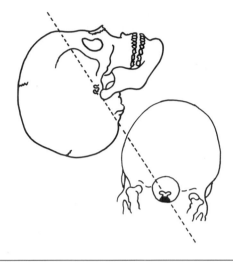

Figure 12-3 The Use of Tube Angulation for Deliberate Anatomical Distortion *Tube angulation (25 to 35 degrees caudad) with the patient in the AP Towne position to project facial structures off the occiput is an accepted technique. Central ray passes through the dorsum sella of the sella turcica, projecting it into the foramen magnum* (right). *Both posterior clinoid processes can be visualized free of superimposed facial structures.*

focal spot size to be used (see Table 4–1)

2 The recommended FFD (see Chapter 11)

3 The projection of central ray, including tube angulation (see Figs. 11–17 to 11–20, 12–2, 12–3, 14–7)

4 Exposure time

5 Screen film combination (Table 12–4; see Chapter 13)

6 Grid ratio and focal range (see Table 5–1)

Technique charts cannot always be followed precisely. They should not be thought of as a prescription or cure-all for technical problems. A standardized technique chart does not take into consideration the nature of patients' pathology or physical conditions. Prior to the making of an exposure, radiographers should review the clinical history on the examination request. A repeat examina-

TABLE 12-3. Cumulative Effect of Variations From Standard*

Error	Density Increase
Overmeasurement	up 30%
Processor temperature elevation	up 30%
mA setting 200 mA; actual mA, 220 mA	up 10%
36-in. FFD used instead of 40-in. FFD	up 20%
Total	up 90%

*In this table, the error in measurement produced a 30% increase in density, which is all that is required to produce a perceivable density change on a radiograph.

In this table, the shortened FFD produces an additional increase of approximately 20% in film blackening.

The elevation of the processor temperature and the increased mA output results in an additional 40% error.

The cumulative effect of errors in technique will result in an unacceptable radiograph. It may be difficult to identify the problem if more than one error occurs at the same time.

TABLE 12-4. Relative Exposure Levels of Some Image Detectors*

Type of Detector	Relative Exposure Level
Detail (rare-earth)	up to 100
Medium (CaWo4)	100
High (CaWo4)	250
Rare-earth (medium speed)	250–300
Rare-earth (high speed)	400–1200

* These screen film speeds are not representative of any manufacturer but are commonly accepted approximations. A medium-speed screen film combination (calcium tungstate) is shown with a representative speed of 100. In practice, most radiology departments use higher screen film combinations, with speed 400 (rare-earth) being the industry standard.

tion can often be avoided if the radiographer is aware of a suspected pathologic condition that could require a change in technical factors.

Radiographers sometimes believe that a specific radiologist has a preference for a particular technique. These assumptions arise when a radiologist requests a repeat examination for a specific reason. For example, if a radiograph were exposed at a lower kilovoltage value, it may not have adequately penetrated a dense osseous structure, and underlying pathology may still be in question. A modification in mAs might be requested with a 10 kVp to 15 kVp increase to image this suspicious area. If this type of request is made with some regularity, a radiographer might assume that the radiologist prefers higher kilovoltage techniques for all examinations. A professional discussion between the radiographer and the radiologist can help to explain why a technical adjustment must be made. Radiographers should not feel that a request for a repeat film is a criticism of their work or the validity of the departmental technique charts.

The Effect of Tissue Density and Pathology on Technical Factors

Some radiographers are reluctant to measure the part under study and prefer a "favorite" technique, substituting a "rule of thumb" for measurement.

The categorizing of patients as to body habitus (size, shape, and tissue density) can be difficult if a patient is seen only in the recumbent position, covered with street or hospital clothing, plaster or mechanical splints, and so

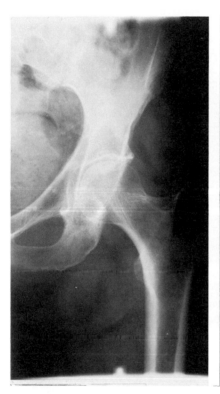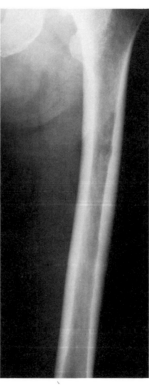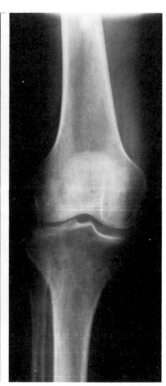

Figure 12-4 Technical Factors Adjustments for Variations in Patient Thickness A representation of the leg from the hip to the lower leg is shown. A single exposure technique would result in over- and underexposed segments of the image. Measurement of each segment of anatomy should be made for proper exposure. One cannot expect to image these differences in tissue thickness with a single exposure. If the entire leg must be visualized, the use of a compensatory filter (see

Fig. 4-9) to overcome variations in density is recommended.

Three separate radiographs of the hip, femur, and knee are shown using 70 kVp and a 12:1 grid for all exposures. As body thickness or density decreased, the milliampere seconds were reduced by one half, with the hip exposed at 100 mAs, the femur at 50 mAs, and the knee at 25 mAs using a 100-speed screen film combination.

on. The recumbent position can cause tissue to spread laterally influencing measurement. The use of measurement calipers with a hands-on approach may help to determine whether one is dealing with muscular or fatty tissue. There must be agreement as to where to measure the part under study (Fig. 12–4). Depending upon where measurement of the shoulder is made, part thickness can vary from 10 cm to 20 cm in the same patient (Fig. 12–5). This could represent more than a 100% change in radiographic density.

Radiographers have been taught that a significant increase in technique is necessary for a wet vs. a dry plaster of Paris cast (calcium sulfate). Recently, Gratale, Turner, and Burns, in an article published in Radiologic Technology, 1986; 57:4 pp 325–329, demonstrated that this is not always a valid rule. The amount of plaster used to reinforce a cast may require an increase in exposure factors (Fig. 12–6).

The type of tissue to be examined can influence the selection of technical factors. A patient may be muscular, obese, or pregnant; may have fluid in the chest (see Fig. 14–17), abdomen, or extremities; or have osteosclerotic or osteolytic tissues. Some diseases or conditions that require an increase in technical factors include ascites, cirrhosis of the liver, osteoarthritis, atelectasis, hydropneumothorax, and cardiomegaly.

An emphysematous patient requires a reduction in technical factors to avoid overexposure of the lung field. (See Fig. 14–17.) An emaciated patient, a withered limb owing to atrophy of disuse, gaseous distention of hollow viscera (see Fig. 14–11), osteoporosis, de-

generative arthritis, pneumothorax (see Figs. 14–25 and 14–26), emphysema, and aseptic necrosis are types of pathologic changes that are radiolucent in nature.

The age and size of the patient must be considered when selecting technical factors.

1 *The neonatal patient.* The osseous structures of a newborn have a low calcium content. With modern neonatal technology, babies weighing 2 lb or less survive and are categorized as newborns. Whereas an average newborn baby can weigh from 6 lb to 7 lb, many newborn babies weigh 10 lb or more. There is a 500% difference in weight between the 2-lb newborn (premature birth) and a large (full-term) newborn. Pediatric technique charts that have been formulated only according to the age of the patient, for example, newborn, 3 months, 6 months, and so on, can be misleading. The weight of the child should influence the selection of technical factors.

2 *The infant and small child.* Pediatric technique charts cannot be adapted from adult charts. The late John Hope, M.D. of Philadelphia was fond of reminding radiographers that "infants are not little people." Infants require special technique charts for quality images. The infant chest is almost round in shape, measuring approximately the same in the anteroposterior (AP) and lateral dimensions, as opposed to the significant difference in adult chest measurements.

3 *The young child/adolescent.* A significant variation in weight, height, and muscularity exists among adolescents. A larger adolescent could require adult techniques.

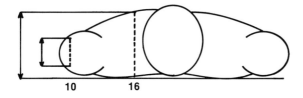

10   16

Figure 12-5 Measurement Concepts
The use of a measurement caliper is essential for conventional variable and fixed kilovoltage techniques. There must be agreement as to where to measure the part under study. In this illustration, the patient was measured over the glenoid fossa, *and a measurement of 10 cm was obtained. If the patient were measured over the center of the clavicle, a significant increase in the measurement (16 cm) would occur. These differences in measurement could produce more than a 100% density change on the processed radiograph.*

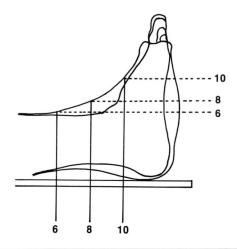

Figure 12-6 Technique Selection for Casted Extremities *It has been traditionally stated that a wet plaster cast required considerably more exposure for adequate penetration than a dry plaster cast. According to Gratale et al, if most of the water has been expressed from the plaster prior to its application, the wet or dry cast should require approximately the same exposure factors. The amount of reinforcement plaster used with the cast must be considered. In this illustration, extra plaster was used to reinforce the cast anterior to the ankle mortise in the AP dimension. Note the configuration of the leg illustrated by the dotted line. A measurement taken just above the ankle joint, measures 6 cm; adjacent to the joint, 8 cm; and above the ankle joint (including the extra plaster), 10 cm. Higher kilovoltage may be necessary to demonstrate the ankle mortise. The use of a grid or Bucky at 80 kVp or greater will result in a high latitude technique with adequate contrast, demonstrating the tibia and fibula as well as the ankle joint. This technique helps to overcome the variations in thickness of plaster used to strengthen casts.*

4 *The geriatric patient.* Special technical consideration must be given to older patients. Atrophic and osteoporotic tissues often require lower kilovoltage to maintain radiographic contrast. (See Fig. 14–10.) Because adequate subject contrast may not be present in severely demineralized structures, radiographic contrast may be difficult to achieve in these patients, regardless of technical factor compensation.

Technical Factors

Milliamperage. Milliamperage determines the quantity of the x-ray to be used for a specific technique and can be described as the current flowing through the x-ray tube. (See Chapter 11.) High mAs techniques, frequently used with low kVp to produce short-scale contrast should not be used as a substitute for scatter control. As mA values are increased, an appropriate reduction in time is possible. Unfortunately, higher mA settings often necessitate the need for a larger focal spot and an increase in the risk of focal spot blooming. (See Chapter 4.) The mA stations must be constantly monitored for mA linearity (Table 12–5). (See Table 3–1.)

Exposure time. The length of the exposure combined with the milliampere value are the major controlling factors of radiographic density (Table 12–1). (See Chapter 11.) In general, shorter exposure times are recommended, because they lessen the possibility of motion (voluntary or involuntary). The use of long exposure times at low mA values help to blur out pulmonary vascular markings when evaluating the sternum or the lateral thoracic spine. (See Figs. 14–4 and 14–5.)

Kilovoltage. Kilovoltage determines the quality of the x-ray beam and influences the amount of scatter generated. (See Chapter 11.) As the wavelength of the beam decreases, the penetration effect increases. When low kilovoltage values are used, portions of the anatomy may not be penetrated and the

TABLE 12-5. Variations in Milliampere Output*

mA Setting			Actual mA		
mA	sec	mAs	mA	sec	mAs
100	1	100	85	1	85
200	1/2	100	220	1/2	110

* Any combination of milliamperage and time that results in the same milliampere second value should yield a radiograph of similar density. In the example shown, the 100 mA station was assigned to a small focal spot, whereas the 200 mA station was assigned to the large focal spot. Although both mAs combinations should result in 100 mAs, a variation in mA output results in about a 30% increase in film blackening at the 200 mA station as opposed to the 100 mA station. The milliampere setting of 100 mA yields a 15% under-the-expected output, and the 200 mA setting yields approximately a 10% over-the-expected output. If it were necessary to change techniques from the 100 (small) to the 200 (large) mA setting, a 25% difference in the expected density would occur.

TABLE 12-6. Typical Kilovoltage Range Selection for Various Body Parts*

55	75	90	120	150
		kVp Range		
Extremities	Abdomen Skull	Thick body parts Lateral LS spine Air contrast studies	Chest Barium studies Pelvimetry	Chest

* Grouping of body parts according to kilovoltage ranges is an accepted approach to a fixed kilovoltage technique chart. When formulating a technique chart using a rare-earth screen film combination, very low or very high kilovoltage values should be carefully evaluated for possible falloff in screen response.

TABLE 12-7. kVp/mAs Adjustments and Their Effect on Heat Units*

kVp	mAs	Heat Units 5Ø	3Ø
53	400	21,200	29,892
61	200	12,200	17,202
70	100	7,000	9,870
80	50	4,000	5,640
92	25	2,300	3,243

* A representative technique, 100 mAs at 70 kVp, is selected as a starting technique (center line). Kilovoltage changes made using the 15% rule are shown with mAs adjustments to maintain a given density. (See Fig. 12–1.) Note the difference in the heat units generated using single-phase equipment, full-wave rectified vs. three-phase, 12-pulse equipment. (See Fig. 2–1, 2–5, and Table 4–2.) An adjustment of 15% in kVp from the original 70 kVp setting (61 kVp or 80 kVp) generates either 17,202 HU or 5640 HU, respectively. This represents more than a 300% increase in heat units at the lower kVp setting.

emulsion of the radiograph may not be adequately exposed. Areas of the film base where unexposed silver compounds were completely removed by the fixing process are devoid of radiographic information.

Kilovoltage controls radiographic contrast. As kilovoltage is raised, the relative absorption differences between structures is lessened, and we can "see through" dense structures. Specific kilovoltage ranges are recommended for certain body parts (Table 12–6).

Single- vs. Three-Phase Equipment

When a technique chart is being developed, generator output must be considered. A single-phase study at 80 kVp, 100 mAs that produces a satisfactory radiographic density can be duplicated at 70 kVp, 100 mAs on a three-phase, 12-pulse unit. There should not be an obvious difference in radiographic contrast between these images, since the effective kVp from the three-phase equipment is higher than the effective kVp generated with the single-phase unit. (See Fig. 2–6 and Table 2–2.) There is, however, a significant reduction in heat units when using three-phase equipment with appropriate technique adjustments (Table 12–7). (See Table 4–2.)

If a similar kilovoltage value (80 kVp) is used for both exposures, approximately a 50% reduction in mAs can be made on the three-phase study. This will produce an image in half the time or perhaps permit the use of a smaller focal spot at a lower mA value to improve image sharpness. The overall contrast of the three-phase radiograph will be of a longer scale, since the effective kVp will be greater.

Standard Positioning and Projection Concepts

Technique charts should contain information regarding radiographic positioning of the patient and the projection of the central ray. One should be familiar with standard terminology for positioning and projections. This information is stated in "Standard Terminology For Positioning And Projections," available from the American Registry of Radiologic Technologists, Minneapolis, Minnesota.

Changes in the position of the patient affect radiographic technique. In the prone position, the weight of the body flattens the abdominal tissues, necessitating a decrease in exposure factors that would be used for the supine position. Decubitus positioning of the patient for an abdominal study can result in uneven tissue thickness in the dependent portion of the abdomen. When a patient is placed in the erect position, there is an increase in tissue thickness in the inferior portion of the abdomen. Patients are also placed in oblique positions of varying degrees. A 15-degree oblique position of the body would require an increase in exposure over the AP position. A 45- or 60-degree oblique rotation of the same body part would require an additional increase in exposure over the 15-degree oblique position.

As the patient position and projection of the central ray are changed, not only should the technique be adjusted, but proper image labeling should be documented on the radiograph.

Types of Technique Charts

The tables presented in this chapter are conceptual. None of the techniques listed is meant to be used with a specific x-ray unit. Some of the standard exposure systems in common use are explained in the following sections.

FIXED MAS, VARIABLE KVP TECHNIQUE

A predetermined fixed mAs value is combined with variable kVp, which is adjusted according to the measured thickness of a part. Centimeter differences of 1 cm to 2 cm in tissue thickness necessitate an increase of 2 kVp to 3 kVp for each increment of tissue thickness (Table 12–8) with a fixed mAs value, regardless of patient size. Some anatomical areas may not be adequately exposed owing to inadequate penetration. As patients increase in size or density, higher kilovoltage values will increase scatter.

FIXED KVP, VARIABLE MAS TECHNIQUE

The fixed kVp technique with varying mAs introduced in the 1940s is often labeled as "optimum kilovoltage" technique. With this method, patients are divided into general categories such as small, medium, large, and extra large, and centimeter measurement groupings are used to determine the mAs settings (Table 12–8).

With the fixed kilovoltage technique, pioneered by the late Arthur W. Fuchs of the Eastman Kodak Company, body parts fall into an average thickness range. In 1955, Fuchs reported in his textbook *Principles of Radiographic Exposure And Processing*, Charles C Thomas, Springfield, Illinois, that the average thickness range of most body parts were similar in approximately 75% of patients. In extremities, thickness is average in almost 100% of the patients.

Fuchs used relatively high kilovoltage values, considering the low ratio grids (6:1 or 8:1) available at that time. The high kilovoltage levels (80 kVp or greater) were probably necessary because of the 100-speed screen film combination used in the 1950s. A fixed kilovoltage was selected to adequately penetrate the part under study, while maintaining adequate contrast. These kilovoltage levels were obtained with single-phase equipment. When reviewing the Fuchs fixed kilovoltage charts, it seems that significantly less kilovoltage is being recommended today than was used by early radiographers for the same body part. Most of today's three-phase equipment will produce radiographs of comparable density and contrast at kilovoltage values approximately 10 kVp below those selected by Fuchs. (See Fig. 2–6.)

Many radiographers state that by using a fixed kilovoltage, radiographic contrast can be maintained throughout a variety of patient sizes. This philosophy does not take into consideration the production of scatter radiation. In practice, there is better exposure latitude at higher kilovoltages, but contrast decreases as patient size or density increases. It is impossible to maintain the same contrast scale in a 15-cm abdomen of an emaciated patient

TABLE 12-8. Variable vs. Fixed Kilovoltage Techniques[*]

mAs	20	20	20
kVp (variable)	62,64,66	72,74,76	80,82,84
cm	17,18,19	20,21,22	23,24,25
(fixed) kVp	76	76	76
mAs	10	20	25

* A representative technique chart for the abdomen is shown with centimeter measurements from 17 to 25. The variable kVp portion (*top*) shows kilovoltage variations of 2 kVp per centimeter measurement with a fixed mAs. The fixed kVp chart lists 76 kVp for all centimeter measurements, with variations in mAs.

as in a 30-cm abdomen of a dense muscular patient with a fluid-filled abdomen.

In support of the fixed kVp values, it should be noted that when a variety of patients are examined with a fixed kilovoltage value regardless of their size, there is less of a variation in the scale of contrast than when variable kilovoltage is used. With a variable kVp technique, a smaller patient may need 60 kVp, whereas a larger patient may need 90 kVp. At 60 kVp, abrupt differences in black and white are seen; at 90 kVp, a longer scale of contrast with many differences in density results. This wide variation in contrast from short scale to long scale is minimized by a fixed kilovoltage technique. Contrast can never be identically matched between similar body parts of different thickness, but a fixed kilovoltage technique will result in images with less variation in contrast over a wider range of patient thicknesses. In practice, kVp may have to be increased for larger size patients (Table 12–9).

Extremity techniques that use low kilovoltage (50 kVp or less) will produce short-scale contrast images with poor soft tissue detail. Rare-earth intensifying screen speed drops off at the lower kVp ranges because of the nature of these phosphors. (See Chapter 8.) With rare-earth screens, the use of modest (65 kVp–70 kVp) kilovoltage values for extremity radiographs with an appropriate decrease in mAs increases soft tissue visualization. Un-fortunately, higher kilovoltage values can require extremely short mAs values. Minor adjustments in exposure time can produce major density changes on the processed image. (See Fig. 14–3.)

Automatic Exposure Device Techniques

Most automatic exposure devices (AED) use fixed kVp techniques. Kilovoltage settings such as 60 kVp, 80 kVp, or 100 kVp are determined by the nature of the part being examined. When the patient is properly positioned to an AED sensor (see Fig. 2–9) and an exposure is made, the length of the exposure is determined by a preselected density setting. Reproducible radiographs should result, regardless of variations in tissue density.

An anatomically programmed unit categorizes the body into several areas and thicknesses. Individual segments of anatomy to be studied are displayed schematically on the AED program selector at the console. The milliampere value can be selected and, on most units, focal spot size can be determined by the radiographer. A kilovoltage value is usually preselected.

Other Types of Technique Charts

A technique chart known as "Supertech" that utilizes a slide rule format was developed by Brice Kratzer and described in "A Technique Computer," Radiol Technol: 45, 1973. This slide rule can be used to compensate for variations in technique, including distance, changes in grid ratio, kVp, mAs, and so on.

Computer software programs permitting the graphic display of technical factors as well as patient and beam positioning could replace the standard technique chart. Elaborate computerized systems permit the radiographer to enter a description of the part to be studied along with patient information such as height, weight, age, and so on to calculate the optimal exposure for the patient and list alternate technique options. Hard copy can be printed for wall chart or classroom use.

Selection of Technical Factors for Use With Contrast Media

Radiographic perception of an object is influenced by the density of the material sur-

---

TABLE 12-9. Fixed vs. Variable Kilovoltage*

	Fixed		Variable	
Size	*mAs*	*kVp*	*kVp*	*mAs*
Small	50	80	70	100
Medium	100	80	80	100
Large	200	80	92	100
Extra large	400/200	80/92	106/92	100/200

* Another approach to a fixed or variable kVp chart is the categorizing of patients as to small, medium, large, and extra large. Centimeter measurements determine patient categories. In this table, a fixed kVp value of 80 is used with variable mAs, and a variable kVp chart is generated for a fixed mAs value. Note the adjustments in factors in both charts for the extra large patient. With the fixed kilovoltage technique, if 80 kVp were to be used for the extra large patient, 400 mAs would be required. An increase in kVp by 15% to 92 kVp would permit the use of a 200 mAs value. For example at 100 mAs, 106 kVp would be required for adequate exposure of the extra large patient. A 15% reduction in kilovoltage to 92 kVp, to reduce scatter, would necessitate the doubling of the mAs to maintain density. (See Fig. 12–1.) It is interesting to note that at this extra large level, the factors needed with either the fixed or variable kVp charts to compensate for body habitus and scatter radiation are the same—200 mAs at 92 kVp.

rounding the object. A body part, when surrounded by a more radiodense material, will appear radiolucent; if surrounded by a radiolucent material, it will appear relatively opaque. Air, fat, water (mostly soft tissue), and bone are naturally occurring tissue densities. Fatty tissue sometimes separates and outlines body structures from one another.

When a survey radiograph of the abdomen is made, the osseous structures of the lower ribs, spine, and pelvis can be seen. The liver and spleen as well as both kidneys are sometimes represented by faint radiolucent outlines owing to fatty tissue envelopment. Gaseous pockets are seen throughout the hollow viscera of the gastrointestinal tract. The lateral margins of the psoas muscles can also be seen.

Pathologic conditions can produce gas, fat, or calcium deposits as well as areas of increased or decreased tissue density.

When significant tissue differentiation does not exist, additional radiographic density can be produced by the introduction of contrast agents into the body. Radiographic contrast is enhanced by the use of radiopaque or radiolucent contrast medium.

The stomach, small and large intestines and biliary, urinary, and vascular systems require a contrast medium for their visualization.

Contrast Agents

POSITIVE CONTRAST AGENTS

Commonly used positive contrast media include:

1 Barium sulfate, which is used to opacify the gastrointestinal tract. Since barium is not absorbed, it does not alter normal physiologic function. It can be used in various suspension weights to fill the esophagus, stomach, small bowel, or colon (single or double contrast study). (See Figs. 5–14 and 14–6.) Barium is also used for mucosal coating studies of the gastrointestinal tract.

2 Iodionated contrast materials

a. Aqueous. Intravenously injected and excreted by the kidneys (intravenous pyelography), or secreted by the liver (intravenous cholangiography). These agents are also used to visualize blood vessels during angiography. A direct injection of aqueous iodine into the hepatic or biliary radicals results in a cholangiographic study (Fig. 12–7).

Aqueous iodine can be used for gastrointestinal studies when the use of barium sulfate would be contraindicated. For example, when a bowel obstruction or perforation of a hollow viscus is suspected.

b. Oil-based iodine. Used for myelography or bronchography. Non-ionic water-soluble contrast agents are also used for myelography.

c. Water-soluble iodinated thickened suspensions, used for hysterosalpinography (see Fig. 5–14); retrograde urethrography; draining sinus injections; and so on.

d. Iodinated pills or capsules used for oral cholecystography.

Studies that use air as a contrast agent in combination with barium require low to moderate kilovoltage values.

There are similarities in x-ray absorption between barium and iodine. (See Fig. 11–1.) Higher kilovoltage values (100 kVp or greater) must be used, however, to penetrate the large, dense barium-filled hollow viscera. Shorter exposure times will help to overcome motion blur resulting from peristalsis or patient motion. (See Chapter 11.)

Some studies, such as the direct injection by means of a urethral catheter into the urinary bladder (cystogram), also require large amounts of aqueous contrast. An opaque-filled dilated bladder is extremely dense and can mask radiolucent or radiopaque calculi or other disease processes. The use of moderate to high kilovoltage (85 kVp–100 kVp) to penetrate the distended opaque bladder produces an image with longer scale contrast.

A low or moderate kilovoltage (70 kVp) should be used when there is an indirect routing of aqueous iodine, such as with intravenous urography or intravenous cholangiography, for optimal visualization of the contrast-enhanced organs. A considerable difference in contrast is evident in a common duct visualized by intravenous cholangiography compared with a direct-injection percutaneous transhepatic cholangiogram (Fig. 12–7). The amount and concentration of the contrast agent delivered by intravenous injection to the biliary system depends upon the function of the liver. A moderate kilovoltage range with tight beam collimation is needed for ad-

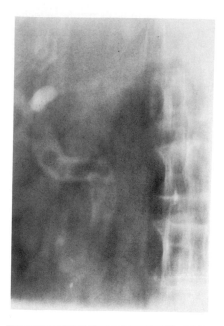 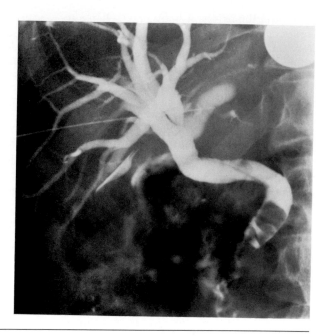

Figure 12-7   The Effect of Kilovoltage on Contrast Media   *The kilovoltage range needed to produce adequate radiographic contrast when using a contrast medium depends upon whether the iodinated media is injected directly or intravenously. The illustration shown is a tomographic section of an opacified biliary system with multiple radiolucent filling defects (left). The iodine (intravenous injection) was diluted by bile. A low kVp/ high mAs technique is required to augment a poorly visualized iodinated shadow.*

A direct injection of undiluted contrast material is shown in a percutaneous transhepatic cholangiogram (right). A needle was passed through the abdomen into the biliary system, bile was withdrawn, and undiluted aqueous iodine was injected directly in the dilated biliary ducts. Note the radiolucent defects near the end of the distal common duct. The high kilovoltage technique (above 90 kVp) will penetrate the dense opacified biliary ducts.

equate radiographic contrast. With the transhepatic cholangiogram (a direct injection of undiluted contrast material), a dense radiopaque shadow is produced. Since non-opaque biliary calculi can be obscured by a dense contrast agent, higher kilovoltage values (85 kVp or greater) are required to penetrate the opacified, often dilated, ductal system.

RADIOLUCENT (NEGATIVE) CONTRAST AGENTS

Radiolucent (negative) contrast agents include gas, air, oxygen, helium carbon dioxide, and nitrous oxide.

Radiolucent contrast agents were initially used for visualization of the ventricles of the brain (pneumoencephalogram or ventriculo-

gram) and injection into the abdomen or retroperitoneal space to outline organ structures in the abdominal cavity. Air is occasionally used as a contrast agent for myelography. Computed tomography (see Chapter 6), which enhances the differences in contrast between soft tissue structures, has replaced most of these examinations.

The use of air or gases in double contrast (air and barium) examinations of the stomach and colon is increasing. Barium sulfate is used to outline the mucosal pattern of the stomach, which is then distended by a gaseous substance, introduced orally or by way of a gastric tube. For the double-contrast barium enema, a dense barium is used to partially fill

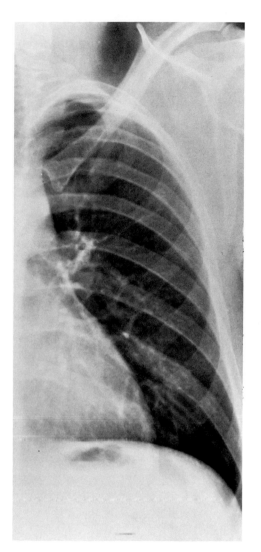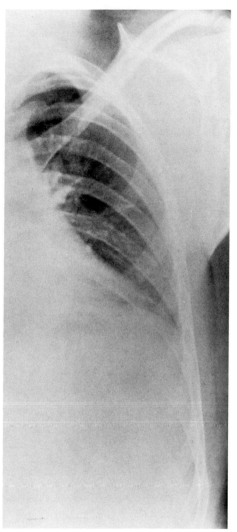

Figure 12-8   The Use of Air as a Contrast Medium for Chest Radiography   *The left side of a PA chest is shown on full inspiration (left) and expiration (right). The difference in radiographic density is due to the degree of inspiration. These exposures were made without an automatic exposure device.*

A fully inspired lung field (left) produces a normal-appearing left lung. The image made on full expiration (right) appears to be significantly underexposed. The elevated diaphragms create the illusion of an enlarged heart. The base of the lung seems congested in the expiratory film. If this examination were made using an automatic exposure device, the densities would be matched, since the AED would permit exposure until a preselected density were reached. The study would not be diagnostic; the heart would be difficult to evaluate. (Modified from Thompson TT: Primer of Clinical Radiology, 2nd ed. Boston, Little, Brown Company, 1980; with permission.)

the colon, and air is then introduced to dilate the hollow viscus. Barium coats the walls of the air-distended colon. (See Fig. 5–14.)

The most common use of air as a contrast medium is for chest radiography. Full inspiration fills the lungs with radiolucent contrast medium (air). The diaphragms are moved downward, and the cardiac shadow assumes its true size and configuration. When an expiratory film is made, the diaphragms are elevated, giving the illusion of an enlarged heart. The right side of the chest is shown after expiration, compared with an image made at full inspiration (Fig. 12–8). The same technical factors were used for both exposures. Note the increase in radiographic density on the inspiration image owing to aeration and separation of the lung tissue.

13 Technical Formulas and Related Data

TECHNICAL information and related data such as mathematics, formulas, and examples, when applicable, are grouped together so that the reader can appreciate the interactive effect of these relationships, one on the other.

The material presented in this chapter should provide an understanding of the basic mathematics and geometry needed for radiographers to modify technical factors. In practice, experienced radiographers, familiar with the principles of radiographic exposure, will not find it necessary to mathematically calculate every change in exposure factors.

Included in this chapter are tables that describe the International System of Measurement (S.I. Units); formulas showing the relationship of electrical current, power, resistance, and transformer operation; and other commonly used principles of exposure.

Basic Mathematics

Mathematics and algebraic functions are performed in terms of their expressed symbols: addition ($+$), subtraction ($-$), division ($\div, :$), and multiplication ($x, \cdot, [x]$, [exponential notations]^x, and placement of letters [ab]).

Decimals and fractions are often used in technical conversions, and some radiologic principles can be stated as ratios, proportions, or percentages. Exponential notations are used to make mathematic operations easier. Formulas relating to image geometry and the measurement of points, surfaces, and angles produced by the object and the x-ray beam can be applied to radiologic principles.

Decimals

Decimals are expressed as follows:

1	= units
0.1	= tens
0.01	= hundreds
0.001	= thousands
0.0001	= ten thousands

CHANGING DECIMALS TO FRACTIONS

Decimals can also be expressed as fractions. A decimal is expressed as a fraction whose denominator is indicated by 10 or some higher power of 10. The number of places to the right of the decimal point indicates the number of zeros in the denominator when the decimal is changed to a fraction.

Examples:

$$0.1 = \frac{1}{10} \quad 0.07 = \frac{7}{100} \quad 0.004 = \frac{4}{1000}$$

CHANGING FRACTIONS TO DECIMALS

It is sometimes easier to use the decimal equivalent of a fraction when computing technical changes.

A fraction can be changed into a decimal by dividing the numerator by the denominator.

Example:

$$\frac{1}{2} = 2\overline{)1.0}^{\,0.5} = 0.5$$

$$\frac{1}{20} = 20\overline{)1.00}^{\,0.05} = 0.05$$

Fractions

If the numerator and denominator of a fraction are both multiplied or divided by the same factor, the value of the fraction is not affected.

Example: In the fraction $^{20}/_{25}$, the numerator and denominator can be reduced by dividing each by 5. The value of the fraction $^{4}/_{5}$ is the same as the fraction $^{20}/_{25}$.

If two similar numbers or letters (not being added or subtracted) are found in the numerator and denominator, the similar items may be cancelled without affecting the value of the fraction.

Example:

$$\frac{AB}{AC} = \frac{\cancel{A}B}{\cancel{A}C} = \frac{B}{C}$$

or

$$\frac{(4)(5)}{(4)(4)} = \frac{(\cancel{4})(5)}{(\cancel{4})(4)} = \frac{5}{4}$$

Note that if the fractions were stated as

$$\frac{A - B}{AC} \text{ or } \frac{5 - 4}{4}$$

the similar items (A or 4) could not be cancelled.

If two fractions have the same denominator, the one with the larger numerator is the greater fraction.

Example: In the fractions $^{1}/_{5}$ and $^{3}/_{5}$, $^{3}/_{5}$ is the greater fraction.

If two fractions have the same numerator, the one with the larger denominator is the smaller fraction.

Example: In the fractions $^{3}/_{9}$ and $^{3}/_{12}$, $^{3}/_{12}$ is the smaller fraction.

In order to add or subtract fractions, a common denominator must be found.

Example:

$$\frac{3}{4} + \frac{5}{8} =$$

$$\frac{6}{8} + \frac{5}{8} = \frac{11}{8}$$

Example:

$$\frac{5}{9} - \frac{1}{3} =$$

$$\frac{5}{9} - \frac{3}{9} = \frac{2}{9}$$

To divide fractions, invert the second fraction and multiply.

Example:

$$\frac{A}{B} \div \frac{C}{D} = \frac{A}{B} \times \frac{D}{C} = \frac{AD}{BC}$$

Proof: Assign an arbitrary numerical value to A B C D

$$A = 2, B = 3, C = 4, D = 5$$

Step 1 $\quad \dfrac{2}{3} \div \dfrac{4}{5}$

Step 2 $\quad \dfrac{2}{3} \times \dfrac{5}{4}$

Step 3 $\quad \dfrac{10}{12} = \dfrac{AD}{BC}$

Ratios and Proportions

A ratio indicates a relationship of one quantity or term to another. It can be expressed with the symbol : or as a fraction. The symbol : is read "is to" or "to."

In determining the efficiency of a grid (its ability to limit the amount of scatter radiation reaching the image detector), it is important that the radiographer know the grid ratio. When a grid is rated at 5:1, it is understood that the height of the lead lines are five times greater than the width of the interspacing material.

PROPORTIONS

Proportions indicate two or more equal ratios that are separated by the symbols = or ::. Proportions can be either directly or inversely related. In a direct proportion, if the factors in the first ratio are changed, a similar change occurs in the second ratio. In an inverse proportion, if the factors in the first ratio are changed, an inverse change occurs in the second ratio.

The symbol :: used to indicate a proportion, is read "equal to."

Example:
   A:B :: C:D is read

   A to B is equal to C to D

   or

   A is to B as C is to D

Radiographers must often calculate for an unknown in a proportion when changing technical factors. When three factors are known, it is easy to solve for the unknown fourth factor. For example, if it is necessary to change the distance at which a radiograph may be taken, the radiographer can determine how the distance change will affect the density on the radiographic image, the intensity of the beam in relationship to patient dosage and exposure, and the amount of mAs needed to maintain the original intensity and/or film density. (See Table 11-1.) The formulas needed to make the above technical adjustments will be presented later in this chapter.

Equations

Equations are mathematical expressions of equality. Two sides of an equation remain equal if similar mathematic or algebraic functions are performed on both sides of the equation at the same time.

Example:
   Given: $3X = 54$.   To solve for X, divide each side of the equation by 3. $X = 18$.

   Given: $X + 3 = 21$.   To solve for X, subtract 3 from each side of the equation.
   $X = 18$.

   Given: $X - 6 = 12$.   To solve for X, add 6 to each side of the equation.
   $X - 6 + 6 = 12 + 6$
   $X = 18$

   Given: $\dfrac{X}{6} = 3$.   To solve for X, multiply each side of the equation by 6.

$$(6)\left(\frac{X}{6}\right) = (3)(6)$$
$$\frac{6X}{6} = 18$$
$$X = 18$$

Percent

Percent can be expressed as a decimal or a fraction.

Example:
   $5\% = 0.05$ or $\dfrac{5}{100} = \dfrac{1}{20}$

To add a percent sign to a number, multiply the number by 100.

Example:
   $3 = 300\%$.

To remove a percent sign from a number, divide by 100.

Example:
   $100\% = 1$
   $10\% = 0.10$

Exponents

Scientific or exponential notation is used to write very large or very small numbers.

Exponents indicate the number of times a base number (usually 10) has been multiplied by itself.

Example:

$$10^1 = 10$$
$$10^2 = 10 \times 10 = 100$$
$$10^3 = 10 \times 10 \times 10 = 1000$$
$$10^4 = 10 \times 10 \times 10 \times 10 = 10,000$$
$$10^5 = 10 \times 10 \times 10 \times 10 \times 10 = 100,000$$

The number of zeros placed to the right of the base number indicates the exponent when scientific notation is used to write a number. A minus exponent indicates a fraction. The $(-)$ exponent indicates the number of zeros placed to the right of the decimal point of the base number.

Example:

$$10^{-5} = \frac{1}{100000} \text{ or } 0.000001$$

$$10^{-3} = \frac{1}{1000} \text{ or } 0.0001$$

To multiply numbers using scientific notation, add the exponents.

Example:

$$10^3 \times 10^5 = 10^8$$

To divide numbers using scientific notation, subtract the exponents:

Example:

$$10^6 - 10^3 = 10^3$$

Similar Triangles

Similar triangles are triangles whose sides and angles are similar in shape. A line drawn parallel to the base of a triangle will produce a similar triangle. The similar sides of similar triangles are proportional to each other.

In radiologic technology, the radiographer uses the principle of similar triangles to solve problems dealing with magnification (enlargement). Collimator opening to field size relationships can also be calculated in this manner. Radiologists use the principle of similar triangles to determine the actual size and location of an object compared to the image (e.g., for fetal maternal measurements or foreign body localization).

Problems can be easier to solve if a rough sketch is drawn and labeled. The information from the sketch can then be stated as a proportion (Figs. 13–1 and 13–2).

Example:

$$\frac{AB}{CD} = \frac{EF}{EG}$$

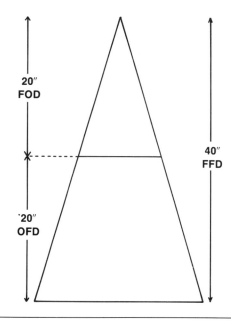

Figure 13-1 Principle of Similar Triangles
The principle of similar triangles can be used to calculate measurements in radiology. The letters used to label the schematic in Fig. 13-2 are arbitrary and do not have to be memorized if the principle is understood. These letters do not constitute a formula for field size dimensions but are used for this illustration to identify the relationship of similar triangles to each other.

It is suggested that when confronted with a problem dealing with a distance-to-size relationship, a rough sketch be made of the stated dimensions. The sketch should be labeled, and the dimensions of the similar triangle should be stated as a proportion.

Using similar triangles, the degree of enlargement of an object can be predicted in its linear as well as area measurements. If all distances, that is, 20 FOD, 20 OFD = 40 FFD are known, the true size of an object recorded on a radiograph can be calculated. The geometric relationship just stated would yield a 2× linear enlargement, 4× area enlargement. (See Figs. 7-12 and 7-15.) See Figure 13-2 for an example of collimator field size determination.

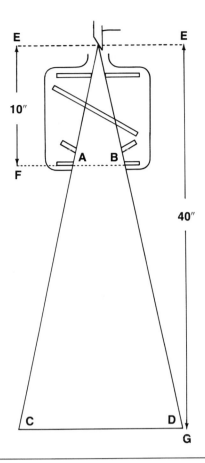

Figure 13-2 Collimator/Field Size Determination *The principle of similar triangles can be used to predict one or both dimensions of a projected field size if the size of the collimator exit shutter opening is known. Conversely, the collimator exit shutter size can be determined if the field size is known.*

The height of the first triangle is measured from the focal spot (E) to the base of the triangle (F) at the level of the exit shutter opening in the collimator (AB).

The height of the second triangle represents the FFD (EG) measured from the focal spot (E) to the base of the triangle (G) at the level of the field size opening (CD).

Temperature Conversion

To convert from Fahrenheit to Celsius (Centigrade) temperature, use the following formula:

$$C = \frac{5}{9}(F - 32)$$

IMPORTANT: Remember to subtract the 32 from the Fahrenheit temperature in the Celsius to Fahrenheit formulas before $\frac{5}{9}$ F is calculated.

Example:
70° F to ° C

$$C = \frac{5}{9}(F - 32)$$
$$\frac{5}{9}(70 - 32)$$
$$\frac{5}{9}(38)$$
$$\frac{190}{9} = 21.1$$

To convert from Celsius to Fahrenheit temperature, use the formula:

$$F = \frac{9}{5}C + 32$$

IMPORTANT: Remember to calculate $\frac{9}{5}$ C before the 32 is added in the Celsius to Fahrenheit conversion.

Example:
21.1° C to ° F

$$F = \frac{9}{5}C + 32$$
$$\frac{9}{5}(C) + 32$$
$$\frac{9(21.1)}{5} + 32$$
$$\frac{189.9}{5} + 32$$
$$37.98 + 32 = 69.98$$
$$F = 70°$$

The Kelvin scale, where Absolute Zero = 0°, is the unit of measure for temperature in the International System of Measurements.

TABLE 13-1.   Wavelength Relationships

Energy	Measured In	Approximate Wavelength
Commercial alternating current	Meters (M)	$\pm 10^6$ M 1,000,000 M
Radio	Meters (M)	$\pm$ 100 M
Television	Meters (M)	$\pm$ 1 M
Visible light	Angstrom units (A)	$\pm 10^4$ A
Medical X-radiation	Angstrom units (A)	$\pm$ 0.1 to 0.5 A

IMPORTANT: The waveform remains the same ($\sim$) in all of the above; however, the penetrating ability of the wave increases as the wavelength become shorter. (See Chapter 1.) Photon energy is not all of the same wavelength; the x-ray beam is heterogeneous, having many wavelengths and energies within the range of medical x-radiation. (See Fig. 1-3.)

39.3 in. = 1 meter
2.54 cm = 1 in.
1 cm = 1/100th meter
1 mm = 1/1000 meter
1 micron (μ) = 1/1000 mm
1 Angstrom unit (A) = 1/10,000 μ (0.1 nm, 1/100,000,000, 10^{-8} cm, 10^{-10} m, or 0.1 nm)
1 nm = 10^{-9} m

TABLE 13-2.   English/Metric Relationships

English			Metric						English	Metric
Weight	Length	Time	Weight	Length	Time	Fraction	Power of 10	Decimal		
							10^3	1000	thousands	kilo
							10^2	100	hundreds	hecto
							10^1	10	tens	deka
pound ounce	yard foot inch	second	gram liter	meter	second		1	1	unit	
						1/10	10^{-1}	0.1	tenths	deci
						1/100	10^{-2}	0.01	hundredth	centi
						1/1000	10^{-3}	0.001	thousandth	milli

Systems of Measure

The three systems of measure used by radiographers in the United States are:

1 The traditional English system
2 The MKS metric system (meter-kilogram-second)
3 The refined modern version of the metric system, known as the International System of Units (SI)

Measurements in the metric system have been used in science, industry, and medicine for many years (Tables 13-1 and 13-2). SI units were introduced as a means of providing a common language for international communications between nations and the sciences. In the 1970s, the International Commission on Radiation Units and Measurements (ICRU) introduced the SI units for measurement of radiation units and suggested replacing the traditional units by the SI units (Table 13-3) over a 10-year period. An understanding of the relationships of SI radiation units of measure is important to radiographers.

TABLE 13-3. Radiation Units of Measure*

Traditional Unit	Symbol	Measure of	SI Unit	Symbol	Relationship
rad	rad	Absorbed dose	Gray	Gy	1 rad = 0.01 Gy Gy/0.01 = 1 rad
rem	rem	Dose equivalent	Sievert	Sv	1 rem = 0.01 Sv Sv/0.01 = 1 rem
Curie	Ci	Radioactivity	Becquerel	Bq	1 Ci = 3.7×10^{10} Bq Bq/3.7×10^{10} = 1 Ci
Roentgen	R	Exposure		C/kg	Measured in Coulomb per kilogram (C/kg) 1 R = 2.58×10^{-4} C/kg C/kg/2.58×10^{-4} = 1 R

* For practical purposes, in radiologic technology, exposure, absorbed dose, and dose equivalent are said to be equal. Exposure is the quantity most easily understood. In diagnostic radiology, however, there is concern for the absorbed dose (the energy transferred per unit mass of matter by the ionizing radiation).
In the SI system, the Gray (Gy), the unit for absorbed dose, has been received when 1 joule (J) of energy has been transferred to 1 kg of mass.

TABLE 13-4. Seven Basic Units of Measure

	Unit	SI Symbol
Length	meter	m
Mass	kilogram	kg
Time	second	s
Electric current	ampere	A
Thermodynamic temperature	Kelvin	K
Amount of substance	mole	mol
Luminous intensity	candela	cd

Size Relationship in Units of Measure

The seven basic units of measure—weight, length, time, current, temperature, substance, and luminescence (Table 13-4)—can be further expanded into many other units (Table 13-5) to measure parameters such as area, volume, density, velocity, mass, electrical force, conductance, and resistance. For example, using the measurement for length, area and volume can be derived. Area is equal to the product of two sides of a surface. This measurement can be expressed in English or Metric units such as square inches or square centimeters (cm²).

The area of a square is calculated by squaring one side

$$A = a^2$$

Example: If a square has the dimension of 3 in. × 3 in., the area of the square will be 3^2, or 9 sq. in.

The area of a rectangle can be calculated by multiplying base times height.
Example: If the base of a rectangle were 5 in. and the height of a rectangle were 4 in., the area of the rectangle would be 20 sq. in.

TABLE 13-5. Some Units Derived From The Seven Basic Units

Quantity	Unit	SI Symbol	Other Units
Acceleration	meter per second squared	—	m/s²
Density	kilogram per cubic meter	—	kg/m³
Electrical capacitance	farad	F	C/V
Electrical conductance	siemens	S	A/V
Electrical potential difference	volt	V	W/A
Electromotive force	volt	V	W/A
Electrical resistance	ohm	Ω	V/A
Energy	joule	J	N·m
Force	newton	N	kg·m/s²
Frequency	hertz	Hz	cycle/sec
Illuminance	lux	lx	lm/m²
Luminance	candela per square meter	—	cd/m²
Power	watt	W	J/s
Quantity of electricity	coulomb	C	A·s
Quantity of heat	joule	J	N·m
Velocity	meter per second	—	m/s
Voltage	volt	V	W/A
Volume	cubic meter	—	m³
Work	joule	J	N/m

The area of a circle is equal to

$$\pi r^2$$

$$\pi = \frac{22}{7} \text{ or } 3.14$$

r = radius of the circle

Example: If the radius of a circle were equal to 5 in., the area of the circle would be:

$$\pi(5)^2 =$$
$$\pi(25) = 3.14(25) = 78.5 \text{ sq. in.}$$

When volume is to be measured, a third dimension must be added.

Example: In a cube, volume is the product of 3 sides and is expressed in cubic units (e.g., cubic inches, cubic centimeters).

Density can be derived by dividing the mass (weight) of an object by its volume. This relationship is often expressed in radiologic technology in reference to tissue density as the mass or amount of tissue per unit of volume.

TABLE 13-6. Electron Shell Arrangement

Spectroscopic Designation	Shell Number	Example $2(N)^2$	Number of Electrons
K	1	$2(1)^2$	2
L	2	$2(2)^2$	8
M	3	$2(3)^2$	18
N	4	$2(4)^2$	32
O	5	$2(5)^2$	50

* See Chapter 1, Figure 1-2.

IMPORTANT: Mass density should not be confused with optical density. (See Chapter 8.)

Velocity can be derived from length and time (wavelength and frequency).

Basic Physics and Electrical Formulas

An awareness of basic physics and electrical formulas is helpful in the appreciation of the physical principles of radiography.

Basic Atomic Structure (See Chapter 1)

The number of protons and neutrons in an atom determines the mass number (A) of the atom. The number of protons in an atom indicates the atomic number of an atom (Z). When represented symbolically, the atomic weight is written in superscript, the atomic number in subscript $^{A}_{Z}X$.

In a stable (non-ionized) atom, the number of protons (+ charges) equals the number of electrons (− charges).

Electrons are arranged in energy shells according to a complex system derived from quantum theory. The relationship of the electron shell number to the maximal number of electrons permissible in a given shell can be expressed by the formula $2(N)^2$ (Table 13-6).

The closer the electron shells are to the nucleus, the greater the binding power and the greater the energy required to dislodge the electron from its shell. Matter and energy are closely related and are interchangeable, as stated in Albert Einstein's Theory

$E = MC^2$
$E = \text{mass} \times \text{speed of light}^2$

Electrical Power

Power, expressed in watts (W), is equal to the electromotive force, expressed in voltage (V), times the current expressed in amperes (I)

$P = VI$

Resistance

There is a relationship between voltage (V), current (I), and resistance (R) as stated in Ohm's law. When resistance opposes the flow of electrical current, the current (I) is equal to the voltage (V) divided by the resistance (R)

$$I = \frac{V}{R}$$

or voltage (V) is equal to current (I) times resistance (R)

$V = IR$

or resistance (R) is equal to voltage (V) divided by current (I).

$$R = \frac{V}{I}$$

The resistance will depend upon the material offering the resistance, the length and cross-sectional area, and its temperature.

Resistance in a wire is directly proportional to the length of the wire. Resistance is inversely proportional to the cross-sectional area of a wire and is increased as temperature increases.

Power Loss or Power Used

To compute for power loss or the amount of power used in an electrical circuit, we must first consider the formula for power

$$P = VI$$

Resistance in a circuit results in some loss of power; therefore, a formula that shows the relationship to voltage and amperage must also be considered. Such a relationship exists in Ohm's law, where $V = IR$. By substituting IR for V in the power formula, power loss can be stated

Power $= VI$
Power Loss $= IR \cdot I$
Power Loss $= I^2R$

Since alternating current permits greater power (wattage) to be transmitted over a given distance with less power loss, power companies usually deliver electrical current in the form of alternating current. The x-ray tube, however, requires direct current for efficient operation. The current is changed from alternating current to direct current by rectification. (See Fig. 2-5.)

With full-wave rectification, both cycles of the alternating current are used.

Rectification

If a test tool (spinning top) is used to check the timer on a single-phase full-wave rectified unit, for each $\frac{1}{120}$ second that the disc revolves, a small black image (dot) will be registered on the film. (See Fig. 2-8.)

Example:

If $\frac{1}{10}$ second were used to expose the film using the spinning top, the number of black dots that should be present on the radiograph could be determined by dividing $\frac{1}{10}$ second by $\frac{1}{120}$ second.

$$\frac{1}{10} \div \frac{1}{120} =$$
$$\frac{1}{10} \times \frac{120}{1} - \frac{120}{10} = 12 \text{ (dots)}$$

If the rectification system failed or if the equipment were not rectified, there would be half the number of dots, because a dot would be recorded every $\frac{1}{60}$ second.

$$\frac{1}{10} \div \frac{1}{60} =$$
$$\frac{1}{10} \times \frac{60}{1} = 6 \text{ (dots)}$$

If the time of exposure is not known, by counting the number of dots on the image (e.g., 12 dots), the time of exposure can be calculated by multiplying the dots by $\frac{1}{120}$ second (full-wave rectified), since there would be one dot for each $\frac{1}{120}$ second.

$$12 \times \frac{1}{120} = \frac{12}{120} = \frac{1}{10}\text{th second}$$

If the equipment is 3∅ rectified equipment, a template test tool is necessary to measure the arc produced by the almost constant voltage. (See Chapter 2.)

Voltage, Current, and Resistance

The voltage measured across a resistor can be calculated if the current flowing through the circuit and the resistance in the circuit are known.

$$V = IR$$

If a series of resistors are connected in a circuit, each resistor lowers the voltage a fraction of the total voltage. There would be only one path for the current flow, and current would be equal at all points.

In a parallel circuit, there are several paths available for current flow to follow. In this situation, each resistor has the full voltage applied to it.

RESISTANCE IN A SERIES CIRCUIT

In a series circuit, the total resistance (R) is equal to the sum of all resistances (r) in the circuit (Table 13-7).

$$R = r_1 + r_2 + r_3 \text{ (and so on)}$$

Example:

If three resistors were wired in series in a circuit with $r_1 = 5$ ohms, $r_2 = 10$ ohms, and $r_3 = 15$ ohms, the total resistance (R) in the circuit would be 30 ohms.

RESISTANCE IN A PARALLEL SERIES

When resistors are wired in parallel in a circuit, the total resistance (R) will be less than the resistance (r) of any single resistor in the circuit, since the current is divided among several branches or paths (Table 13-7).

There is a reciprocal relationship of the re-

TABLE 13-7. Current–Voltage–Resistance Relationships In Circuits*

Series	Parallel
$R = r_1 + r_2 + r_3$	$\dfrac{1}{R} = \dfrac{1}{r_1} + \dfrac{1}{r_2} + \dfrac{1}{r_3}$
$I = i_1 = i_2 = i_3$	$I = i_1 + i_2 + i_3$
$V = v_1 + v_2 + v_3$	$V = v_1 = v_2 = v_3$

* In a series circuit, the connections are in a line along the same conductor. In a parallel series, the connections bridge the conductor.

sistance in a parallel series to the total resistance.

$$\frac{1}{R} = \frac{1}{r_1} + \frac{1}{r_2} + \frac{1}{r_3} \text{ (and so on)}$$

Example:

If two 8-ohm resistors are wired in parallel in a circuit, the total resistance would be

$$\frac{1}{R_T} = \frac{1}{8} + \frac{1}{8} = \frac{2}{8}$$
$$R_T = \frac{8}{2} = 4 \text{ ohms}$$

TOTAL VOLTAGE IN A SERIES CIRCUIT

The total voltage (V) in a series circuit can be calculated by adding the voltage input at each terminal junction.

$$V = v_1 + v_2 + v_3$$

CURRENT IN A PARALLEL SERIES

In a parallel series, the current flowing through the main branch (I) is equal to the sum of the current in all other branches (i).

$$I = i_1 + i_2 + i_3$$

Current in a parallel circuit follows several paths and is divided among the paths. The voltage applied in the parallel circuit is equal at all points (Table 13-7).

IMPORTANT: Total resistance takes into consideration several forms of resistance (inductive, capacitive, and electrical) and is known as impedance.

Transformer Principles

A transformer is used to step up or step down voltage in an electrical circuit. (See Chapter

2.) Transformers require alternating current for their operation and operate on the principle of mutual induction.

The electromotive force (voltage) induced in the secondary coils of the transformer is directly proportional to the number of turns in the coils in the secondary side of the transformer. If the turn ratio is increased on the secondary side, the transformer will step up voltage. If the turn ratio is decreased on the secondary side, the voltage will be decreased. (See Fig. 2-4.)

V_S = secondary voltage
V_P = primary voltage
N_S = number of turns in secondary
N_P = number of turns in primary

$$\frac{V_P}{V_S} = \frac{N_P}{N_S}$$

Example:

If the primary coil of a transformer has 10 turns and a potential of 100 volts and the secondary coil has 5000 turns, the potential in the secondary can be calculated.

$$\frac{100}{V_S} = \frac{10}{5000}$$
$$10V_S = 500,000$$
$$V_S = 50,000 \text{ or } 50 \text{ kVp}$$

This would be a step-up transformer. The current (amperage) induced in the secondary coils of a transformer is inversely proportional to the voltage applied to the primary coils of the transformer. As voltage in the secondary is increased, amperage decreases; as amperage is increased, voltage decreases.

$$\frac{I_P}{I_S} = \frac{V_S}{V_P}$$

The efficiency of a transformer is determined by the ratio of the amount of power outgoing to the incoming power.

$$\text{Transformer efficiency} = \frac{\text{power out}}{\text{power in}}$$

$$\text{Percentage of efficiency of transformer} = \frac{\text{power out}}{\text{power in}} \times 100$$

Formulas as Applied to Principles of Exposure

X-Ray Tube Heat Units

Heat units (see Chapter 4) generated for a single exposure with single-phase equipment are the product of mA · time · kVp. The heat units generated by 3-phase, 6-pulse equipment can be determined by multiplying the single ∅ heat units by the factor 1.35. For 3∅ 12-pulse equipment, the 3∅ multiplication factor is changed to 1.41.

Example:

$$\text{HU (3∅, 6-pulse)} = \text{mA} \cdot \text{time} \cdot \text{kVp} \cdot 1.35$$
$$\text{HU (3∅, 12-pulse)} = \text{mA} \cdot \text{time} \cdot \text{kVp} \cdot 1.41$$

To determine total heat units (when multiple exposures are made in sequence), multiply the heat units per single exposure times the number of exposures in the series.

Grids

GRID RATIO

Grid ratio is expressed as the relationship of the height of the lead grid lines (h) to the distance between the lead lines (d). (See Chapter 5.)

$$\text{Grid ratio} = \frac{h}{d}$$

Grid Selectivity

Grid selectivity is the relationship of the amount of primary radiation to the amount of secondary radiation transmitted through a grid.

$$\text{grid selectivity} = \frac{\text{primary transmitted}}{\text{secondary transmitted}}$$

GRID FREQUENCY

Grid frequency indicates the number of lead lines per inch in the grid. If efficiency is to be maintained, as grid frequency increases, the grid ratio also increases.

RADIOGRAPHIC CONTRAST WITH A GRID

The relationship of contrast achieved with a grid to contrast without a grid can be ex-pressed as the contrast improvement factor (CIF).

$$\text{CIF} = \frac{\text{contrast with grid}}{\text{contrast without grid}}$$

MAS AND GRIDS

To make changes in mAs to compensate for changes in grid ratio: list the grid ratio from a non-grid to 16:1 grid, and assign correction factor value to each grid.

non grid = 1
5:1   = 2
6:1   = 3
8:1   = 4
12:1   = 5
16:1   = 6

To determine new mAs find:

1 Grid correction factor of new grid
2 Grid correction factor of original grid

Divide:

$$\frac{\text{new grid correction factor}}{\text{original grid correction factor}}$$

Multiply the above result by the original mAs to determine new mAs needed to maintain a given density.

Example: If 100 mAs is required for a given technique using a 5:1 grid, the exposure required for use with an 8:1 grid can be determined by placing the grid correction factor assigned to the 8:1 grid (4) over the grid correction factor assigned to the 5:1 grid (2) and arriving at a correction factor of 2. When the correction factor is multiplied by the original mAs (100), the new mAs is obtained.

$$2(100) = 200 \text{ mAs}$$

KVP AND GRIDS

Since the relationship of kVp to density is not linear, changes made with kilovoltage to compensate for grid conversions are approximations (Table 13-8).

Radiographers rarely change technique from non-grid to a high-ratio grid; however, it may be necessary to perform one part of an examination without a grid and another part

TABLE 13-8. kVp/Grid Conversions*	
Grid Ratio	**Add**
5:1	8 kVp
6:1	8 kVp
8:1	15 kVp
12:1	20–25 kVp
16:1	20–25 kVp

* The kilovoltage values listed above are theoretical. In practice, conversion from a non-grid technique to a grid technique rarely occurs.

of the series with a low to moderate ratio grid.

Radiographic Density

Density is determined by the log of the light incident to the radiograph (from the viewbox) to the light transmitted through the radiograph (from the viewbox). (See Chapter 11.)

$$D = \log \frac{\text{incident light}}{\text{transmitted light}}$$

Since radiographs are transparencies, a density of 1 indicates that for every 10 units of light that fall upon the film, only 1 unit, or 10%, is transmitted through the film.

An area on the radiograph with a density of 2 would permit only 1/100th, or 1%, of the incident light to be transmitted through the film.

mA and Time Relationship

$$mA \cdot T = mAs$$

The product of milliamperage and the time factor expressed in seconds results in mAs (milliampere seconds). (See Chapter 11.)

Example:
$$\left.\begin{array}{l} 100 \text{ mA at } 0.1 \text{ sec} = \\ 100 \ (0.1) = \end{array}\right\} \ 10 \text{ mAs}$$

mAs and Time Relationship

mA is inversely proportional to time. If a given density is to be maintained, an inverse amount of mA is required as the length of exposure (time) is changed.

$$\frac{mA_1}{mA_2} = \frac{T_2}{T_1}$$

Example: If 100 mA is used for $\frac{1}{10}$ (0.1) second to produce an acceptable radiographic density, 50 mA would be required to produce the same density at $\frac{1}{5}$ second (0.2).

$$\frac{mA_1}{mA_2} = \frac{T_2}{T_1}$$

$$\frac{100}{X} = \frac{0.2}{0.1}$$

$$0.2X = 100 \ (0.1)$$

$$0.2X = 10$$

$$X = \frac{10}{0.2} = 50 \text{ mA}$$

mAs_1 (100) = mAs_2 (100); therefore, density remains unchanged.

mAs and Density

Radiographic density is directly proportional to mAs. This relationship is linear. A doubling of the mAs factor results in a doubling of radiographic density. Since mAs is the product of mA and time (mA · T = mAs), an increase or decrease in either factor results in a corresponding density change on the radiograph. (See Table 11-1.)

IMPORTANT: At least a 30% change in mAs is required for a change in density to be perceived on a radiograph.

Density and Distance

Changes in focal film distance produce changes in radiographic density (Fig. 13-3). (See Chapter 11.)

The Inverse Square Law is used to compute the intensity of the beam (amount of radiation that will cause exposure to the patient and/or film blackening). (See Table 11-2.) The change in beam intensity and/or radiographic density varies inversely with the square of the distance.

$$\frac{I_1}{I_2} = \frac{D_2^2}{D_1^2}$$

I = intensity of beam
D = focal film distance

Example:
If the amount of radiation reaching a patient at 40 in. is 3 R and the distance were

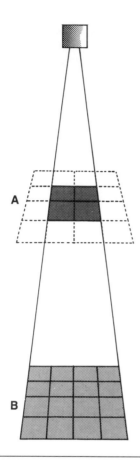

Figure 13-3 **The Effect of Focal Film Distance on the Radiographic Image** *Changes in focal film distance will produce visible changes in radiographic density and the size of the field covered by the beam. The intensity of the x-ray beam (relative to the exposure to the image receptor [film blackening] and dosage to the patient) will also be affected by changes in distance.*

A 36-in. FFD is shown (A) compared to a 72-in. FFD (B). Note the size of the x-ray field at 36 in. (A) compared to that at 72-in. (B). There is a 2× linear, 4× area enlargement, with the x-ray intensity of B reduced to one fourth the intensity of A.

When a change in the FFD is made, the change in radiographic density and beam intensity varies inversely with the square of the distance.

increased to 60-in., the dosage would be reduced to 1.33 R.

$$\frac{3R}{X} = \frac{60^2}{40^2}$$
$$\frac{3R}{X} = \frac{3600}{1600}$$
$$3R(1600) = 3600X$$
$$X = \frac{4800}{3600}$$
$$X = 1.33 \text{ R}$$

This same reasoning can be applied to the amount of radiation that will cause a film to exhibit a radiographic density. As distance is increased, radiographic density decreases in proportion to D^2. (See Table 11-1.)

mAs and Distance and Density

The amount of milliamperage and time needed to produce a given radiographic density varies directly with the square of the distance. (See Table 11-1.)

$$\frac{mAs_1}{mAs_2} = \frac{D_1^2}{D_2^2}$$

Since $mA \cdot T = mAs$, the relationship of mA or time to distance is also directly proportional.

$$\frac{mA_1}{mA_2} = \frac{D_1^2}{D_2^2}$$

and

$$\frac{T_1}{T_2} = \frac{D_1^2}{D_2^2}$$

Example:

If 100 mA were used at 40-in. FFD and it were necessary to decrease the FFD to 36 in., 81 mA would be needed to maintain density.

$$\frac{100}{X} = \frac{40^2}{36^2}$$
$$\frac{100}{X} = \frac{1600}{1296}$$
$$1600X = 129600$$
$$X = 81 \text{ mA}$$

If 0.5 second were used at 40-in. FFD and it were necessary to increase the FFD to 48 in., 0.72 second would be required to maintain density.

Example:

$$\frac{T_1}{T_2} = \frac{D_1^2}{D_2^2}$$

$$\frac{0.5}{X} = \frac{(40)^2}{(48)^2}$$

1600X = 1152

X = 0.72

A short formula can be used to calculate changes in mAs (mA or Time) and distance. If the new distance is divided by the old distance and the resultant conversion factor is then squared, this factor multiplied times the original mAs will yield the new mAs required at the new distance. (See Table 12-2.) This method permits the radiographer to work with smaller numbers, since only one factor will be squared.

Example 1:

Using the factors in the previous example:

Step 1 $\dfrac{36 \text{ (new distance)}}{40 \text{ (old distance)}} = 0.9$

Step 2 $(0.9)^2 = 0.81$
Step 3 $0.81 \times 100 \text{ mA} = 81 \text{ mA}$

Example 2:

Step 1 $\dfrac{48 \text{ in.(new distance)}}{40 \text{ in.(old distance)}} = 1.2$

Step 2 $(1.2)^2 = 1.44$
Step 3 $1.44 \times 0.5 \text{ sec} = 0.72 \text{ sec}$

Reciprocity Law (mAs Density Relationship)

When equal products of mA and time are used to produce two radiographs (e.g., 100 mA at 1 second or 200 mA at 0.5 second) and all other factors remain unchanged, the radiographic density should be equal, since $mAs_1 = mAs_2$.

In theory, reciprocity may fail when using

intensifying screens at extremely long or extremely short exposure times. In practice, reciprocity law failure can occur with exposures such as those used for the PA chest (10 msec or less) or with pluridirectional tomographic studies (6 seconds to 9 seconds).

Photographic Effect

Milliamperage, time (in seconds), kilovoltage, and distance produce a photographic effect on the radiograph. This relationship can be stated in the formula

$$PE = \frac{mA \times T \cdot kV^2}{D^2}$$

kVp and Density

Changes in kVp are not linear in their effect on radiographic density. Changes in the lower and higher kilovoltage ranges have a greater effect on density than changes at moderate kilovoltages. (See Fig. 11-4.)

If a 15% change (increase or decrease) in kVp is made at any kilovoltage range, the effect should be a doubling or halving, respectively, of the radiographic density.

Example to reduce density to ½:

Given 40 kVp:
$40 \times 0.15 = 6.00$
$40 - 6 = 34 \text{ kVp} = ½$ density of image produced at 40 kVp

To increase density:

$40 + 6 = 46 \text{ kVp} =$ double density of image produced at 40 kVp

Given 100 kVp. To decrease density to ½:

$100 \times 0.15 = 15 \text{ kVp}$
$100 - 15 = 85 \text{ kVp} = ½$ density of image produced at 100 kVp

To double density:

$100 + 15 = 115 \text{ kVp} =$ double density of image produced at 100 kVp

Radiographers often substitute ± 10 kVp in the 60 kVp to 70 kVp range to change density (see Chapter 12), since 60 kVp at 0.15 = 9 kVp and 70 kVp at 0.15 = 10.5 kVp. A ± 10 kVp change is not acceptable across the entire kilovoltage range used for medical radiography. (See Fig. 11-4.)

Kilovoltage and Milliamperage Compensations

If a change in kVp is required but density must remain the same, the mAs must also be simultaneously adjusted. Since a 15% change (increase) in kVp results in two times increase in density, by adjusting the mAs factor to half the original mAs, radiographic density can be maintained. If kilovoltage must be decreased by 15%, a doubling of the mAs will produce a radiograph of comparable density. (See Fig. 11-4.)

Intensifying Screens and Density

When a change in intensifying screen speed is made, the effect on radiographic density can be predicted if each screen speed is assigned a conversion factor. Medium or average speed screens are assigned a value of 1. Faster or slower systems are assigned numbers relative to the average screen (Table 13-9).

Intensification Screen Relationships

INTENSIFICATION FACTOR (IF) AND INTENSIFYING SCREENS

The relationship of the radiation needed to obtain the same film blackening with and without intensifying screens can be expressed in the following manner:

$$IF = \frac{\text{exposure without screens}}{\text{exposure with screens}}$$

TABLE 13-9. mAs/Screen Conversions

Screen Type	Conversion Factor
Direct exposure (medical film)	50 × mAs
Detail or slow	2–4 × mAs
Medium	1
High speed (fast)	½ × mAs
Rare earth	¼ (or less) × mAs

THE CONTRAST IMPROVEMENT FACTOR

The relationship of contrast on a radiograph obtained with intensifying screens compared to a direct exposure radiograph is known as the contrast improvement factor (CIF).

$$CIF = \frac{\text{contrast with screens}}{\text{contrast without screens}}$$

INTENSIFYING SCREENS—ABSORPTION CONVERSION RATIO

Intensifying screen effectiveness relies on the absorption of radiation by the screens and the converting of the absorbed energy into light (fluorescence) that is capable of exposing radiographic film. (See Fig. 8-7.)

IMAGE-INTENSIFIED BRIGHTNESS GAIN (INTENSIFICATION)

With the image intensifier, the intensification factor depends upon the relationship of the gain in light achieved by the reduction in size of the output phosphor from the input phosphor size (minification factor) and the gain achieved by acceleration of the photons to the output phosphor (flux gain).

$$\text{brightness gain} = \text{minification} \times \text{flux}$$

Flux gain occurs from the acceleration of electrons striking the output phosphor. Minification gain (MG) is achieved by electronically focusing the light from the input phosphor to a smaller area (output phosphor). (See Chapter 6.)

$$MG = \left(\frac{\text{diameter of input phosphor}}{\text{diameter of output phosphor}} \right)^2$$

Example: The minification achieved with an input phosphor of 6 in. on an output phosphor of 1 in. would be $(6/1)^2 = 36$. If the flux gain for each electron ejected from the photocathode surface produced 50 light photons for each electron accelerated, the brightness gain on the 6-in. intensifier would be:

$$50 \times 36, \text{ or a gain of } 1800$$

For a 9-in. input phosphor with a flux gain of 50 and a minification gain of 9^2, a brightness gain of 4050 would be achieved:

50 × 81, or a gain of 4050

Collimation and Field Size

It is possible to determine field size of a collimated area by using the principles of similar triangles. The sides of similar triangles (equal in shape, but not size) have a direct relationship to each other (see Fig. 13-2).
Example:
Determine the collimator opening size required to cover a 10-in. × 12-in. field size if the collimator opening is 10 in. from the source.

$$\frac{AB}{CD} = \frac{EF}{EG}$$

Side 1) $\frac{X}{12} = \frac{10}{40}$ Side 2) $\frac{X}{10} = \frac{10}{40}$

$X = 3$ in. $X = 2.5$ in.

The collimator opening should be 2.5 in. × 3 in. to cover a 10 in. × 12 in. field.

Recorded Detail

Geometric principles influence the edge sharpness on an image. (See Chapter 11.)

FOCUS FILM DISTANCE; OBJECT FILM DISTANCE; FOCAL SPOT SIZE; AND DETAIL

The smaller the focal spot size, the less geometric unsharpness.

P = penumbra (area of unsharpness)
FS = focal spot size (see Fig. 11-10)
FOD = focus object distance (see Fig. 7-14)
OFD = object film distance (see Figs. 11-11 and 11-12)
FFD = focal film distance

Penumbra (P) = $\frac{\text{effective FS} \times \text{OFD}}{\text{FOD}}$

Geometric detail is increased whenever unsharpness can be decreased.
Example: When a 0.6-mm focal spot is substituted for a 1.2-mm focal spot for an examination made at a 40-in. FFD with a 10-in. OFD, 30-in. FOD (see Fig. 11-12), unsharpness will be significantly decreased.

$$P = \frac{1.2 \times 10}{30} = 0.4$$
$$P = \frac{0.6 \times 10}{30} = 0.2$$

IMPORTANT: Remember that FOD = FFD − OFD.

Example: When the focal film distance is increased from 40 in. to 72 in. as in bedside radiography compared to conventional chest radiography, the unsharpness of the image approximates the image made at the shortened FFD using the same factors except for the FOD,

$$P = \frac{1.2 \times 10}{62} = 0.193$$

Geometric unsharpness caused by penumbra is diminished, and the sharpness of the small focal spot is approximated.

The location of the source and the part to the image detector greatly influences the degree of penumbra on the image. (See Fig. 11-10.) If the OFD could be reduced, unsharpness would also decrease.
Example: Using the same factors as stated in the original example except for the OFD, which was reduced to 5 in.,

$$P = \frac{0.6 \times 5}{35} = 0.085$$

In the best situation, the smallest focal spot, the shortest OFD, and the longest FOD would result in the least amount of unsharpness:

$$P = \frac{0.6 \times 5}{67} = 0.045$$

IMPORTANT: These examples do not take into consideration other influences on unsharpness, such as motion or the use of intensifying screens. (See Chapters 4 and 8.)

IMPORTANT: Although the formula stated for unsharpness is universally accepted, it must be noted that in the examples given, the factors are expressed in millimeters and inches and have not been converted to a common unit of measure, such as millimeters. Most textbooks use this conceptual approach when explaining how to calculate geometric unsharpness.

Magnification

MAGNIFICATION AND OBJECT FILM DISTANCE

Geometric principles can be used to solve problems dealing with magnification and distance or determine the size of an object or the size of the resultant image. (See Chapter 7.) The width of the image and the width of the object are related to the distance of the image and the distance of the object from the source. In radiography, the FFD is the distance from the focal spot to the film, and the FOD is the distance from the focal spot to the object.

MAGNIFICATION (M)

$$M = \frac{FFD}{FOD}$$

PERCENTAGE OF MAGNIFICATION

To compute the degree to which an object is magnified, subtract the object width from the image width, divide by the object width, and multiply by 100.

$$\% \text{ of mag} = \frac{\text{image width} - \text{object width}}{\text{object width}} \times 100$$

AREA ENLARGEMENT

Enlargement (magnification) occurs in linear and area dimensions. In enlargement techniques, a distance that produces a $2\times$ linear enlargement produces a $4\times$ area, since the area of a square or rectangle is the product of 2 sides (base $\times$ height). (See Fig. 7-12 and Table 11-1.)

Stereo Shift

The interpupillary distance and the distance at which stereo images are viewed have a direct relationship to the degree of stereo shift and the FFD.

$$\frac{\text{interpupillary distance}}{\text{viewing distance}} = \frac{\text{tube shift}}{\text{FFD}}$$

The distance between the pupils of the eyes is approximately 2.5 in.; the viewing distance for stereo radiography is usually about 25 in. This is a 1:10 ratio.

Example: If a 40-in. FFD were used, the total tube shift required to produce stereo images would be 4 in. Each exposure must be made 2 in. either side of midline:

$$\frac{1}{10} = \frac{X}{40}$$
$$10X = 40$$
$$X = 4$$

IMPORTANT: The tube shift must be in the direction of the grid lines to avoid grid cutoff; there must be no change in the position of the part or degree of inspiration between images; and the collimator shutter pattern must be open to a greater degree in the dimensions of the tube shifts to avoid image cutoff.

Technical Conversion Exercises

The radiographer can predict the outcome of radiographs made with various exposure factors under given conditions.

This type of problem is usually presented as an exercise to determine whether the application of the principles of radiographic exposure are understood. In practice, problems of this type will not be encountered, since it is not advisable to simultaneously make several changes in technical factors. (See Chapter 12.)

Problems should be written with significant differences in mAs, kVp, time, or distance to make the mathematical operations meaningful.

Contributing Factors

Fact to remember Re DENSITY

1 The highest mAs = greatest density
2 The fastest screen film combination = greatest density
3 The lowest grid ratio = greatest density
4 Direct exposure techniques = least density
5 The shortest distance = greatest density
6 The longest time = greatest density

7 The highest kVp = greatest density

8 The smallest area of collimation = the least density (conventional techniques)

Facts to remember Re CONTRAST

1 The lowest kVp = greatest contrast (short scale)

2 The highest grid ratio = greatest contrast (short scale)

3 The smallest area of collimation = the greatest contrast (short scale)

Facts to remember Re DETAIL (geometric)

1 The smallest focal spot = greatest detail

2 The shortest object film distance = greatest detail

3 The greatest focal film distance = greatest detail

4 The shortest time = greatest detail if motion is a consideration

5 The slowest screen film system = the greatest detail (when comparing the same phosphor type)

6 Direct exposure technique = the greatest detail

To determine the effect of technical changes:

1 Evaluate and determine the number of distractor groups in each item, for example,
a.
b.
c.
d.
e.
number of distractor groups = 5

2 Consider each similar factor in the groups, and evaluate against other factors, determine which factor would produce the greatest density, and assign a number value to that factor (e.g., 200 mAs would produce the greatest

density; therefore, it would be assigned the highest number value (5), 150 mAs (4), 100 mAs (3), 75 mAs (2), 50 mAs (1).
a. 100 mAs (3)
b. 200 mAs (5)
c. 150 mAs (4)
d. 50 mAs (1)
e. 75 mAs (2)

3 If two or more factors in the group are similar, assign them the same numerical value starting with the number of distractor groups in the problem, for example,
a. 100 mAs (5)
b. 100 mAs (5)
c. 50 mAs (3)
d. 75 mAs (4)
e. 100 mAs (5)
The greatest density would be achieved with 100 mAs; therefore, a, b, and e would be assigned the number 5; d should be assigned number 4; and c should be assigned number 3.

4 Proceed to next factor group and, using the same procedure, assign numerical factors.

5 Add the assigned values ACROSS each distractor group.

6 The distractor group with the highest total will be the option that will produce the greatest density.

7 If two distractor groups have the same total reevaluate them using the procedure described above.

See examples below.

IMPORTANT: *This same logic can be used to determine the greatest detail, contrast, and so on. Consider only those factors that have a noticeable effect on the result being evaluated. It is not necessary to consider focal spot size when evaluating contrast or density; however, it certainly must be considered when evaluating detail.*

Example:

	mA	Time	kVp	Screens	FFD	mAs	kVp	Screens		
A.	100	⅓ second	100	Medium	30 in.	33 (3)	100 (3)	Medium (3)	30 in. (4)	= 13
B.	200	⅛ second	85	High	45 in.	25 (2)	85 (2)	High (4)	45 in. (1)	= 9
C.	50	1 second	115	Medium	36 in.	50 (4)	115 (4)	Medium (3)	36 in. (3)	= 14
D.	400	½₀ second	100	High	40 in.	20 (1)	100 (3)	High (4)	40 in. (2)	= 10
						C = greatest density				

Example: Consider the factors listed below. Which radiograph would exhibit the shortest scale of contrast?

	mA	Time	kV	Grid	FFD
A.	600	⅕ second	80	8:1	30 in.
B.	200	½ second	92	6:1	50 in.
C.	500	¼ second	80	12:1	30 in.
D.	300	⅕ second	116	5:1	72 in.

Remember to assign the highest value to the shortest scale of contrast achieved with each factor.

A. 80 kVp = (4)   8:1 grid (3) = 7
B. 92 kVp = (3)   6:1 grid (2) = 5
C. 80 kVp = (4)   12:1 grid (4) = 8
D. 116 kVp = (2) 5:1 grid (1) = 3

80 kVp with 12:1 grid will produce the shortest scale of contrast.

14 Image Evaluation and Application of Radiographic Principles

THE previous 13 chapters of this textbook were devoted to information needed to produce a quality radiograph. This chapter will be devoted to the clinical application of previously stated radiographic principles.

Information needed for the optimal operation of x-ray equipment can be found in Chapter 3.

Image quality depends in part upon the skill level and attitude of the radiographer.

Radiographic techniques should constantly be reviewed and improved to produce "state-of-the-art" images reflecting the technical skills of the radiographer. The more clearly the tasks and departmental standards are defined, the closer one comes to achieving image quality.

The examination of the chest will be used whenever possible to illustrate the application of principles of radiographic exposure and radiographic evaluation.

The value of learning is the application of acquired knowledge. A systematic approach to image evaluation must be applied in a reasonable, logical manner when evaluating a radiograph. Identifying a problem is essential to solving it.

A radiograph should be systematically analyzed to determine:

1 Whether a problem exists (e.g., Is the radiograph technically acceptable?)

2 Whether there is enough information available to make a decision? (e.g., Are there other factors that, if known, would enter into the decision-making process?)

3 The nature of the problem (e.g., Is the radiograph overexposed, underexposed, or fogged?)

4 Whether the problem is due to something other than a technical error (e.g., patient condition, processor malfunction, equipment miscalibration)

5 The alternatives and possible course of action (e.g., Is a shorter exposure time needed? Will a change in patient position improve the image?)

6 What considerations must enter into the changes to be made (e.g., If the FFD is changed, will the grid remain in focus? Will an increase in kVp generate an unacceptable amount of scatter?)

7 Whether a repeat examination is indicated or advisable (e.g., Is the repeat radiograph of importance to the overall study? What is the department policy regarding authorization for a repeat study?)

The approach just described can be implemented with either a printed (Table 14-1) or a mental checklist.

Technical Considerations

IMPORTANT: If filtration is removable, the radiographer must be certain that the filter has been reinserted into the collimator prior to the exposure of a patient.

The arbitrary disposal of a radiograph prior to the evaluation of the entire study should be avoided. Whenever possible, a quality control radiographer or radiologist should review a less than optimal image. The radiologist may find some information on the image that might be helpful in diagnosis; the quality control technologist can sometimes include these images in a technical teaching file.

A poor quality radiograph should not be accepted for interpretation unless the patient's condition or age contraindicates re-examination.

Before repeating a radiograph, one should determine whether proper technical factors were used. If it can be established that the technical factors were correct and the cause of the poor radiograph cannot be identified, a consultation with a supervisor or radiologist is in order before the study is repeated.

Just as a clinical history is necessary when ordering a radiographic examination, a technical history is needed before a repeat examination is attempted. A review of the previously used technical factors is important. If previous radiographs are available, they can be used to establish an alternate technique if needed. Good technical practice dictates that the number of variables in the repeat study be limited. If possible, repeat examinations should be made using the same equipment, under the same conditions, by the same radiographer.

Part of the radiographic evaluation should be to determine whether the correct size cassette was used for the view. For example, a film that is too small for an extremity examination may not permit at least one joint to be included on the radiograph. Cassettes that are

too small will exclude areas of adjacent anatomy that may be needed for diagnosis, necessitating a repeat examination. The size of the cassette, when used with positive beam limiting devices, will determine the size of the patient area that is exposed. (See Chapter 5.) Cassettes that are too large for the study increase the potential for scatter radiation and increase patient dosage.

TABLE 14-1. Film Evaluation Checklist

Density

Overall density

Acceptable _____yes _____no

  Due to:

    _____technique   _____processing

Change density by adjusting

    _____mAs _____kVp _____screens

    _____film _____grid ratio _____distance

    _____position of patient to AED

    _____collimation _____other

Contrast

Long-scale _____ Short-scale _____

Acceptable _____yes _____no

  Due to:

    _____technique   _____processing

Change contrast by adjusting

    _____kVp _____grid

    _____beam restriction

    _____grid ratio _____other

Recorded Detail and Visibility of Detail

_____excellent _____adequate

_____poor

Poor detail caused by:

_____lack of penetration of part

_____patient motion

    _____voluntary   _____involuntary

_____fog

    _____chemical   _____radiation

    _____white light   _____safelight

Quality assurance testing of x-ray equipment and processors is a prerequisite for the making of quality radiographic images. (See Table 3-1.)

TABLE 14-1 *Continued.*

Image geometry

_____OFD _____FFD

_____focal spot size

_____distortion due to

_____part angulation

_____tube angulation

_____receptor angulation

_____screen type

_____screen film contact

Scatter Control

Grids

_____required _____not required

Collimation

_____evident _____not evident

_____extra focal radiation

_____image undercutting

_____backscatter

Radiation Protection

Collimation

_____evident _____not evident

Shielding

_____evident _____not evident

_____not possible, area of interest in field

Intensifying screens

_____type _____speed

Distance

_____FFD _____FOD

Technique

_____kVp range _____mAs

Positioning

Departmental routine _____yes _____no

Supplemental views _____yes _____no

Patient centering

_____excellent _____acceptable

_____poor

Correct by:

_____adjusting film position into alignment with central ray and or patient area of interest

Anatomy

Area of interest demonstrated

_____yes _____no

Correct by adjusting:

_____central ray _____tube angle

_____collimation _____patient position

Identification

Patient name _____yes _____no

Patient age _____yes _____no

ID number _____yes _____no

Radiographer ID _____yes _____no

Student ID _____yes _____no

Markers used _____yes _____no

Markers correct _____yes _____no

Artifacts or Foreign Bodies

_____increased density

_____decreased density

Caused by:

_____film _____grid

_____screen _____patient

_____cassette _____internal

_____tabletop _____external

_____processor _____other

Extremity examinations are usually made on a single cassette divided into multiple segments by lead rubber sheeting or tight beam collimation. Multiple images exposed on the same cassette should be oriented in the same direction to make comparison of the views easier.

The selection of the grid ratio and focal range is generally predetermined for the radiographer. The centering of the x-ray beam to the grid at proper focal range by the radiographer is critical. The use of an improper FFD, for example, 40-in. FFD instead of 72-in. FFD for a chest radiograph will produce bilateral grid cutoff on the image. Both costophrenic angles may appear underexposed with a loss in recorded detail (Fig. 14-1). This loss of density and detail should not be at-

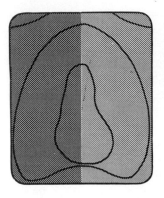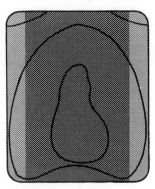

Figure 14-1 Grid Cutoff
When an x-ray tube is positioned off-center to a focused grid, a difference in radiographic density can be noted on one side of the radiograph (left). In the illustration on the left, the tube was positioned off-center to the left side of the patient.

If an improper FFD were used, for example, a 40-in. FFD with a grid focused at 72-in. FFD (right),

there would be a loss of radiographic density, bilaterally. One-to 2-in. segments of both lateral aspects of the chest radiograph would appear underexposed.

The shaded areas represent the portions of the radiograph that received an adequate amount of x-ray exposure. The lighter areas represent the effect of grid cutoff.

tributed to poor screen contact (see Fig. 8-14) or pathology.

Grid damage or the capturing of a grid in motion by short exposure times (see Fig. 5-15) can produce changes in the radiographic image that blend into the superimposed radiographic anatomy. These subtle changes can mask normal radiographic anatomy or pathology. To evaluate the image when grid artifacts are suspected, the radiograph should be positioned so that the image of the grid pattern is viewed horizontally. By stepping away to view the image, it may be easier to identify grid stripping artifacts. A simple test for grid damage is suggested in Chapter 5. (See Fig. 5-15.)

Viewing conditions influence the evaluation of an image. Viewboxes at the quality control station or automatic processor should be similar in light intensity to the viewboxes used for interpretation. Ambient light reflecting off the surfaces of the images on the viewbox can influence the perception of technical quality.

Image unsharpness is easy to identify when a radiograph appears blurred at a normal viewing distance (Fig. 14-2); however, the source of unsharpness may be difficult to identify. Tube crane vibration, faulty Bucky

locks, and cassette vibration in the Bucky tray (see Fig. 5-17) or cassettes not securely fastened in the Bucky tray when used for upright radiography should be considered.

Cardiac and peristaltic motion also influence image sharpness. The ability of the patient to cooperate often determines the length of the exposure. The use of short exposure times, with high-speed intensifying screen technology requires strict adherence to a technique chart. The selection of a screen film detector is determined by departmental policy. Occasionally, a higher speed system may be necessary to reduce radiation or patient motion. Minor adjustments in exposure times can result in significant changes in density (Fig. 14-3).

Immobilization techniques can help to overcome motion, although compression may be contraindicated in selected examinations.

Motion can be used to advantage with certain body parts (Figs. 14-4 and 14-5).

If a magnifying glass is used to view a radiograph, an image may appear to be unsharp. This is due in part to the parallax effect of dual emulsion film and is particularly obvious with tube-angled techniques. Whenever possible, minimal tube angulation should be used to avoid the parallax effect associated

(Text continues on p. 244.)

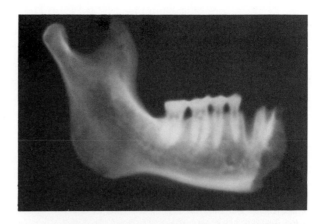

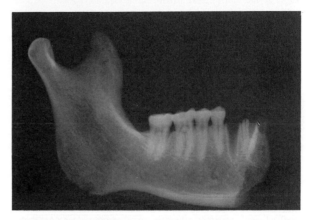

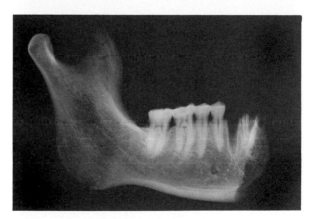

Figure 14-2   Image Unsharpness
Three radiographs of a dry mandible are shown. The unsharp image is easy to identify since the radiograph appears blurred at a normal viewing distance (top). *A low-contrast image minimizes the differences between densities, reducing visibility of detail* (center).

Appropriate geometric considerations combined with adequate contrast results in a visibly sharp image (bottom). *(Courtesy of Eastman Kodak Company, Rochester, New York)*

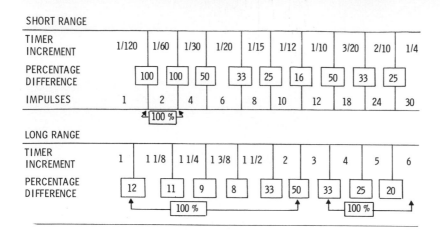

SHORT RANGE

TIMER INCREMENT	1/120	1/60	1/30	1/20	1/15	1/12	1/10	3/20	2/10	1/4
PERCENTAGE DIFFERENCE		100	100	50	33	25	16	50	33	25
IMPULSES	1	2	4	6	8	10	12	18	24	30

100 %

LONG RANGE

TIMER INCREMENT	1	1 1/8	1 1/4	1 3/8	1 1/2	2	3	4	5	6
PERCENTAGE DIFFERENCE	12	11	9	8	33	50	33	25	20	

100 %   100 %

Figure 14-3 Radiographic Density and Timer Increment Variations Minor changes in exposure times can cause major changes in radiographic density.

In the short-exposure range, a "time step" adjustment, that is, 1/120th second to 1/60 second results in 100% increase in exposure length, with a corresponding 100% increase in radiographic density. A high-speed screen film combination selected to reduce radiation or patient motion compounds this problem.

With exposures of longer times, that is, 1 second or greater, a timer increment change of one "time step" is not as critical.

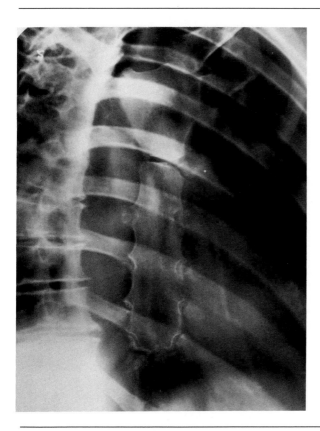

Figure 14-4 The Use of Motion During Radiography of the Sternum The sternum is difficult to image radiographically because of superimposed pulmonary structures. The patient in a prone oblique position is instructed to breath rhythmically during the exposure. An extended exposure time (5 seconds or greater) is used with a low mA setting to erase pulmonary vasculature on the image.

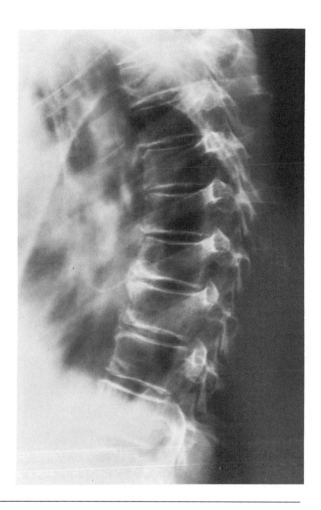

Figure 14-5 The Use of Motion During Radiography of the Thoracic Spine The thoracic spine is difficult to image radiographically in the lateral position, because of superimposed pulmonary structures. The patient is instructed to breath rhythmically during the exposure. An extended exposure time (5 seconds or greater) is used with a low mA setting to erase pulmonary vasculature on the image. Note that the ribs moved during the exposure and are almost completely blurred out.

with dual emulsion film. Sharpness will also vary from cathode to anode in an angled projection as a result of the change in the shape of the projected focal spot. (See Fig. 11-15.)

The distortion of anatomical structures may sometimes be necessary. The barium-filled colon is used as a clinical example. On the conventional anteroposterior (AP) projection, there is a foreshortening of the sigmoid portion of the colon. When the tube is angled 35 degrees cephalad in the AP projection, the rectosigmoidal area is distorted (elongated) to better visualize this area (Fig. 14-6).

The examination of the abdomen for an opaque foreign body (Fig. 14-7) demonstrates the divergent effect of the x-ray beam (see Fig. 11-19) on the foreign body, even though the x-ray tube is not angled. The radiographic image must be evaluated for scatter radiation or other types of fog, including the identifi-

cation of all sources of extra density (fog), such as image undercutting. (See Figs. 5-3, 5-4, and 9-4.)

Collimation should be evident in the form of unexposed borders on the radiographic image. Extraneous unsharp radiographic images that often appear outside the shutter pattern are generally due to extrafocal radiation (see Fig. 5-10) and should not be attributed to scatter radiation. Changes in shutter pattern (degrees of collimation) have a major effect on radiographic density.

IMPORTANT: When conventional techniques are used, an adjustment must be made in exposure factors to compensate for tight beam collimation (Table 14-2).

The radiographic image should be evaluated for evidence of radiation protection of

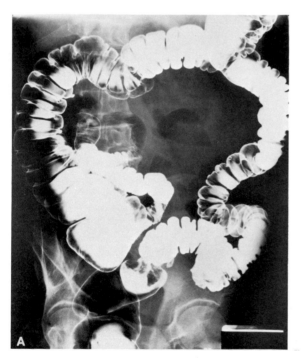
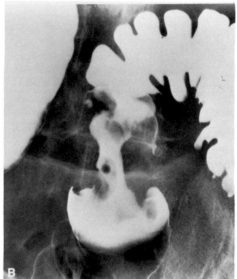

Figure 14-6 Deliberate Distortion of Anatomical Structures *A barium-filled colon is shown, with narrowing of the colon at the distal end, near the rectum (A). Foreshortening of the rectosigmoidal area in this projection makes a tube angle technique necessary.*

A 35-degree cephalad tube angle is used to distort (elongate) the rectosigmoidal colon (B).

Note that the angled projection adequately demonstrates the disease process. The remaining segments of the colon are underpenetrated and are of marginal diagnostic value.

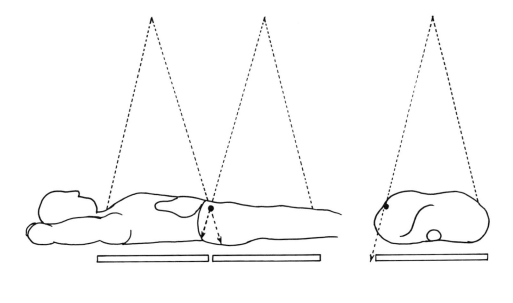

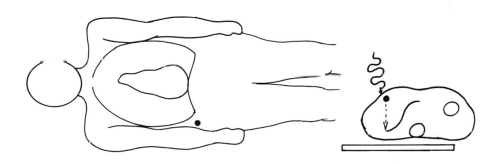

Figure 14-7 The Effect of the Divergent Beam on the Radiographic Image *An illustration of a patient with a foreign body* (filled-in circle) *in the anterior right upper quadrant of the abdomen is shown. This represents a bullet lodged near the upper anterior portion of the liver. An entrance wound was noted in the anterior portion of the thorax; no exit port was evident. Since it was impossible to determine the path of and location of the foreign body, survey radiographs of the thorax and abdomen were required. Note that the divergent effect of the x-ray beam used for the thorax examination projected the foreign body caudally. When the abdominal image was obtained, the divergent beam projected the foreign body cephalad* (top, left). *A transverse section of the abdomen is shown* (top, right), *with the diver-*gent effect of the x-ray beam projecting the foreign body laterally away from the detector.

The patient is shown in the supine position, demonstrating the relationship of the foreign body to the abdomen and thorax (bottom). *If this metallic structure were to be visualized, central ray must pass through the object, with the cassette appropriately placed to avoid the divergent effect of the x-ray beam* (bottom, right).

AFter survey images of the thorax and abdomen are made, radiographs of the thoracolumbar junction must be considered. The cassette must be placed at the level of the right diaphragm, with the patient positioned so that central ray enters the right upper quadrant just below the right costophrenic angle.

TABLE 14-2.   The Effect of Collimation on Technical Factors

Size	Sq. in.	Field size	Timer adjustments	Heat units
14 × 17	238	full	1/10 sec	2400
8 × 10	80	one third	2/10 sec	4800
4 × 5	20	one twelfth	3/10 sec	7200

Starting factors: 300 mA; 1/10 sec; 80 kVp (single-phase, full-wave rectified). The timer adjustment factors are approximations and are presented for the purpose of illustration only. No consideration was made for screen film speed, kilovoltage, and so on.

When shutter patterns are reduced to a smaller field size (see Fig. 5-2), an adjustment in one or more technical factors is required to maintain the original radiographic density. Because 50% or more of a full-field (238 sq. in.) radiograph is comprised of scatter, an adjustment in technical factors must be made to compensate for the decrease in radiographic density owing to the reduction in scatter radiation. Conversely, if field size is increased, a reduction in technical factors is necessary to maintain the original radiographic density.

When evaluating a radiograph made with a conventional technique, if a repeat examination is necessary, any one of several technical adjustments can be selected by the radiographer. A change in exposure time only increases the possibility of patient motion, may necessitate the need for a large focal spot, and may tax the anode thermal capacity of the x-ray tube. (See Fig. 4-8.)

When an automatic exposure device (AED) is used with a reduction in field size, if the mA or kVp settings are not adjusted, the exposure time will be prolonged until a preselected density is reached. Note the increase in heat units associated with an increase in exposure times.

patient and operator. Information needed to protect patients, radiographers, or associated personnel from radiation can be found in Chapter 3. The radiograph should be evaluated for evidence of collimation as well as for appropriate shielding of the gonads, if applicable (Fig. 14-8). It may be impossible to evaluate patient protection from the radiographic image. For example, for a study of the hand or wrist with the patient seated at the edge of the x-ray table, the x-ray beam passes through the cassette and tabletop and can strike the gonadal area of the patient. Gonadal protection in the form of lead shielding or a lead apron would not be evident on the radiographic image.

The processor temperature should not be lowered to minimize the effect of an inherent high-contrast radiographic film or to compensate for a film with a high gross fog. When the processor temperature is lowered, an increase in exposure factors is needed to make up for inadequate film processing, increasing dosage to both patient and operator.

Radiographic contrast is subjective. Although overall density and contrast should be adequate, it is important to evaluate the specific part or segment of the area under study. For example, a 35-degree cephalad-angled exposure of the sigmoidal area may adequately demonstrate disease of the colon near the rectum but not penetrate adjacent portions of the colon (Fig. 14-6). Although this radiograph is of excellent quality for its intent, an additional radiograph would be needed to adequately

visualize the remainder of the barium-filled colon.

When a unique radiographic position is requested (Fig. 14-9), a positioning guide or textbook should be consulted for tube angulations or part positioning, since a minor error in tube/part alignment may fail to produce the intended image.

Some density or contrast limitations are the result of pathologic conditions and are not technical errors.

It is impossible to evaluate a radiograph unless one is aware of the conditions present when the study was made. When the technical factors selected for the study are not consistent with the recommended factors on the technique chart, these changes should be documented. For example, if the lumbar spine was evaluated and it has been determined radiographically that the spine is osteoporotic (Fig. 14-10), a lower kVp value could be used with increased mAs to augment subject contrast. If the radiograph were to be repeated for a positioning error, a second radiographer assigned to the repeat examination may correct the positioning error but, if he or she is unaware of the previous technique adjustment, may make an improper technical factor selection.

Pathology or tissue detectability is often limited by superimposed skeletal and soft tissue structures. Pathologic changes can be absorptive or nonabsorptive (Fig. 14-11) and can assume unusual shapes.

Technical information should be docu-

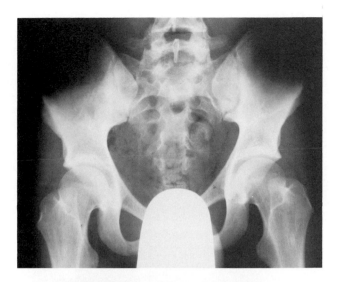

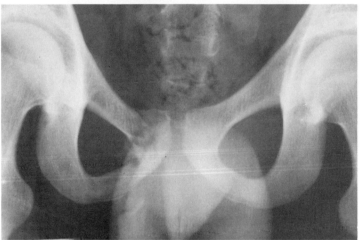

Figure 14-8   The Use of Gonadal Shielding
Since a fracture was not suspected in the pubic area, the gonadal area of an 18-year-old male was appropriately shielded from radiation during an x-ray exposure of the pelvis (top), masking a fracture. A repeat examination of the pubic area demonstrated fractures of the pubic bones on the right side (bottom).

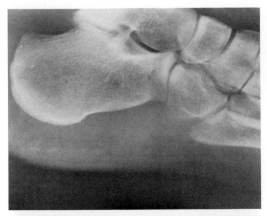

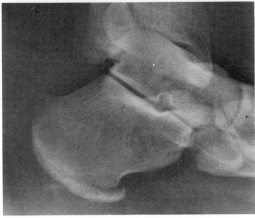

Figure 14-9 *Perpendicular vs. Angled X-Ray Beam Study* *A conventional radiograph of the calcaneous demonstrates normal anatomical relationships (top). A dual tube angulation technique (25 degrees caudad, 25 degrees to the toes) with the foot in the lateral position distorts the osseous structure of the foot and ankle while demonstrating the talocalcaneal joint (bottom). Of interest, there is a fracture of the inferior portion of the calcaneous, demonstrated only on the dual tube projection.*

mented using precise technical and medical terminology. The labeling of the radiographs and documentation of technical factors can become a medicolegal issue. Radiographers may be called upon to substantiate their role in the making of a radiograph.

Jargon is not appropriate on a medicolegal document. For example, when examining the

supine abdomen in the AP position, the term *flat plate of the abdomen* or *KUB* is often used. Flat plate of the abdomen is a term derived from the use of emulsion-coated glass plates prior to the development of cellulose acetate film base (mid 1920s). The term *KUB* refers to an evaluation of the kidneys, ureters, and bladder. A more descriptive term is *scout* or *survey radiograph of the abdomen.*

Two lateral views of the skull are shown for image evaluation. Both short-scale and moderate-scale contrast are evident in these images (Fig. 14-12).

Application of Principles of Exposure to Chest Radiography

Since the posteroanterior (PA) projection of the chest is the most frequently performed radiologic examination, the remainder of this chapter will be devoted to the application of radiographic principles of exposure to chest radiography.

Radiographic Positioning of the Chest

Information regarding positioning of a patient for chest radiography is available in many textbooks. Because stability of the patient during the procedure is essential, the use of an overhead arm support for the lateral position is helpful. A laser positioning device can also be helpful.

For the PA erect chest examination, the patient should be positioned with the body weight distributed equally on both feet. The back of the hands should be placed on the hips, with the elbows flexed slightly and the shoulders rotated forward, against the image receptor. If the shoulders have not been rotated sufficiently, the scapulae will be superimposed on the lung fields. The chin should be raised and placed at the top of the image receptor. If the chin is markedly elevated, however, the occipital portion of the skull can be projected into the apical area of the chest. The chest of a kyphotic patient should be centered with the chin elevated as high as possible, even though the inferior portion of the mandible may appear on the radiograph.

More of the contents of the thoracic cage

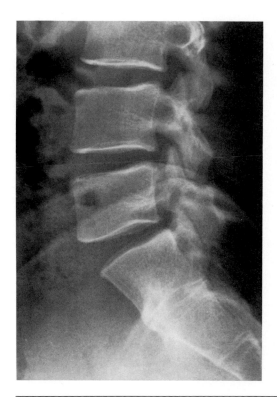 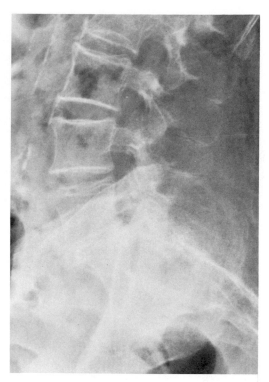

Figure 14-10   The Effect of Pathology on Subject Contrast   *A lateral lumbar spine view demonstrates the normal osseous anatomy of a young patient. Excellent radiographic contrast and detail can be seen (left).*

An osteoporitic lumbar spine of an 85-year-old patient is shown in the lateral position (right). Note the lack of subject contrast. Osseous detail is difficult to demonstrate in an osteoporitic spine unless low kVp-high mAs technical factors are used to augment subject contrast. Note the presence of calcification in the abdominal aorta.

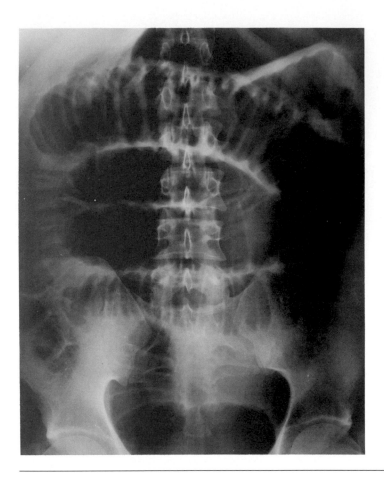

Figure 14-11 The Effect of Air-Distended Hollow Viscera on Radiographic Technique *A survey film of the abdomen with distended loops of small bowel is shown. The dilated radiolucent loops of bowel are easily penetrated. Since the abdomen of the patient is visibly distended, centimeter thickness measurements can be misleading. If factors suggested on the technique chart for a routine survey radiograph of the abdomen were used, the image would be overexposed.*

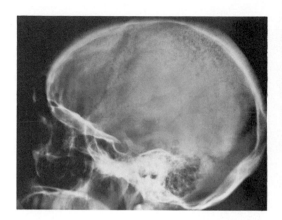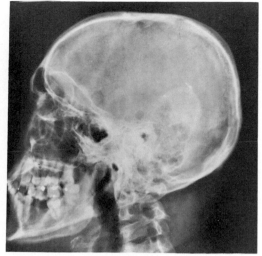

Figure 14-12 Evaluation of Lateral Skull Radiographs *Radiographs should be systematically analyzed to determine whether they are technically acceptable.*

Using the checklist provided in Table 14-1 and the limited information that follows, the reader is asked to critique the above images.

A lateral skull view is presented for evaluation (left). *A second image is presented for evaluation and comparison* (right).

The radiograph on the left was made with a 400-speed screen film combination, a 0.6-mm focal spot, a 40-in FFD, a 12:1 ratio moving grid, and

80 kVp at 20 mAs. Factors required to expose the vault of the skull will overexpose the aerated sinuses and soft tissue of the scalp.

The lateral skull view on the right was made on a dedicated head unit with a 200-speed screen film combination, a 2.0-mm focal spot, 36-in. FFD, and an 8:1 ratio moving grid. A kVp value of 75 at 20 mAs (400 mA at 1/20th second) was used.

Note that the sinuses and facial bones are not overexposed. A faint "corduroy" pattern caused by the capturing of the grid in motion can be seen superimposed on the bony vault of the skull. (See Fig 5-15.)

can be seen with the patient in the erect position. The patient is able to cooperate, particularly with regard to breathing. The abdominal organs do not press against the diaphragms, causing compression of the lung fields, and the heart is shown in its normal configuration. In the AP projection, the heart, which is primarily anterior, appears enlarged and is superimposed on adjacent pulmonary structures. The PA projection permits rotation of the scapulae, taking advantage of the divergent effect of the x-ray beam to project the scapulae off the lung fields. Large-breasted females can be asked to displace their breasts laterally to lessen the filtering effect of breast tissue.

Comparison films of the chest are often difficult to evaluate unless images of comparable quality are available. In facilities where

the chest is examined for specific diseases such as pneumoconiosis, the quality of chest images is almost always consistent. Every effort must be made to follow established chest techniques since technical changes made by the radiographer may affect the treatment of the patient.

The making of a chest radiograph requires careful attention to the basics, from focal spot selection to processor control. The "simple" PA chest examination utilizes a high level of technology. When evaluating the PA chest radiograph (Figs. 14-13 and 14-14), the following questions should be asked and answered:

1 Are the densities of both lung fields equal? If not, is this due to pathology, unilateral grid cutoff (see Fig. 5-16), or some type of artifact?

(Text continues on p. 254.)

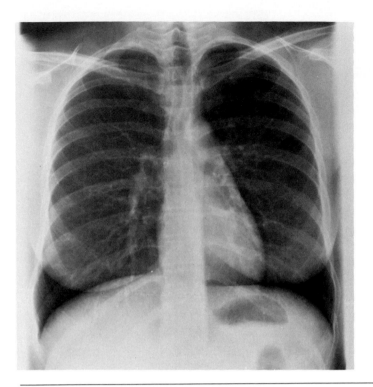

Figure 14-13 Evaluation of a Conventional PA Chest Radiograph   *Using the checklist provided in Table 14-1 and the suggestions in the text, the reader is asked to critique the above image.*

This PA view of the chest was made in the erect position with a 72-in. FFD. A 250-speed screen film (latitude film, Fig. 14-21B) combination and a 1.2-mm focal spot was used with a 12:1 stationary grid, 140 kVp (three-phase, 12 pulse), and automatic exposure timing.

Note: *Compare the osseous details at the lateral aspect of the ribs bilaterally near the costophrenic angles. One of the internal shutters of the collimator is out of alignment. An internal shutter above the mirror is protruding into the x-ray field, causing an image "cutoff" on the right side of the chest, even though the exit shutters were restricted to the cassette in use. (See Fig. 5-7.)*

As part of the chest evaluation process, compare this image to that in Figure 14-14, a bedside chest examination.

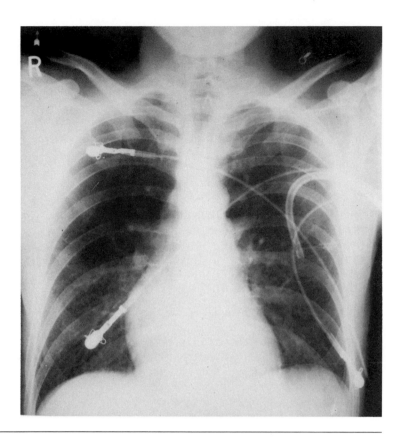

Figure 14-14 Evaluation of a Bedside Chest Radiograph *Using the checklist provided in Table 14-1 and the suggestions in the text, the reader is asked to critique the above image.*

A PA chest in the upright position was made at the bedside using a 72-in. FFD. The increased FFD was made possible because of a 400-speed screen film (high contrast film Fig. 14-21A) combination and a 1.2-mm focal spot. A non-grid exposure at 85 kVp (full wave rectified) was used.

Compare this image to a conventional chest radiograph in Figure 14-13.

2 Are the scapulae clear of the lung fields?

3 Are the clavicles horizontal? Are the medial ends of the clavicles symmetrical? Is the patient rotated?

4 Is the relationship of the sternoclavicular joints to the thoracic spine symmetrical?

5 Was the exposure made on full inspiration?

6 Is there evidence of motion?

7 Is there evidence of beam collimation?

8 Is the radiograph properly identified?

9 Are the apices and costophrenic angles imaged?

10 Is there tracheal displacement?

Air as a Contrast Medium

Radiography of the chest should be made on full inspiration. When the lungs are completely expanded, vascular markings are easier to see and small lesions may be demonstrated. Since the expanded lungs are more radiolucent, less exposure is required than for an image obtained during an expiration phase. There is an increase in subject contrast, and the mediastinum is well outlined.

Valsalva's maneuver, which consists of forced expiration against a closed glottis, should be avoided. This maneuver lowers the flow of venous blood to the heart, reducing cardiac output and producing changes in the appearance of the heart size and vascular markings of the lung. If an enlarged lymph node is suspected in the hilar area, it should be more obvious on the image made with Valsalva's maneuver, since the hilar blood vessels decrease in size. Occasionally, a radiograph may be requested using Valsalva's maneuver.

The cardiothoracic ratio changes on expiration. The heart will appear wider, and the lung markings will be compressed closer together; the lung fields will appear to be more radiodense (Fig. 14-15). (See Fig. 12-8.)

Two PA views of the chest are shown for evaluation by the reader (Figs. 14-13 and 14-14).

Application of Technical Factors

When technical factors are considered for a radiographic examination, kVp and mAs se-lection are the first priority. With chest radiography, the choice of a grid or non-grid technique will influence the choice of kVp and mAs. A grid is not ordinarily used for body parts measuring less than 10 cm in thickness. The chest, owing to its radiolucent nature, is an exception to this rule, and an acceptable image can be obtained with or without a grid. The use of lower kVp values (approximately 85 kVp) for non-grid chests produces a high-contrast image. Although the lung fields are often satisfactorily exposed, mediastinal details are difficult to demonstrate. Non-grid techniques are popular for mobile or bedside radiography because of grid focusing difficulties (see Table 5-1) and the limited output of mobile units. (See Chapter 3.)

There is a growing tendency toward high kVp and high-ratio grid techniques for chest radiography. High kVp used with chest radiography accentuates the differences between the heart and the lung. Soft tissues of the thorax are well visualized, particularly structures in the retrocardiac area or those that are superimposed on vertebral or rib shadows.

For chest radiography, the grid should be positioned with its lines running perpendicular rather than parallel to the floor. When a smaller patient is centered to the grid or Bucky, the x-ray beam can be positioned to the patient without fear of grid cutoff. If the grid were positioned with its lead lines running parallel to the floor, the x-ray tube would have to be centered equidistant from the top to the bottom of the grid. The center of every chest examined would have to be exactly 8.5 in. from both ends of the cassette. (See Fig. 5-18.)

Single- vs. Three-Phase Kilovoltage Values

There is a considerable difference in radiographic density and contrast when three-phase equipment, rather than single-phase equipment, is used. Since three-phase x-radiation is almost ripple free as opposed to single-phase x-radiation (100% ripple), technique adjustments are often required to maintain image quality, particularly if a specific radiographic density and scale of contrast is to be maintained. Identical kVp values (single-phase vs. three-phase) will produce visi-

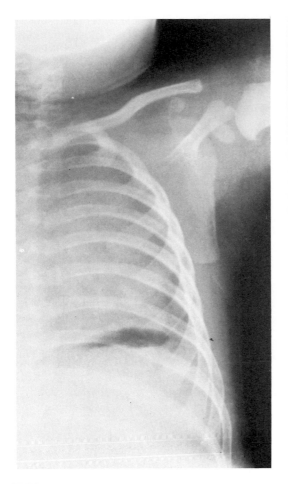
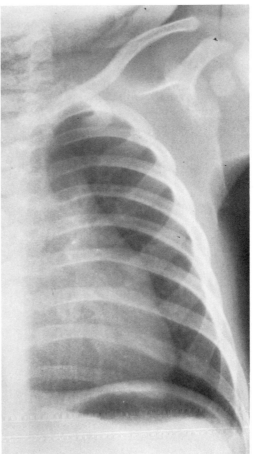

Figure 14-15 Inspiration vs. Expiration, Pediatric Chest Study The left side of a chest radiograph of an infant is shown at full expiration. Note the lack of normal lung markings and the appearance of massive pulmonary disease. The diaphragm is not seen, and the heart appears enlarged (left)

A repeat radiograph of the same infant was made at full inspiration, with the left diaphragm visualized at the level of the 10th posterior rib.

The same technical values were used for both exposures. (Courtesy of the Department of Radiology, Rochester General Hospital, Rochester, New York)

ble differences in density and in the scale of contrast. The three-phase image will exhibit a longer scale of contrast than the single-phase image when the same kVp setting is used. (See Fig. 2-6 and Table 2-2.) The use of three-phase radiographic equipment for chest radiography will shorten exposure time compared with single-phase equipment if the same kVp and mA settings are used. This shortening of exposure time can affect the minimal response time of the automatic exposure device (AED), requiring an adjustment in the mA value. (See Fig. 2-11.)

Selection of Grid Ratio to Match Kilovoltage Range

The proper grid ratio (including proper focal range) must be matched to the kVp level used for chest radiography. When a high-ratio grid is used with a low to moderate kVp value, the mediastinum may not be penetrated. The lucent lungs and opaque mediastinum and osseous structures can mask a small pulmonary nodule that may be superimposed on a rib or "lost" in the blackened lung fields associated with low-kVp, high-mAs techniques. As kVp is lowered, a lower ratio grid should be used (Table 14-2).

With an air-gap chest radiograph, the patient is positioned 10 in. or 12 in. (OFD) from the image receptor; an increased FFD (10 feet or 12 feet) is necessary.

The use of an air gap for scatter cleanup for chest radiography is an acceptable substitute for a high-ratio grid in most situations unless the chest is abdominal-like in thickness and density (Fig. 14-16). If a patient with an enlarged heart or a fluid-filled chest were examined using an air gap, the scatter radiation produced by the chest would be difficult to overcome.

J. McInnes, in "The elimination of scatter radiation," Radiography 36:141–142, 1970, states that a 6-in. air gap is roughly equivalent to a 6:1 radio grid.

The use of a grid technique at a standard 72-in. FFD is more effective in controlling this increase in scatter radiation.

Exposure Times for Chest Radiography

Short exposure times to stop motion are especially important in chest radiography. The use of an exposure time of 10 msec or less is recommended for the examination of the chest.

The limitations of an AED must be considered when evaluating a radiograph. An AED can produce images of comparable density, regardless of the degree of inspiration or expiration.

Careful attention must be paid to the degree of inspiration, particularly when using an AED. The radiograph made with poor inspiration may give the illusion of an enlarged heart (Fig. 14-15). (See Fig. 12-8.) For example,

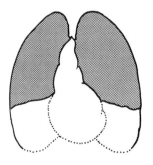 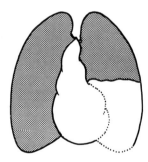

Figure 14-16   A Limitation of the Air Gap Technique   *Schematic representations of the chest include enlarged hearts with diffuse pulmonary disease bilaterally (left) and fluid in the left thorax (right). The use of an air gap technique for chest radiography is usually an adequate replacement for a grid technique. When an enlarged heart or fluid constitutes a major part of the thorax, a high ratio grid or Bucky is recommended.*

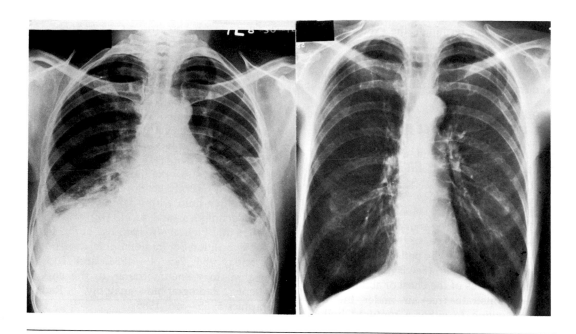

Figure 14-17 The Effect of Pathology on the Radiographic Image *Pathological changes can influence radiographic density. A chest radiograph of a patient in congestive heart failure with bilateral pleural effusion is shown (left). Note the prominent pulmonary vessels in the hila and upper lung fields. (Courtesy of Thompson TT: Primer of Clinical Radiology Boston, Little, Brown and Company, 1973; with permission.)*

A second chest image is shown of a patient with pulmonary emphysema (right). Note the elongation of the heart, causing a disproportionate cardiothoracic ratio. Nipple shadows can be seen in both long fields. A nipple localization technique is described in this chapter. (Courtesy of the Department of Radiology, Rochester General Hospital, Rochester, New York)

an enlarged heart or bilateral pleural effusion may cause the AED to stay activated until a preselected degree of film blackening is produced (Fig. 14-17). The increase in radiographic density associated with pulmonary emphysema resulting from a marked increase in the retrosternal air space with the diaphragms pushed downward by air trapped within the lungs (Fig. 14-17) may necessitate an exposure shorter than the minimal response time of the AED. (See Chapter 2.) An adjustment in mA can sometimes overcome the limitations of the minimal response time. One should avoid the lowering of kVp, since the lungs will blacken, osseous structures will be enhanced obscuring vascular details, and mediastinal structures may not be adequately penetrated.

IMPORTANT: If an image is of poor quality because of an improperly functioning AED, a repeat examination will yield a film of equally poor quality.

Evaluation of Patient Positioning Relative to AED Sensor

When a radiographic image of the chest is not acceptable because of improper density (under- or overexposed), the position of the patient relative to the AED sensor should be considered. An incorrect sensor may have been selected, or the patient may be positioned off-center to the selected sensor. Image undercutting occurs in the lateral position when the unattenuated primary beam strikes a major portion of the receptor surface, caus-

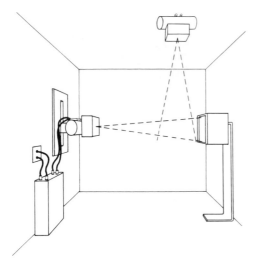

Figure 14-20 Ceiling-Mounted Tube for Recumbent Radiography of the Chest *A ceiling-mounted x-ray tube permits the examination of the chest of critically ill patients in the recumbent position. The increased FFD combined with a low ratio grid results in a radiograph that approximates the quality of a conventional chest image.*

A lateral view of the chest with the patient in the supine position can also be made with a horizontal beam projection. (See Fig. 14-18.) (Courtesy of Cullinan, JE: A Perfect Chest Radiograph—Or A Compromise? Radiol Technol 53: 2, 1981; with permission)

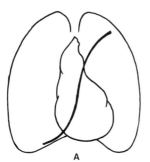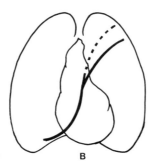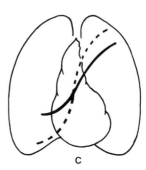

A   B   C

Figure 14-21 Sensitometric Representation of Films Used for Chest Radiography *A latitude or extended latitude film is recommended with a high kVp technique for chest radiography.*

Sensitometric representations of three types of radiographic film available for radiography of the chest are illustrated. A high contrast film (A) will image vascular details within the darkened lung fields but will often fail to demonstrate mediastinal structures (imaged near the toe of the sensitometric curve). A latitude x-ray film (B) can be used to reduce film blackening of the radiograph in the areas of the lungs. The dotted extension of the curve represents a high contrast film (A). An ex-tended latitude film (C) will also minimize blackening of the lung fields. Note the filled-in toe of the sensitometric curve, which permits imaging of the mediastinal structures without an increase in x-ray exposure to the patient. This film was designed specifically for chest radiography. (See Fig. 14-23.) An extended scale of contrast is seen when evaluating a radiograph made with extended latitude film (C). This type of film is not recommended for iodinated contrast studies or osseous evaluation.

The dotted representation is used for comparison to the high contrast film (A).

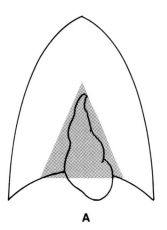
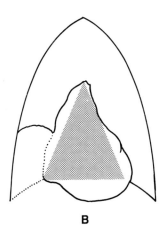
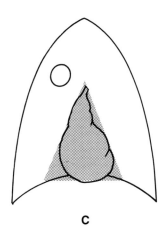

A   **B**   **C**

Figure 14-22   The Use of a Compensatory Filter for Chest Radiography to Demonstrate Mediastinal Densities   *It is difficult to produce adequate film blackening in the mediastinal area with conventional PA chest techniques. A compensatory filter is occasionally used to image the mediastinum without compromising the lung fields. Metallic or lead acrylic filters, shaped to conform to a typical PA chest configuration, are used in the external tracks of a collimator. (See Fig. 4-9.) The filter in this illustration permits more x-ray to pass through its triangular opening.*

A single-size opening in a filter is not adequate for all types of body habitus or disease processes. With an emphysematous chest (A), the opening in *the filter does not permit proper exposure of the inferior portion of the heart. When an enlarged heart (B) is evaluated with this filter, much of the cardiac silhouette extends beyond the filter opening. In this example, there is a significant amount of fluid in the right lung, which requires additional penetration rather than filtration of the x-ray beam. Even if the filter were to match the mediastinal configuration (C), a lesion in the right upper lung may not be adequately penetrated by the x-ray beam. Most filters of this type require an increase in 2× or greater in the amount of exposure ordinarily needed for a conventional PA chest to adequately penetrate the mediastinum. (See Fig. 14-24.)*

tracks of the collimator. (See Fig. 4-9.) Most filters used for chest radiography differ from wedge or trough filters in that the filter has an opening in its center to permit the full x-ray exposure to penetrate the dense mediastinum while attenuating the radiation used to image the lung fields. Since the opening in the filter is a predetermined size, it does not match the mediastinal configuration of every patient examined. One filter cannot be designed to accommodate the narrow cardiac silhouette often associated with the emphysematous chest, the enlarged heart (Fig. 14-17), fluid in the lung, or a pulmonary mass (Fig. 14-22).

Sensitometric characteristics of x-ray film can be modified specifically for chest radiography (Fig. 14-23), lessening the need for compensatory chest filters. A conventional high-contrast sensitometric curve is shown compared to latitude and extended latitude sensitometric curves. Structures are demonstrated on a radiograph if they are adjacent to tissues of differing densities (contrast). The cardiac shadow is easily visualized because it is silhouetted against the lung fields. The dense blood-filled heart is similar in radiopacity to the descending aorta and thoracic spine. These structures are imaged on conventional radiographic film at or near the toe of the sensitometric curve (Fig. 14-24) where very little separation of the superimposed tissues can be demonstrated. (See Fig. 8-5.) The use of an extended latitude film with a sensitometrically "filled-in toe" can help to demonstrate the air–soft tissue interface of the mediastinum (Fig. 14-24).

A 400-speed screen film combination may require exposure times shorter than the minimal response time of the AED. The use of

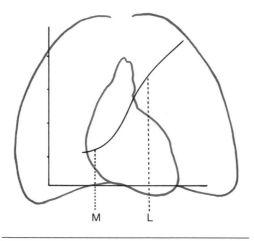

M L

Figure 14-23 Sensitometric Characteristics of X-Ray Film Specifically Designed for Chest Radiography *A schematic of a chest x-ray is superimposed on a sensitometric curve. The vertical axis illustrates increased density; the horizontal axis illustrates increased exposure. Exposure is expressed logrithmically. (See Fig. 11-4.) The letter M is used to illustrate the portion of the sensitometric curve that images the mediastinum. The letter L is used to illustrate the portion of the sensitometric curve that typically images the blackened lung fields. Note that the mediastinum is imaged near the toe (inferior portion) of the sensitometric curve. The lungs are imaged in the ascending (straight line) portion of the curve. Density differences in the mediastinum should be better visualized with this film.*

high kVp values (up to 150 kVp) can further complicate this problem.

IMPORTANT: The light output of the intensifying screens used for chest radiography must be matched to the spectral sensitivity of the film. (See Chapter 8.)

Patient Pathology

An overexposed radiograph may be necessary to demonstrate the position of a pacemaker lead, to evaluate the battery of a pacemaker, or to determine the location of gastric tubes within the esophagus, superimposed upon the mediastinum.

Special positions or projections are required for certain disease processes. When free air is present in the pleural cavity as the result of a pneumothorax, there is an absence of lung markings in the space between the visceral pleura and the parietal pleural. Air can enter the pleural space in several ways, for example, a penetrating injury from a sharp edge of a fractured rib, a spontaneous pneumothorax, and so on. The presence of free air in the pleural space can cause collapse of the lung. The use of expiration radiography of the chest is of value when a pneumothorax is suspected. A radiograph made during expiration in the lateral decubitus position with the suspected side elevated can be helpful when evaluating the chest for a minimal pneumothorax.

IMPORTANT: Expiration images should be made using manual technical factors. If an AED were used, the predetermined density generated by the AED could mask a minimal pneumothorax (Figs. 14-25 and 14-26). A skin fold may give the impression of a pneumothorax or pleural thickening (Fig. 14-26). Loose skin folds can produce this edge effect when a patient is moved across the tabletop. Breast shadows in younger patients can also simulate a pneumothorax.

The nipples of a patient can simulate a pulmonary lesion (Fig. 14-17). External markers should be applied to the chest before a repeat film is made to identify the nipple shadows. A paper clip straightened full length and then formed into a circle (approximately 1-in. in diameter) can serve as a marker, with the nipple positioned in the center of the circle. If the suspected lesion is the nipple, it should appear in the center of the metallic ring on the repeat radiograph. Slight oblique projections (5 degrees–10 degrees) are sometimes requested, since a slight rotation of the thorax would cause a pulmonary mass to shift right or left in relation to the metallic ring. This localization technique can also be used to radiographically identify moles or warts on the surface of the body that may be projected into the lung fields, giving the illusion of pulmonary lesions.

Occasionally lead shot is taped to a patient's skin to radiographically identify an area of interest, for example, a suspected rib fracture or a mass.

(Text continues on p. 266.)

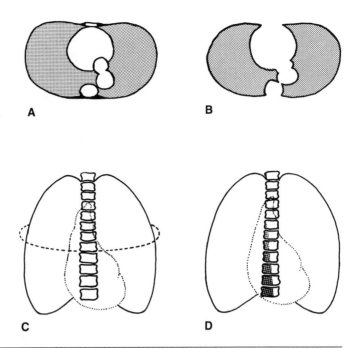

Figure 14-24   Mediastinal Air/Soft Tissue Interface   Using conventional radiographic film, it is difficult to demonstrate mediastinal air/soft tissue interfaces because of sensitometric limitations. (See Fig. 14-21.) A transverse anatomical section of the chest is illustrated (A). For a PA examination, the x-ray beam enters the posterior portion of the thorax and passes through the ascending aorta and the blood-filled muscular heart and exits through the sternum. In the PA projection, the mediastinal structures approximate the absorption characteristics of the abdomen.

The lung fields are shaded in A and B. Note the amount of air in the right lung field, behind the heart anterior to the thoracic vertebrae. An outline of the lung fields is shown in B. The transverse section (C) is represented by a dotted oval pattern.

When evaluating a conventional PA chest image, it is often suggested that the vertebral bodies should be visible through the dense cardiac silhouette. As the heart widens at its inferior portion, the vertebral bodies and interspaces become more difficult to visualize. Aerated lung tissue behind the heart, adjacent to the soft tissue structures (air/soft tissue), interface should be visible within the mediastinum. Since there is lung tissue on the right side of the chest between the cardiac silhouette and thoracic spine, more x-radiation should pass through the aerated lung, imaging the right side of the vertebral bodies to a greater degree than the left (D). This air/soft tissue interface is difficult to demonstrate with conventional x-ray film, because it is imaged near the toe of the sensitometric curve. The use of an extended latitude x-ray film helps to overcome the differences between the aerated lungs and the dense mediastinum. (See Fig. 14-23.)

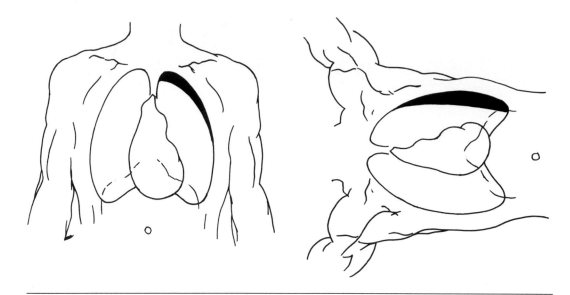

Figure 14-25 Demonstration of a Minimal Pneumothorax *Schematic representation of the chest in the PA erect position (left) as well as the lateral decubitus position (right) is shown. On the PA projection, a dotted line represents a minimal pneumothorax; the space between the distal and parietal pleura is occupied by free air. A small pneumothorax can be easier to visualize when the patient is placed in the decubitus position with the suspected side elevated. Radiographs should be taken on expiration, since free air trapped within the thorax will maintain its radiolucency while the lungs will become relatively radiodense (owing to the effect of expiration).*

The use of an automatic exposure device with the expiration technique is not recommended, because an AED is calibrated to produce a preselected film blackening, which may mask a minimal pneumothorax.

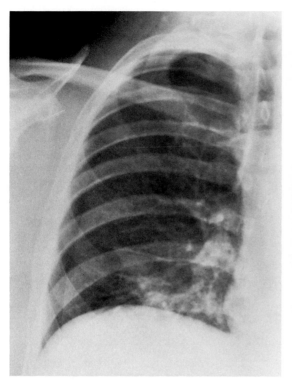 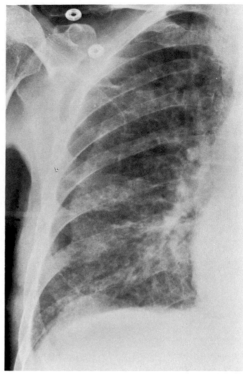

Figure 14-26 Pneumothorax vs. Skin Fold
The right side of the chest is shown (left) *with an x-ray exposure made at full expiration, demonstrating a pneumothorax. Note that the lung has decreased in size and that the diaphragm is elevated. There is an absence of peripheral lung markings in the area of the collapsed lung. A radiograph made at expiration in the lateral decubitus position with the suspected side elevated can be helpful when a minimal pneumothorax is suspected. (See Fig. 14-25.) The right side of a chest is shown* (right) *with a patient in the AP supine position. Note the thickened edge of a skin fold. (Courtesy of the Department of Radiology, Rochester General Hospital, Rochester, New York)*

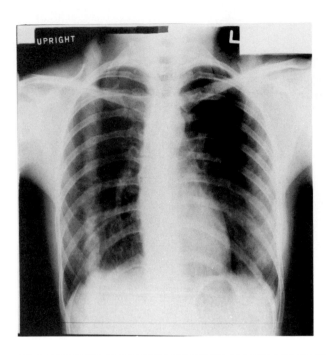

Figure 14-27 The Effect of an External Artifact on a Radiographic Image *Hair, ribbons, rubberbands, externally applied medications, oils, powder, or an excessive amount of deodorant may be imaged on the radiograph.*

A PA chest is shown, with hair braids superimposed on the lung fields. The braids were concealed by the patient's gown and were not appar- *ent to the radiographer. The right braid was anterior to the chest, in contact with the image receptor; the left braid was draped over the posterior chest (increased OFD).*

The braid on the right side of the chest is obvious, but the braid artifact on the left side of the radiograph simulates a unilateral grid cutoff. (See Fig. 5-16.)

IMPORTANT: Some patients are reluctant to remove any type of identification marker applied in a radiology department. The metallic markers, if left in position for an extended period of time, may break through the skin, causing an inflammatory process. It is important to remove localization markers from the patient's skin after it has been determined that the radiographs are technically acceptable.

Clothing artifacts can produce confusing radiographic densities. Some synthetic fibers can simulate the small rounded opacities associated with pneumoconiosis. An artifact-free gown should be substituted for patient clothing. Flame-retardant children's sleepwear may contain changes in the surface properties of the fabric that may produce radiographic artifacts. Laundering processes, including starch, may also produce artifacts in clothing. These external artifacts should be considered when evaluating a radiograph.

Hair should be raised away from the shoulders to avoid extraneous shadows in the upper portions of the lungs (Fig. 14-27). Ribbons, rubberbands, externally applied medications, oils, powder, or an excessive amount of deodorants may appear as external artifacts on the image.

A detailed description of radiographic artifacts is beyond the scope or intent of this textbook. A book by Richard J. Sweeney, entitled "Radiographic Artifacts: Their Cause and Control," J. B. Lippincott, Philadelphia, 1983, is recommended.

15 Related Terminology

RADIOLOGIC technology has its own unique language by which members of the profession communicate with each other. Radiographers must be familiar with two forms of terminology. The first, medical terminology, which deals with the terms used to describe the anatomy and pathology of the human body, have been well documented. The second, the terms associated with the principles of radiographic exposure, are not found as readily. Whenever an unfamiliar term or word is encountered by a radiographer, several reference books must often be consulted before an adequate explanation can be found. Many textbooks fail to explain the differences or similarities of the terms used in radiologic technology. For example, *incandescence, fluorescence, luminescence,* and *phosphorescence* all emit a form of light, but their meanings are distinctly different. The terms *accommodation* and *adaptation* are not interchangeable, although both terms refer to the response of the eyes. There is a difference in how this response is achieved.

Approximately 250 terms and items related to radiologic technology are explained in this chapter. Much of this material is cross referenced, and the reader is referred to the text and illustrations for additional information.

The definitions in this chapter are those most commonly used in the clinical setting and are not necessarily those found in a standard or medical dictionary. For example, when radius is listed, no mention is made to its medical use where radius would refer to a bone in the forearm.

A list of abbreviations associated with radiographic principles of exposure is presented on the inside front cover of this book.

Absorption the process by which an x-ray beam gives off all or some of its energy as it passes through matter. (See Chapter 11 and Differential absorption.)

Accommodation automatic adjustment of the lenses of the eyes to various distances. (See Chapter 3.)

Actual focal spot see *Focal spot.*

Adaptation the process of adjustment of the eyes to various intensities of light in order to increase sensitivity to low light levels; in radiology, dark adaptation of the eyes requires approximately 20 minutes either in a darkened room or by the wearing of light adaptation red goggles; adaptation is necessary before the eyes can see a dimly illuminated conventional fluoroscopic image. (See Chapter 3.)

Afterglow a persistence of image (lag) after the activating force has ceased; common to low-light level conventional fluoroscopic screens; not acceptable in intensifying screens or image intensifiers. (See Phosphorescence.

Alignment the act of arranging the central ray, patient, and image detector in a straight line.

Alternating current see *Current.*

Aluminum equivalent the thickness of any absorbing material that would attenuate the x-ray beam to the same degree as a given thickness of aluminum.

Amp a unit of electrical current.

Ampere a rate or measure of electrical current; produced by 1 volt acting upon the resistance of 1 ohm. (See Chapter 2.)

Amplitude a term related to conventional tomography; defined as the motion of the x-ray tube during an exposure; a pluridirectional tube cassette motion has approximately a five times increase in amplitude compared with a linear motion. (See Figs. 7-1 and 7-6.)

Angstrom the internationally accepted measurement of wavelength. (See Fig. 1-3 and Table 13-1.)

Anode the positive electrode or pole of an x-ray tube, valve tube, or any diode tube; when rapidly moving electrons interact with the target of the anode, as in an x-ray tube, x-radiation is produced. (See Chapter 4.)

Anode heel effect see *Heel effect.*

Anode thermal capacity the capacity of the anode of the x-ray tube to tolerate and store large amounts of heat. (See Fig. 4-8.)

Artifact (1) undesirable markings on radiographs that are produced in handling, storing, or processing of radiographic film (see Fig. 8-6); (2) superfluous images (see Figs. 14-26 and 14-27) on the radiograph, including snaps on gowns, pins, metal sutures, or clips; (3) phantom imaging artifacts are peculiar to conventional tomography; a linear movement of the tube and cassette will produce linear striations or streaking of anatomical structures positioned parallel to the tube cassette trajectory; complex tube motions produce artifacts peculiar to their trajectories. (See Fig. 7-4.)

Atom the smallest part of an element that still retains its chemical and other physical properties. (See Fig. 1-1.)

Atomic mass number the total number of protons and neutrons in the nucleus of an atom.

Atomic number the number of protons in the nucleus of an atom (see Fig. 1-1); the number of electrons in orbit around the nucleus of a stable atom are equal to the number of protons in the nucleus.

Attenuation the decrease in intensity and the change in quality of a beam of x-radiation as it passes through matter (see Figs. 1-9, 9-21, and 11-1 and Chapter 13); filtration can be used to attenuate the beam (see Figs. 4-9 and 14-22); tungsten on the tube window and absorptive cassette fronts and tabletops can also attenuate the x-ray beam (see Fig. 9-6).

Automatic brightness control an automatic exposure device that senses the light output from the output phosphor of the image intensifier; the ABC adjusts either kVp and/or mA to produce a predetermined fluoroscopic density. (See Chapters 2 and 6.)

Automatic exposure device see *Timer.*

Autotransformer an electrical device with a single coil of wire wound around an iron core; part of its turns are common to both the primary and secondary circuit; the primary and secondary windings are connected in series with no electrical insulation between the primary and secondary sides. (See Figs. 2-2 and 2-4.)

Average gradient the slope of the characteristic curve of a radiographic film in the useful density range of diagnostic medical imaging. (See Figs. 8-5 and 11-4.)

Backscatter see *Radiation.*

Back-up time represents the maximal exposure that an automatic exposure device will permit with given mA and kVp values. (See Fig. 2-11.)

Beam radiant energy (x-rays) moving in a straight line from a source; since the x-ray beam starts from a small, almost point source, a divergent effect occurs; anatomical structures at the outer edges of this divergent beam can be distorted (see Figs. 12-2 and 14-7); the central portion of the beam produces images with minimal distortion; angulation of the path or the beam relative to the object can produce elongation or foreshortening of the image. (See Figs. 11-15–11-20, 14-6.)

Beam splitter an optical system consisting of lenses and mirrors used to reflect a predominent percentage of the light from the output phosphor of an image intensifier toward a photographic recording device. (See Figs. 6-1 and 6-2.)

Blooming a change in values (usually increased) in focal spot dimensions; high mA, low kVp techniques may cause a focal spot to bloom. (See Chapter 4.)

Blur used most often to describe image unsharpness owing to patient motion; see Detail and Resolution.

Body section common term used for tomography; other synonyms include planigraphy, laminagraphy, ordography, stratigraphy; see *Tomography*. (See Chapter 7.)

Bremsstrahlung radiation "braking radiation" is a literal German translation; a heterogeneous beam of radiation created as electrons interact with the target; the attraction between the negatively charged electrons and the positively charged nuclei cause the electrons to be deflected and decelerated from their original path, with some loss of energy. (See Fig. 1-5.)

Bucky diaphragm a grid that is made to move before, during, and after the x-ray exposure to obliterate grid lines and grid artifacts (see Fig. 5-15); the grid is suspended beneath the table but above the x-ray cassette; see Grid.

Calcium tungstate a type of phosphor that emits primarily blue violet light when activated by x-radiation (see Fig. 8-2); used in the manufacture of intensifying screens; because of its poor absorption/conversion ratio (see Fig. 8-7), calcium tungstate was rarely used for intensifying screens greater than 200 speed.

Calibration the determination of accuracy of equipment operation by comparing results to a known standard or value. (See Chapter 3.)

Caliper a measuring device, usually divided into centimeters, used to measure part thickness; used in conjunction with a technique chart. (See Figs. 12-5 and 12-6.)

Canting the manufacturing process of inclining grid lines uniformly and bilaterally; the canting process determines the grid focal range. (See Figs. 5-11 and 5-12 and Table 5-1.)

Capacitor a device able to hold and store an electric charge; often used with a type of mobile radiographic unit. (See Chapter 3.)

Cassette (1) a light-tight holder for x-ray film; usually contains two intensifying screens (see Fig. 8-13); (2) a light-tight take-up container for roll or strip photographic film (see Chapter 9); (3) a light-tight container for electrostatic imaging plates (see Figs. 9-19 and 9-20).

Cathode the negative electrode or pole of an x-ray, valve, or any diode tube; when heated, the filament of the cathode emits electrons; this effect is known as thermionic emission. (See Figs. 4-1 and 4-2.)

Central ray center of the x-ray beam emanating from the focal spot of the x-ray tube.

Characteristic curve see *Sensitometric curve*.

Characteristic ray see *Ray*.

Cineradiography motion picture recording of the fluoroscopic image (see Figs. 9-12 and 9-13) from the output phosphor of an image intensifier. (See Figs. 6-1 ad 6-2.)

Collimator a device with a series of lead shutters used to confine a beam of radiation to the field of interest; usually square or rectangular in shape (See Figs. 5-6 and 5-7.)

Compton effect when kVp is increased, the incoming x-ray photon has increased energy and can strike an electron in an outer shell and be deviated from its original path with a reduction in energy (see Fig. 1-8); commonly referred to as *scatter*.

Conductor a medium that can be used to transmit or carry electricity, heat, or sound.

Cone a beam-restricting device in common use before the design of the collimator; the beam-restricting pattern may be circular, square, or rectangular; occasionally used in conjunction with a collimator. (See Fig. 5-6.)

Constant potential electric current with a constant direct voltage. (See Chapter 2.)

Contrast (1) differences between adjacent densities on a radiograph; the number of tonal differences visible on a radiograph determines the scale of contrast; short-scale contrast is demonstrated by abrupt difference in density; longer-scale contrast is presented as a greater range of tones with more shades of gray (see Figs. 11-7–11-9); contrast is primarily controlled by kilovoltage (see Fig. 11-5 and Table 11-2); (2) radiographic contrast consists of both film contrast and subject contrast (see Chapters 8, 11, and 12); (3) the term *contrast* is also used in reference to opaque or radiolucent media introduced into the body to enhance subject contrast (see Figs. 5-14, 9-3, 9-7, 9-17, 12-7, 12-8, and 14-15.)

Coulomb   a quantity of electricity equal to 1 ampere/sec. (See Table 13-5.)

Current   (1) the movement or flow of electrical charges (electrons) by means of a conductor; (2) alternating—a regular reversal of direction and speed of electrons (see Fig. 2-1); (3) direct—a continuous flow of current in one direction (see Fig. 2-1); direct current is required for the operation of an x-ray tube.

Densitometer   a device for determining the degree of blackening of photographic or radiographic film owing to the amount of light or x-radiation received (see Fig. 8-4); quantitative measurements, known as *sensitometry,* can be made of the response of the film to exposure and development. (See Fig. 8-5.)

Density   (1) optical or radiographic density; degree of blackness on a radiographic image; measured by the log of the light incident to the radiograph to the light transmitted through the radiograph (see Fig. 11-2); (2) the mass/cm^3 of a substance or tissue density affects optical density (see Figs. 11-1 and 11-6 and Chapter 13) by its absorption of x-radiation.

Detail   the sharpness of the structural edges of the radiographic image, often referred to as *recorded detail;* sometimes referred to as *umbra, sharpness, definition,* and *resolution;* usually measured in line pairs per millimeter (see Chapters 8 and 11); affected by focal spot size, intensifying screens, and changes in geometry; when patient motion is involved, it is usually referred to as *blur.*

Diaphragm   (1) aperture; a primary source beam-restricting device; usually mounted as close to the source of x-radiation as possible (see Fig. 5-6); (2) keyhole; a beam-restricting device usually added to the external tracks of a collimator; the opening is often formed to the shape of the part being examined; when used for cerebral angiography, the shape of the skull and cervical area results in a keyhole-like opening. (See Fig. 5-6.)

Differential absorption   the relative differences in attenuation of x-radiation by air, fat, water (soft tissue), bone, and metal (see Fig. 1-9); the degree of absorption is influenced by the atomic number and thickness of the absorber; equal thickness of dissimilar materials may have different degrees of absorption. (See Figs. 11-1 and 11-6.)

Diode   any vacuum tube with two electrodes (positive and negative); such as an x-ray or valve tube.

Direct current   see *Current.*

Direct exposure technique   a cardboard or plastic film holder, often with a thin lead foil backing to minimize backscatter; used with x-ray film sensitive to the direct action of x-radiation (see Fig. 8-1); screen-type radiographic film when used without intensifying screens in a direct exposure holder requires up to four times more radiation than do direct exposure films for the same examination. (See Chapter 8.)

Distortion   the size and shape of the radiographic image compared to the size and shape of the object being radiographed; overall equal size distortion is referred to as *magnification* (see Fig. 11-16); shape distortion results in elongation or foreshortening (see Fig. 11-17); there is some degree of enlargement present in all radiographs. (See Chapters 11 and 13.)

Divergent   see *Beam.*

Dose   the amount of radiation received as radiation absorbed; expressed in terms of the traditional unit of the rad; the international unit of measure of absorbed dose is the Gray (See Table 13-3.)

Dose equivalent   a unit used to express an estimation of biological effects upon people who have been exposed to various qualities of radiation; the traditional unit of DE is the rem; the international unit, the Sievert; in diagnostic radiology, the rad, rem, and roentgen are said to be equivalent. (See Table 13-3.)

Dosimeter   a direct-reading miniature ionization chamber, usually pencil size; used in personnel monitoring for measuring accumulated dosage of radiation.

Duplication   the process of copying a radiograph. (See Fig. 9-16.)

Dynamic   moving; as with fluoroscopy, a dynamic image. (See Chapters 3 and 6.)

Edge gradient   a term sometimes used to define the area of unsharpness or penumbra seen on a radiograph caused by the shape of an object and its relationship to the central ray. (See Fig. 11-14.)

Electromagnet   a magnet produced in a core of iron when an electric current is passed through the coils of wire wound around it (see Chapter 2); unlike a permanent magnet, an electromagnet can be turned on and off.

Electromagnetic induction   with an electromagnet, a magnetic field exists only while the current is flowing; current can be induced in a second wire if the wires cut through the magnetic field lines produced by an electrical current; since both coils are not electrically connected, the first coil induces an electrical current in the second coil by mutual induction; the force in the second wire is directly proportional to the number of turns in the first wire. (See Chapter 2.)

Electromagnetic spectrum   bundles of electrical and magnetic fields arranged in nature in an orderly fashion according to the wavelength of their energies. (See Fig. 1-3.)

Electron   a negative atomic charge that revolves around the nucleus of the atom; in a stable atom, the number of electrons is equal to the number of protons in the nucleus; when there is an excess or deficiency of electrons, the atom is ionized. (See Fig. 1-1.)

Element   the simplest substance composed of atoms of the same atomic number.

Emulsion   the radiation-sensitive portion of film that contains the latent image prior to development and the visual image after development of the exposed film (see Chapter 8); composed of a gelatin mixture containing a silver halide compound; emulsion is coated on one or both sides of the film base. (See Fig. 8-1.)

Energy   the ability to perform work; exists in nature in many forms such as kinetic energy, potential energy, magnetic energy, and molecular energy. (See Chapter 1.)

Enlargement   increase in size; generally associated with unsharpness; affected by FFD, FOD, and OFD (see Figs. 7-12, 7-13, and 11-16 and Chapter 13); direct roentgen enlargement requires a 0.3-mm focal spot or smaller to minimize image unsharpness. (See Chapter 7.)

Exponent   scientific notation used to write very large or small numbers; may be expressed as either a positive or negative number. (See Table 13-2.)

Exposure   (1) a measure of the ionization produced in air by x-rays or gamma rays; (2) subjection of sensitized film to light or x-rays, either directly or with intensifying screens.

Exposure angle   the angle through which the x-ray beam moves during a tomographic exposure; determines the thickness of a tomographic section. (See Figs. 7-5 to 7-7.)

Exposure rate   exposure expressed in R (roentgen) divided by T (time in minutes).

Exposure time   a measure of time of x-ray exposure expressed in seconds or fractions of a second.

Field size   the area and shape of the segment to be exposed to x-radiation.

Film badge   a dental film in a special holder usually worn by personnel who may be exposed to ionizing radiation; the degree of blackening on the processed film is used to determine the amount and quality of radiation exposure received.

Filter   any obstacle removing low-energy quanta (photons) from the x-ray beam through which x-rays pass from the focal spot to the object under study (see Figs. 4-9 to 4-12, 14-22); total filtration includes added and inherent filtration.

Fluorescence   a form of luminescence that emits light only when subjected to an activating force. (See Chapter 8.)

Fluoroscope   a device used for dynamic evaluation of organs and structures; radiation from an x-ray tube usually mounted beneath an x-ray table passes through the patient to produce a visual image on the fluoroscopic screen; zinc cadmium sulfide is the basic phosphor used for conventional fluoroscopic screens. (See Figs. 3-2 and 3-9 and Chapter 8.)

Focal spot   (1) actual—the section on which the anode of an x-ray tube intersects with an electron beam emanating from a filament (see Figs. 4-2, 4-3, and 4-5); (2) effective—the size of the projected focal spot in a specified direction; measured with the slit camera method (see Chapter 4); (3) projected—the projection of the actual focal spot along the central ray, perpendicular to the x-ray port plane and passing through the center of the focal spot; often referred to as the *focal spot* (see Fig. 4-2).

Generator   a device that can be used to convert mechanical energy into electrical energy.

Gonad   a generic term used to describe male and female reproductive organs.

Grid   (1) a radiographic accessory designed to minimize the effect of scatter radiation (see Fig. 5-11); (2) radius or focus—an imaginary point in space where imaginary lines drawn from the outer aspects of the grid would intersect (see Fig. 5-12); (3) ratio—the height of the lead lines of the grid to the width of the interspaces between the lead strips (see Fig. 5-11).

Ground   an electrical connection of an electrical conductor to the earth.

H & D curve   see *Sensitometric curve.*

Half-value layer   the amount of any material (e.g., lead, copper, cement, or aluminum) that will reduce the intensity of a beam of radiation by 50%; also known as half-value thickness.

Half-value thickness   the thickness of an absorptive material that, when placed in the x-ray beam, will lower the beam intensity by one half its original value; also known as half-value layer.

Heat units   a heat unit (HU) is the energy produced in the form of heat by 1 kVp and 1 mA for 1 sec (single-phase, fully rectified radiographic equipment); a multiplication factor is used to calculate heat units generated by three-phase equipment. (See Table 4-2 and Chapter 13.)

Heel effect   a variation in intensity of x-radiation from cathode to anode; sometimes referred to as anode heel effect; the projected focal spot size is also affected by the heel effect. (See Figs. 4-3 and 4-4.)

Helix   a cylindrical coil of wire.

Heterogeneous   x-ray energies of varying wavelengths and intensities. (See Chapter 1.)

Homogeneous   x-ray energies of similar wavelengths. (See Chapter 7.)

Image detector   the term often used for any recording media; used to image radiation for direct viewing or hard copy; also known as *image receptor;* in addition to radiographic and photographic film and conventional fluoroscopes, the image may be recorded on Polaroid film (see Figs. 6-10 and 9-18); image-intensified fluoroscopic screens (see Figs. 6-1 and 6-2); motion picture film (see Figs. 9-12 and 9-13); cathode ray tubes (see Figs. 6-5, 6-7, 6-8, 6-10–6-14); and electrostatic recording media (see Figs. 9-21–9-23).

Image distributor   see *Beam splitter.*

Image intensifier   electronic-enhanced fluoroscope with a brightness gain as much as 10,000 times greater than a conventional fluoroscopic screen; makes television viewing, motion picture recording, and strip film recording possible (see Figs. 6-1 and 6-2).

Impedance   total resistance, which includes inductance, capacitance, and electrical resistance.

Impulse   1/120th second of a commercial 60-cycle alternating current; see *Timer, impulse.*

Incandescent   glowing, white hot; usually refers to the illumination of the filament of the x-ray tube: see *Thermionic emission.* (See Chapter 4.)

Incident light   see *Density.*

Index   a factor used to measure a ratio against a given standard. (See Chapter 13.)

Induction   the generation of an electrical current in a second coil by close subjection to another coil bearing an electrical charge; electrical current can be induced in the second wire if the wires cut through the magnetic field lines produced by the current flowing in the first wire. (See Chapter 2.)

Inertia   a property of matter that causes a body at rest or in motion to remain at rest or in motion until an external force changes its state.

Instantaneous load   the maximal kVp and mAs values that can be used for a given length of time for a single exposure. (See Fig. 4-7.)

Insulator a material (nonconducting) that resists the conduction of electrical current.

Intensifying screen fluorescent crystals coated on a paper or plastic base; used in conjunction with single emulsion film (one screen) or duplitized x-ray film (two screens) to convert x-radiation into light. (See Figs. 8-8 and 8-13).

Inverse square law a law expressing that the intensity of radiation is inversely proportional to the square of the distance from the source of radiation. (See Fig. 13-3.)

Ionization chamber (1) an automatic exposure timer used to achieve reproducible radiographic densities over a wide range of body sizes and thicknesses (see Fig. 2-10); (2) a radiation-sensing device (such as a geiger counter) used to detect and measure ionizing radiation.

Joule a derived unit of work or energy in the SI system of measure where 1 watt per second is equal to 1 joule.

KeV the effective voltage value; the direct current voltage required to generate the same amount of energy as an alternating current with a given resistance; eV = 0.7 pV; pV = 1.41 eV.

Kilovolt 1000 volts.

Kilovoltage (1) optimum—a radiographic technique using a fixed kVp with variable mAs (see Tables 12-8 and 12-9); (2) variable—a radiographic technique using a variable kVp with a fixed mAs (see Tables 12-8 and 12-9).

Kilovolt peak the highest kilovoltage that occurs during an x-ray exposure; the peak voltage is not present throughout the entire exposure with single-phase equipment; the beam contains photons of various energies.

Kilowatt 1000 watts.

Lag afterglow; light from a fluoroscopic screen after the activating force has ceased; see *Phosphorescence*. (See Chapters 6 and 8.)

Laminagraphy see *Tomography*.

Laser L(ight) A(mplification) by S(timulated) E(mission) of R(adiation); a laser beam is used to "write" directly on photographic film in laser printing devices to eliminate the electronic interference and raster lines associated with cathode ray tube imaging. (See Chapter 6.)

Latitude this term has several applications in medical radiography: (1) film latitude is a design parameter using sensitometry to define the range of contrast possible in an image, with a given film product; multiple tonal shades (long-scale contrast) represent extended latitude; abrupt black and white changes in density are associated with lower-latitude, high-contrast film products (see Figs. 8-5, 14-21 and 14-23); (2) technical latitude is generally described in terms of the high kVp and lower mAs values that result in a longer scale of contrast on the image; changes at higher kVp are more easily tolerated than changes at lower kVps (see Figs. 11-4 and 12-1); slow screen film combination speeds making larger changes more tolerable (increased exposure latitude).

Light adaptation see *Adaptation*.

Linear energy transfer the measurement of the amount of energy transferred from x-radiation to the soft tissues of the body.

Line spread function a test used to measure the light diffusion (blurred or unsharp edges of the image) associated with intensifying screens; this information is then used as the basis for determining the modulation transfer function of a screen film combination.

Luminescence the production of energy in the form of light without producing heat. (See Chapter 1.)

Magazine a take-up cassette for exposed strip, roll, or cut film. (See Chapter 9.)

Magnetic field the area of magnetic influence in space around a current carrying wire; the magnetic force only exists while current is flowing through the wire.

Magnification see *Distortion, size, shape;* and *Enlargement*.

Mass the amount of matter in a body as measured by its inertia; the weight and compact nature of a substance.

Matter any substance composed of atoms that occupies space. (See Chapter 1.)

Milliampere 1/1000 ampere.

Milliampere second product of the milliampere value times the length of exposure expressed in seconds (mA × T). (See Chapters 11–13.)

Minimal reaction time See *Minimal response time*. (See Chapter 2.)

Minimal response time represents the time

Radiolucent permits the passage of x-rays; a structure or object that does not appreciably attenuate the x-ray beam.

Radionuclides atomic structures that emit radiation and, in so doing, disintegrate; radionuclides are used in nuclear medicine for diagnosis and treatment. (See Figs. 6-8 and 6-9.)

Radiopaque stops radiation; dense bone or metal objects absorb x-radiation in the medical diagnostic range; also refers to radiopaque contrast media; see *Contrast*.

Radius (1) a line extending from the middle of a circle to a point on its circumference (see Chapter 13); one half the diameter of a circle; (2) grid radius—see *Grid*.

Range the difference between the smallest and largest set of variables in a series.

Ray (1) a beam emanating from a focal area such as the actual focal spot in an x-ray tube (see Figs. 4-1–4-3); (2) cathode ray— negatively charged electrons emanating from the cathode or filament of a vacuum tube (see Fig. 4-2); (3) characteristic ray— occurs as electrons collide with the atoms of the target and displace structural electrons from any inner shell of the target atom (see Figs. 1-6 and 1-7 and Tables 1-1 and 1-2); can also be produced as a secondary effect when x-rays interact with the subject being radiographed; characteristic radiation produced by the interaction of x-rays with matter is usually referred to as *secondary radiation* and is a form of scatter (see Chapter 5); (4) hard—x-rays produced by higher kilovoltage values; hard rays are capable of increased penetration and possess shorter wavelengths (see Fig. 11-5); filtration can remove softer (often non-image-forming), less-penetrating waves (see Chapter 4); (5) primary—x-ray beam emanating from the actual focal spot; radiation discharged directly from a radioactive substance; (6) roentgen—as a courtesy to Wilhelm Conrad Roentgen, who discovered x-radiation on November 8, 1895, the term *roentgen ray* is sometimes substituted for x-ray; (7) scatter ray—see *Radiation, scatter*; (8) secondary ray—see *Radiation, secondary*.

Receptor see *Image detector*.

Rectification the changing of alternating electrical current to direct electrical current; early rectification units were mechanical switches that controlled the flow of current in a given direction; inefficient when compared with valve tubes or solid state rectifiers. (See Figs. 2-3 and 2-5 and Chapter 13.)

Rectifier a valve tube or a solid state device used to transform alternating current into direct current. (See Figs. 2-3 and 2-5.)

Reflection (1) turned back; the term *reflection* is used in intensifying screen design when the posterior surface of a screen is reflective in nature (see Fig. 8-11); (2) reflection is also encountered in ultrasonography (see Fig. 6-11) where high-frequency sound waves are emitted from a transducer; when the boundary edges or surfaces of internal structures are encountered by the sound waves, they are reflected back to the transducer, which acts alternately as a transmitter or receptor.

Rem term used to describe radiologic dose equivalent in traditional units; Sievert in SI units. 1 rem = 0.01 Sv. (See Table 13-3.)

Resistance the impedance effect of conductor atoms to the flow of electrons; there is resistance to the electron flow in all circuits, with some absorption and, thus, loss of energy. (See Chapters 2 and 13.)

Resolution recorded detail; the appearance of well-defined structural edges of the radiographic image; affected by sharpness and contrast. (See Fig. 11-14.)

Rheostat an electrical control (resistor) used to vary the amount of current entering a circuit; used to control current to the primary of the step-down transformer. (See Figs. 2-2 and 2-3.)

Roentgen see *Ray*.

Schematic usually a drawing of an electrical circuit; can be an abstract or conceptual outline or plan.

Screen see *Fluoroscope* and *Intensifying screen*.

Secondary radiation see *Radiation*.

Section, body section see *Tomography*.

Semiconductor a silicon or selenium device that has inherent low resistance to the flow of current in one direction; used in modern rectifying systems. (See Figs. 2-3 and 2-5.)

Sensitometer a device used to expose a radiograph to produce a stepwedge of photographic densities used to make qualitative measurements of the response of the film to exposure and development; the exposed stepwedge is evaluated by the use of a densitometer, and sensitometric curves are generated. (See Figs. 8-4 and 8-5.)

Sensitometric curve   a graphic representation used to describe the photographic characteristics (e.g., speed, contrast, latitude) of a radiographic film product; also referred to as a characteristic curve or H & D curve (after Hurter and Driffield). (See Fig. 8-5.)

Sensitometry   a qualitative measurement of the response of film to exposure and development. (See Fig. 8-5.)

Shield   a protective device such as lead sheeting, gonadal coverings, and eye lens shields used to protect patient and/or operator from unnecessary exposure to ionizing radiation.

SI units   the refined modern version of the metric system known as the International System of Measure, introduced as a means of providing a common language for communications between nations and the sciences. (See Tables 13-4 and 13-5.)

Sinewave   an oscillating curve that is used to diagram the flow of alternating current (see Fig. 2-1) or the change in electrical and magnetic fields of electromagnetic radiations (see Fig. 1-4.)

Slit camera   a quality assurance test tool used to measure the size of the projected focal spot in a specified direction; resulting in the effective focal spot. (See Chapter 4.)

Solenoid   a coil of wire with current flowing through it. (See Chapter 2.)

Solid state   electronic devices such as silicon diode rectifiers used to rectify alternating current; see *Semiconductor.*

Solution   liquid-containing substances with water used as a solvent, that is, developer, fixer, and replenishments solutions. (See Chapter 10.)

Source   often substituted for focal spot, that is, source image receptor distance (SID).

Spatial   pertaining to an extension in space; as in scatter radiation emanating in all directions.

Spectrum   electromagnetic radiations arranged in the order of their wavelengths.

Spinning top   a rotating metallic disc used to check the timer of single-phase x-ray equipment. (See Fig. 2-8.)

Static   (1) at rest, not moving; in a fixed or stationary position; (2) a form of artifact seen on a radiograph, caused by a discharge of electricity caused by friction.

Stem radiation   see *Extra-focal radiation.*

Stereo shift   a predetermined change in the location of the x-ray tube in relationship to the part for the purpose of producing a three-dimensional effect on a radiographic image. (See Chapters 3 and 13.)

Subtraction   photographic or electronic process of removing overlying structures from a radiographic image. (See Figs. 6-5, 9-16, and 9-17.)

Technique chart   a guide for the selection of exposure factors needed to produce a radiographic image; formulated after consideration for radiographic image; formulated after consideration for radiographic equipment calibration and limitations, automatic processor control, use of radiographic accessories, patient habitus, positioning, and pathology. (See Tables 12-8 and 12-9.)

Teleroentgenogram   a radiograph obtained using an extended FFD, usually 6 in. as with a chest radiograph to overcome image enlargement. (See Fig. 14-13.)

Thermionic emission   the "boiling off" of free electrons by the heating of a filament within the vacuum of a glass tube. (See Chapter 4.)

Thermoluminescent dosimeter   a personal monitoring device that stores energy caused by x-radiation; when the crystals in the device are heated, the stored radiation can be measured, since the thermal luminescent crystals give off light proportional to the radiation exposure received by the TLD.

Timer   (1) a mechanism used to initiate and terminate an exposure of a predetermined time; (2) automatic exposure device—an automatic timer in which the exposure is initiated by the radiographer, but the length of the exposure is automatically terminated after a preselected density has been reached; can be either a phototimer or ionization chamber (see Figs. 2-9–2-12); (3) cumulative—indicates the lapsed times of a fluoroscopic examination; usually a preset time that shuts off the machine automatically; must be reset before fluoroscopy can begin again; (4) impulse—a conventional electronic timer, usually reliable to 1/120th second; (5) synchronous—a conventional motor-driven timer, not reliable for exposure shorter than 1/20th second.

Tomography the generic term selected by the International Commission of Units and Standards to designate all systems of body section radiography; includes planigraphy, stratigraphy, ordography, and laminagraphy. (See Chapter 7.)

Transformer an induction apparatus used to change electrical energy at one voltage and current to electrical energy at another voltage and current through magnetic induction. (See Figs. 2-3 and 2-4.)

Umbra geometric sharpness at the edges of a structure on a radiograph; true or sharply defined as opposed to penumbra.

Unit smallest standardized measure of size, weight, or other quality.

Valve tube a vacuum tube rectification device used to change alternating current into direct current. (See Fig. 2-3.)

View the body part as seen on a radiograph or other recording media; refers to the actual radiograph or medical image.

Vignetting a lower intensity of light at the periphery of the field than at the center of the fluoroscopic image on an image intensifier.

Volt unit of electrical pressure. (See Chapter 13.)

Voltage the electromotive force or difference in potential when a current of one ampere flows through a conductor that has a potential difference of one volt, the power consumed equals one watt. (See Chapter 13.)

Watt unit of electrical power; measured in ohms. (See Chapter 13.)

X-ray tube (1) a vacuum tube (diode) designed especially for the purpose of producing x-rays; (2) grid-controlled—an x-ray tube with a third electrode near the filament; the potential may be varied to turn the x-rays on or off for percision x-ray exposure timing. (See Chapters 4 and 6.)

Zero potential having neither positive nor negative voltage or pressure.

Index

The letter *f* following a page number indicates a figure; the letter *t* following a page number indicates a table.